TAKING THE FIRST STEP:

DAILY MEDITATIONS FOR

TWELVE STEP PROGRAMS

By Tony Caetano

Westland Park Press

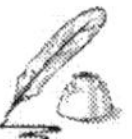

Published by Westland Park Press. Not to be reproduced or reprinted without written consent of the publisher.

First Edition June 2015

ISBN: 978-0-9884444-9-2
ISBN 10: 0988444496

10 9 8 7 6 5 4 3 2 1

Printed in the United States of America

ACKNOWLEDGEMENTS

I would like to gratefully acknowledge all of the writers I have quoted from in these daily meditations for their wisdom and inspiration. An exhaustive search was done to determine whether previously published material included in this book required permission to reprint. If there has been an error, I apologize and a correction will be made in subsequent editions.

The following authors, their agents, and publishers have graciously granted permission to include excerpts from the following:

The Language of Letting Go: Daily Meditations for Codependents, copyright 1990 by Melody Beattie. Reprinted by permission of the Hazelden Foundation.

Tough Minded Faith for Tender Hearted People, copyright 1983 by Robert H. Schuller. Reprinted by permission of Thomas Nelson, Inc.

The Good Sex Book: Recovering and Discovering Your Sexual Self, copyright 1992 by Sherry Sedgwick, M.Ed. Reprinted by permission of CompCare Publishers.

The Answer to Addiction: The Path to Recovery from Alcohol, Drug Food and Sexual Dependencies, copyright 1996 by John Burns. Reprinted by permission of East Ridge Publishers.

Power Through Constructive Thinking, copyright 1968 by Emmet Fox. Reprinted by permission of Harper Collins Publishers.

Discover the Power Within You, copyright 1989 by Eric Butterworth. Reprinted by permission of Harper Collins Publishers.

Legacy of the Heart: The Spiritual Advantages of a Painful Childhood, copyright 1992 by Wayne Muller. Reprinted by permission of Simon & Schuster publishers.

The Power of Hope: The One Essential of Life and Love, copyright 1995 by Maurice Lamm. Reprinted by permission of Rawson Associates.

Stake Your Claim: Exploring the Gold Mine Within, copyright 1992 by Emmet Fox. Reprinted by permission of Harper Collins Publishers.

The Twelve Steps for Christians, copyright 1989 by Friends in Recovery. Reprinted by permission of Recovery Publications, Inc.

DEDICATION

"There is an instinct for newness, for renewal,
for a liberation of creative power,
We seek to awaken in ourselves a force,
which really changes our lives from within.
And yet the same instinct tells us that this
change is a **RECOVERY** of that, which is deepest,
most original, most personal in ourselves.
To be born again is not to be somebody else,
but to become ourselves. -- Thomas Merton, **Love and Living**

"<u>**Taking the First Step**</u> with a good thought, the second with a good word, and the third with a good dead, I entered Paradise." James Allen, **From Poverty to Power**

Seek first God's kingdom and His righteousness, and all these things shall be yours as well. (Matthew 6:33)

This book is dedicated to everyone who is in a Twelve Step program as a thank you for sharing your experience, strength, and hope with the author for the past twenty-five years.

A special thank you to my wife Deborah Wilson who first introduced me to the Steps, and to my children and step-children who helped me appreciate my need to work the Steps on a daily basis and to my mother who showed me the meaning of Serenity.

An extra special thanks goes to Laura Wagner for her tireless editing and to Brian Ward for his support, work on the cover design and his marketing efforts.

PREFACE

"This life therefore, is not righteousness but growth in righteousness, not health but healing, not being but becoming, not rest but exercise. We are not yet what we shall be but we are growing toward it, the process is not yet finished but it is going on, this is not end but it is the road." -- Martin Luther

The road to Recovery is a process. It take time to regain, reclaim, and recoup all that was lost while we tried on our own to cope with the many forms of addiction we may have encountered. Building trust takes time, change takes time, healing old wounds takes time, and there are no immediate, ready-made solutions. But the tools and principles of "The Program" can lead us to the answers that are right for us.

- Recovery comes through the healing of the spirit.

- Recovery comes a little at a time.

- Recovery is not a place to be reached or a goal to achieve, but an experience you can choose to be in for the rest of your life.

"If as Herod, we fill our live with things, and again with things. If we consider ourselves so unimportant that we must fill every moment of our lives with action, when will we have time to make the long slow journey across the desert, as did the magi? Or brood over the coming of the child as did Mary? For each one of us there is a desert to travel, a star to discover and a being within ourselves to bring to life." – Anonymous

Hopefully by reading these daily meditations and by working "The Program", our journey through the desert will be shorter; we will discover the power and divinity within us; and, our life will be filled with the peace and joy described in the **Serenity Prayer –**

"Living one day at a time;
Enjoying one moment at a time;
Accepting hardship as the pathway to peace;
Taking, as **He** did,
This sinful world as it is,
Not as I would have it;
Trusting that **He** will
Make all things right
If I surrender to **His Will**;
That I may be reasonably happy in this
Life and supremely happy with **Him**
Forever in the next."

INTRODUCTION

This book is designed to help persons in Twelve Step Programs to daily experience the new philosophy of life which Recovery represents, and to recognize the benefits of discovering and expanding spiritual awareness.

The basic principles of Twelve Step Programs, like Alcoholics Anonymous, Co-Dependents Anonymous, Al-Anon, Narcotics Anonymous, Over-Eaters Anonymous, etc., are as old as recorded history. They are the same concepts on which <u>all</u> spiritual philosophies and mythical literature are based. These elements are found in the Bible as well as Oriental and Hindu religions. They are the very substance of the Ten Commandments, the Sermon on the Mount, the Golden Rule, the TAO, and the Upanishads. They include the following:

- Acknowledgment of our dependency on a Supreme Being.

- Love of our fellow man and recognition of human dignity and value.

- Awareness of the need to improve ourselves through self-appraisal and admitting to our faults.

- Belief in the effective spiritual power of true personal humility and conscious gratitude.

- Willingness to help others.

These principles not only form the working philosophy of Twelve Step Programs, but they provide a pattern for (1) Right living, (2) Overcoming difficulties, and (3) Helping us to achieve our aspirations. By working "The Program" at our own pace and in our own way; relying on the help and support of our Higher Power and others who also work "The Program", we can change and be transformed.

As newcomers to "The Program" we often have difficulty in identifying addiction in ourselves or in our families as the cause of our problems. We see ourselves reflected in our parental mirrors and we adopt beliefs that are not okay. By doing so, we give up our identity and begin searching for ways to feel good about ourselves.

As adults, we often continue this pattern by allowing others to influence our self-image, self-esteem, and happiness. Our self-defeating beliefs about ourselves lead us to make self-destructive choices. Because we grow up in chaos, we do not learn appropriate interpersonal or decision-making skills. And because of our denial we continue to resist recognizing these limitations in ourselves.

Denial is our defense against the reality of our condition. It keeps us unaware of our compulsive behaviors which manifest themselves through various means, such as: (1) the need to be in control, (2) the lack of self-confidence or personal esteem, (3) being victims or martyrs, (4) an inability to express our needs and feelings and, (5) Being unaware of our repressed feelings of pain, resentment, shame, fear and rage.

When life's circumstances force us to come to terms with ourselves, we start looking for explanations. We try self-help books, therapy groups and other forms of consciousness raising. After exhausting these resources, we come to the realization that the peace we seek is not to be found in these sources. When we reach this point, we are ready to accept the support and guidance of a Higher Power. As we work the Steps "One Day at a Time" we will experience the Miracle of the restoration of trust, dignity, courage and faith in the newness of life.

As newcomers we have a great deal to learn. We need to be willing to change. We also need to be committed to working the Steps on a **daily** basis – only then will we receive the priceless gift of Serenity.

The material in this book is designed to help us on our daily journey in Recovery. Each month is dedicated to one of the Twelve Steps. Each day in the month contains information and stories, which relate to issues and/or suggestions for working the Step.

For optimum results it is necessary to work through all of the Steps. Many of us have found that we may continue to revisit one Step or another as the events in our lives prescribe. The **INDEX** is arranged alphabetically by topic so when we need help with a particular problem, issue or character defect we can look at the **Where to Turn List** and find the guidance, strength and comfort we are seeking.

In addition, daily quotations, meditations, affirmations and scriptural passages are provided for personal reflection and inspiration. Finally, **TODAY'S STEP** helps us to keep the focus on ourselves and to change our thinking and attitudes in relation to others in a positive way.

Appendix A: The Twelve Steps And Twelve Traditions adapted from AA.
Appendix B: Daily Affirmations and Selected Prayers contains some popular affirmations and helpful prayers.

Appendix C: Suggested Reading provides a list of books, publications, and references for further reading.

CONTENTS

<u>Step One</u>

<u>*We admitted we were powerless over the effects of addiction – that our lives had become unmanageable.*</u>

The idea in Step One is overwhelming to most of us until we begin to accept the reality of our lives as they actually are. It is humiliating to admit we are powerless and our lives have become unmanageable. We have spent a major portion of our lives attempting to manage the behavior, thoughts and feelings of others so we could feel safe and secure. Some of us may strive for control by appearing weak and incapable, thereby manipulating others to perform for us. We may be obsessed with achieving a superior status in life, and we find it difficult to acknowledge we could actually be powerless. We may be preoccupied with being the smartest or the fastest, or with having the best job. Whatever we do, no matter how hard we try to make it appear okay, some of our behavior puts our health and wellbeing at serious risk. Step One brings us to the threshold of identifying the causes of the obsessive and compulsive behavior we cannot control.

We realize, in this life, we have the power to make choices about matters which affect us. In attempting to influence and manage the outcomes of these choices, we may sometimes experience conflict. Prior to becoming aware of our problem, we sense that something is wrong because life is unfulfilling in many ways. As a natural result, we desperately try to right the wrong by "fixing" things. No matter what we do or where we turn, we continue to suffer acute anxiety attacks or experience episodes of bizarre and compulsive behavior. When we finally are forced to look closely at ourselves and see that we have exhausted all other possibilities, we are ready for Step One. At this point, we have no alternative but to admit we are powerless and our lives have become unmanageable. For the first time, we begin to alter the course of our lives, and strive for healing.

Step One is the foundation for all the Steps. When working this Step, we begin to acknowledge the reality of our life experiences. We see our behavior, thoughts and feelings as they really are, and recognize the need for greater honesty with ourselves and others. It is through confronting and admitting our powerlessness that we begin to risk being honest about our limitations.

Step One consists of two distinct parts: (1) admitting we are powerless over the effects of addictive or dysfunctional behavior, and (2) admitting our lives have been, and will continue to be, unmanageable if we do not change.

FIRST STEP PRAYERS

"We admitted we were powerless over the effects of addiction – that our lives had become unmanageable."

Today, I ask for help with my addiction. Denial has kept me from seeing how powerless I am and how my life is unmanageable. I need to learn and remember that I have an incurable illness and abstinence is the only way to deal with it.

In this moment I do not have to control anyone, including me. And if I feel uncomfortable with what another person is doing or not doing, I can remind myself, I AM POWERLESS over this person and I AM POWERLESS over my compulsion to act in inappropriate ways.

MEDITATIONS

This day, dear Lord, my needs weigh heavy, filling my heart and mind with apprehension. There is so much I want to accomplish and I am in need of Thy divine strength. I know all I have to do is to reach out and let Thy love permeate my whole being, and all is mine. If I forget, dear Father, let me feel the comfort of Thy everlasting love, let me recognize Thee in everyone I see today. When I am called upon to make decisions that affect not only myself, but others, let me first come to Thee for heavenly reassurance. May I ever be conscious that success is only of this earth and all I do should be with Thee in mind. Thou art ever with me, in every decision, every hope, and every hurt. I pray that Thy presence bless all I do today.

AFFIRMATIONS

Problems are my teachers. They help me to learn and grow. Without them, I would be going nowhere. With them, I am moving forward in the direction of my goals.

There is no problem which I cannot conquer. I am strong in mind, body and spirit. My will, my strength, and my determination are always greater than any problem I face.

Having problems is not a problem for me. I am confident, self-assured, positive, and determined. I always know I am going to overcome any problem I encounter – and I always do.

"They know and do not know, what it is to act or suffer. They know and do not know, that acting is suffering." - T.S. Eliot, *Murder in the Cathedral*

I Didn't Know, I Didn't Know

Newcomers to Twelve Step recovery programs will frequently hear speakers say, "I didn't have a clue how to live **before** I got into a program; I didn't know I was in prison until I broke out; and I didn't know, I didn't know."

Dysfunctional living, for many of us, is so habitual and familiar we don't recognize that we have choices and that there **is** a better way to live. We get so wrapped up in **self** and the pursuit of our needs for success, wealth, love, etc., that we loose sight of our spiritual needs. Soon our lives rapidly become more and more "unmanageable," our compulsive behaviors take over, and we become "powerless" over our addictions.

Admitting powerlessness runs contrary to many of our cultural messages that say, "Be strong! Be the master of your own destiny!" The admission of powerlessness also conflicts with the addictive message, because the addiction itself tells us, "Use more of me! You can handle it!"

Nevertheless, the central paradox of Step 1 is that the admission of complete defeat permits a life-transforming victory through Recovery. The admission of powerlessness over an addiction actually becomes the foundation for the strength to eventually overcome the dependency.

Admitting powerlessness is absolutely essential to breaking the addiction cycle, which includes:
- Pain.
- Reaching out to, or escaping with, an addictive **substance**, such as food, drugs alcohol, or addictive **behavior**, such as sex, gambling, work, shopping, dependent relationships to ease our pain.
- Temporary anesthesia.
- Negative consequences.
- Shame and guilt, which result in more pain or low self-esteem.

And ye shall know the Truth, and the Truth shall make you free. (John 8:32)

TODAY'S STEP: I pray my Higher Power gives me the courage and strength to recognize the Truth about myself and to help me accept that I am powerless.

"Everything is funny as long as it is happening to somebody else." - Will Rogers,
The Illiterate Digest

<u>A Sense of Humor</u>

At a very large discussion meeting one Sunday evening, the topic was Gratitude. The Chairperson randomly asked people to share their "experience, strength and hope."

A woman who was a Newcomer to the group was asked to share. It was her first time at the podium and she was very nervous. She kept saying just how nervous she was and this was her first time speaking before a large group.

We all identified with her feelings and intuitively knew what research has found – "People are more afraid of speaking in public than they are of facing death."

The woman said, "Hi my name is Marie, and I'm an alcoholic." She laboriously told her story of addiction, substance abuse, divorce, and entering and leaving numerous treatment programs. She was very confused and frequently stumbled over her words. More than once she hesitated and apologized for her lapses of memory.

During a particularly long lapse she again said, "I've lost my train of thought." One of the regular group members seated in the front row innocently spoke out and commented, "That's OK; Marie another train will be along soon."

Everyone had a good-natured laugh. But more importantly, Marie was able to laugh too.
She immediately relaxed and gained her self-confidence. Effortlessly she completed her story and sat down to the applause of the entire group.

For two years I watched Marie continue to come to meetings every Sunday. She made this her "home group" and she got involved. She started being a "greeter", then she sold tickets, and eventually she was elected Secretary. On her second anniversary of being "clean and sober", she again related her story, but this time she didn't have any difficulty keeping her train of thought. In fact, she was right on track!

Thou wilt show me the path of life: in thy presence is fullness of joy... (Psalm 16:11)

TODAY'S STEP: My sense of humor helps me to carry – and to get – the message of the Twelve Steps. I will laugh more.

"It is not the critic who counts; not the man who points out how the strong man stumbled, or where the doer of deeds could have done them better. The credit belongs to the man who is actually in the arena." -- Theodore Roosevelt

<u>Working Through a Problem, Conflict Or Issue</u>

The "core-issues" approach to Recovery can help us apply a name to our particular problems or conflicts instead of blaming persons, places or things. Once we name an issue, we can begin to focus on it and then we can concentrate on working to resolve it using experiential techniques. Experiential techniques involve four characteristics: (1) Being real, (2) Being focused on our inner life, (3) Being structured and (4) Doing our healing work. As we name and work through our core issue(s), we go through the following steps:

1. **Identify** and **name** our **specific problem** or **conflict.**

2. **Reflect** upon it from our powerful **inner life.**

3. **Talk about** it with safe people (that is, tell that specific part of our story).

4. Ask for **feedback** from them.

5. **Name** the core issue.

6. Select an appropriate **experiential technique.**

7. **Use** that **to work** our specific conflict and feelings at a **deeper** level.

8. **Talk** and/or **write some more** about it.

9. **Meditate** or **pray** about it.

10. Consider **how** we might **learn** from it.

11. If we still feel incomplete, **repeat** any of the above.

12. Whenever we are ready, **let it go.**

Not returning evil for evil or insult for insult, but giving a blessing instead; for you were called for the very purpose that you might inherit a blessing. (1 Peter 3:9)

TODAY'S STEP: I face my problems squarely and without blame.

"We, ignorant of ourselves beg often our own harms, which the wise powers deny us for our good; so we find profit by losing our prayers." -- William Shakespeare, **Anthony and Cleopatra (II, I, 5)**

Hitting Bottom

Cleopatra may have been the queen of the Nile, but I was the king of **DENIAL.** When I first came into The Program I denied everything. I denied I had any problems. I denied my feelings of hopelessness and helplessness. I denied I was "powerless" over people, places and things. I denied that my life had become "unmanageable", even though I quit my job, filed for divorce and claimed bankruptcy – all in the same day!

Breaking out of denial often requires a painful encounter with the consequences of our addictions, called "hitting bottom." "Hitting bottom" forces us to admit our powerlessness over our addictive life-styles. The three major "bottoms" we may hit are:

1. A physical bottom;
2. An emotional bottom; and,
3. A spiritual bottom.

After hitting an emotional and spiritual bottom, I finally came to recognize the importance of Step 1 and the need to live "Life on Life's Terms." Now, I constantly rely on the wisdom of **The Serenity Prayer** to help me:

1. **Accept** the things that I cannot change;

2. **Change** the things I can;

3. **Accept** hardship as a pathway to peace;

4. **Take**, as He did, this rebellious world, as it is, not as I would have it; and,

5. **Trust** that God will make all things right if I surrender to His will.

If I follow this prescription for living, I can confidently be assured that I may be reasonably happy in this life and supremely happy with God in the next.

Do not conform to the pattern of this world, but be transformed by the renewing of your mind. (Romans 12:2)

TODAY'S STEP: I let go of denial and accept responsibility for myself and my life.

"All discovery is self-discovery and all knowledge is self-knowledge. Thus the greatest discovery in science is not the outward accomplishments, but the inward revelation and the Truth that sets us free to take the outer step." -- Eric Butterworth, **Discover the Power Within You**

<u>The Slogans</u>

Alcoholics Anonymous, Al-Anon and all the other Twelve Step programs embrace a set of principles that are at once simple and profound. As a Newcomer in a recovery program we are often in such confusion and deep pain about our (or someone else's) addictive behavior that we are unable to grasp a complicated philosophy. Usually we are desperately searching for relief from suffering. What we discover when we enter a Twelve Step program (beyond the warmth, caring and understanding offered by other members) is a number of simple phrases known as the "slogans".

The slogans are often the first tools we are able to hear and hold on to. They have often opened many a closed mind and have given suffering family members the first ray of hope that life can be different. Once we discover our capacity for change, a slogan once accepted for its simplicity often takes on deeper and deeper meaning.

Each of the slogans represents a particular spiritual discipline and provides a logical starting point for dealing with many situations. They are also easy to recall in times of stress and can be used as a measuring stick in evaluating our progress along the road to personal recovery. Refer to the pages in parenthesis for detailed descriptions of each of the following slogans (and to page 400 for a complete list of slogans):

        (1)   **"Easy Does It"** (page 18)

        (2)   **"Let Go and Let God"** (page 71)

        (3)   **"First Things First"** (page 140)

        (4)   **"Live and Let Live"** (page 202)

        (5)   **"One Day at a Time"** (page 300)

        (6)   **"Let It Begin with Me"** (page 345)

For God gives wisdom and knowledge and joy to a man who is good in His sight.... (Ecclesiastes 2:26)

TODAY'S STEP: I visualize myself achieving my goal of changing for the better.

"Not in the clamor of the crowed street, not in the shouts and plaudits of the throng, But in ourselves, are triumph and defeat." -- Henry Wadsworth Longfellow, **The Poets**

<u>Abraham Lincoln Didn't Quit</u>

T – Teach ability. Truthfulness. Tolerance. Temperance

R – Rationality. Reasonableness. Responsibility.

I – Integrity. Intelligence. Intuition. Introspection.

U – Understanding. Usefulness. Uncritical ness.

M – Mastery. Motivation. Morality. Mental Health.

P -- Patience. Persistence. Playfulness. Pleasantness.

H -- Hopefulness. Heart. Humility. Happiness. Hard Work. Humor. Honesty. Healthy Habits. Help.

Nothing pays off like perseverance. Probably the greatest example is Abraham Lincoln. Born into poverty, Lincoln was faced with defeat throughout his life. He lost eight elections, failed in business twice and had a nervous breakdown.

Lincoln could have quit many times – but he didn't and because he didn't quit, he became one of the greatest presidents in the history of our country. Here is a brief description of his journey to the White House:

1816	His family was forced out of their home. He had to work to support them.
1818	His mother died.
1831	Failed in business.
1832	Ran for state legislature - lost.
1833	Borrowed money from a friend to begin a business and went bankrupt within a year. Spent the next 17 years paying off his debt.
1835	Engaged to be married, and his sweetheart died.
1836	Had a total nervous breakdown.
1843	Ran for Congress – lost.
1846	Ran for Congress again – this time he won.
1848	Ran for re-election to Congress – lost.
1854	Ran for the Senate of the United States – lost.
1858	Ran for the U.S. Senate again – again he lost.
1860	Elected 16th president of the United States.

Let me not grow weary while doing good, for in due season I shall reap if I do not lose heart. (Galatians 6:9)

TODAY'S STEP: There are many things I can do to improve my life and to further my Recovery, but I cannot heal myself. I need to continually ask God's help in becoming free of all that blocks me from my true self.

"Let me not pray to be sheltered from dangers but to be fearless in facing them. Let me not beg for the stilling of my pain but for the heart to conquer it. Let me not look for allies in life's battlefield but to my own strength. Let me not crave in anxious fear to be saved but hope for the patience to win my freedom. Grant me that I may not be a coward, feeling your mercy in my success alone; but let me find the grasp of your hand in my failure." Rabindranath Tagore, **Fruit-Gathering**

<u>Never, Never Give Up</u>

If an old problem continues to stick – pray for inspiration and intelligence. Stop struggling and thank God constantly for setting you free.

If nervous or frightened – throw the responsibility on God, and tell Him that you know you are safe in His hands.

If someone is being troublesome – see only the Presence of God where the troublesome person seems to be.

If you want faster progress – claim understanding and affirm that divine Love is working through you.

To recognize failure intelligently is the first step toward building success.

Recognize success with thanksgiving, and build more success on that.

You can have anything in life you really want in God's will, but you must be prepared to take the responsibility that goes with it.

God is bigger than any problem.

God in you is greater than any difficulty that you have to face.

God will help you in proportion to the degree in which you revere Him.

You revere God by really putting your trust in Him instead of in outer conditions, or in fear, or in depression, or in seeing dangers, etc.

Casting all your care upon Him; for He cars for you. (1 Peter 5:7)

TODAY'S STEP: By calling on my Higher Power for help daily, I can turn failure into success.

"Courage is fear that has said its prayers." -- Anonymous

Definition of Alcoholism

Alcoholism is a **primary**, chronic **disease** with genetic, psychosocial and environmental factors influencing its development and manifestation. The disease is **often progressive and fatal**. It is characterized by continuous or periodic: **impaired control** over drinking, **preoccupation** with the drug alcohol, despite **adverse consequences**, and distortions in thinking, most notably **denial.**

- **Primary** refers to the nature of alcoholism as a disease; it suggests that alcoholism, as an addiction, is not a symptom of another disease, but a disease in and of itself.

- **Disease** means an involuntary disability, one which an individual is unable to control.

- **Often progressive and fatal** means the disease persists over time and that physical, emotional, and social changes are often cumulative and may progress as drinking continues.

- **Impaired control** means the inability to limit alcohol use, the quantity consumed, and the behavioral consequences.

- **Preoccupation** or association with alcohol use indicates excessive, focused attention given to the drug alcohol, its effects, and/or its use.

- **Adverse consequences** are alcohol-related problems or impairments in such areas as physical health; psychological functioning (e.g., impairments in cognition, changes in mood and behavior); interpersonal functioning (e.g., marital and relationship problems); occupational functioning (e.g., job or scholastic problems); and financial, legal, or spiritual problems.

- **Denial** reduces an individual's awareness of the fact that alcohol use is the cause of, rather than, the solution to the alcoholic's problems. Denial is also an integral part of the disease and a major obstacle to recovery.

. . . Awake you who sleeps, arise from the dead, and Christ will give you light. (Ephesians 5:14)

TODAY'S STEP: I am finding the courage to face the truth about myself.

"The time will come when the sight of this wretchedness, which horrifies you now, will fill you with joy and keep you in a delightful peace. It is only when we have reached the bottom of the abyss of our nothingness and are firmly established there that we can walk before God in justice and truth . . . The fruit of grace must, for the moment, remain hidden, buried as it were in the abyss of your wretchedness underneath the most lively awareness of your weakness." -- Simon Tugwell, O. P., ***Ways of Imperfection***

Six Steps That Turn Desire into Gold

Dr. Napoleon Hill, in his book ***Think and Grow Rich!,*** sets out six principles Andrew Carngie used to build his own personal success philosophy, which earned him $100,000,000. The method by which desire for riches can be transmuted into its financial equivalent consists of the following definite specific steps:

1. Fix in your mind the **exact** amount of money you desire. It is not sufficient merely to say I want plenty of money." Quantify the amount.

2. Determine exactly what you intend to **give** in return for the money you desire. (There is no such reality as "something for nothing.")

3. Establish a specific date for when you intend to **possess** the money you desire.

4. Create a specific plan for carrying out your desire and begin **at once**, whether you are ready or not, to put this plan into **action**.

5. Write out a clear, concise statement of the amount of money you intend to acquire, name the time limit for its acquisition, state what you intend to give in return for the money, and describe clearly the plan through which you intend to accumulate it.

6. Read your written statement aloud twice daily, once just before retiring at night, and once after arising in the morning. As you read – see, feel and believe yourself already in possession of the money.

. . . but with God all things are possible. (Matthew 19:26)

TODAY'S STEP: I trust my truth, my instincts, and my ability to ground myself in reality.

"Freedom is the will to be responsible to ourselves." -- Anonymous

<u>SOBRIETY</u>

The authors of AA's "**Big Book**" talk of principles, and in their wisdom, they leave it to each of us to discover what these principles are. However, the overriding principle is **SOBRIETY**, which encompasses eight other principles:

HONE<u>S</u>TY   - The first principle of honesty is given in chapter three: "We learned we had to fully concede to our innermost selves that we were an alcoholic."

H<u>O</u>PE   - We experience a new hope in Step Two when we come to believe That a "Power greater than ourselves" can restore us to sanity.

RESPONSI<u>B</u>ILITY - Steps Eight, Nine, and Ten help us to accept responsibility for our actions now and in the past and to make amends to those we have harmed.

COU<u>R</u>AGE - The Fourth Step requires courage to do a "fearless moral inventory" to discover who we are and then to continue in the Fellowship.

FA<u>I</u>TH   - Faith is the principle in Step Three which allows us to turn our will and life over to God's care.

LOV<u>E</u>   - Love, as exemplified in the Twelfth Step, is the most godly of the principles. It is the one principle that makes AA what it is, a Fellowship of the Spirit.

PA<u>T</u>IENCE - Steps Six, Seven, and Eleven teach the value of patience and tolerance, which brings us into harmony with God.

HUMILIT<u>Y</u>   - In Steps Five, Six and Seven we must humbly admit our defects to ourselves, God, and another person; become ready to have God remove them; and humbly ask Him to remove them.

But my God shall supply all your need (Philippians 4:19)

TODAY'S STEP: I do not run myself, my circumstances, or my feelings. I am open to myself, others, my Higher Power, and to loving myself unconditionally.

"What we cannot control, and by undertaking, one day at a time, the monumental task of setting our world in order through a change in our thinking." -- One Day at a Time in Al-Anon

Learning to Surrender

It seems everywhere we go these days, we hear people talking about the Twelve Steps or "The Program." Some social commentators have called the Twelve Step groups the most significant spiritual movement in the twentieth century.

The primary reason for the popularity of the Twelve Steps is that more people than ever are being exposed to them through addiction/treatment programs. Virtually all addiction therapists recommend follow-up participation in a Twelve Step program for their clients.

Most of us working the Twelve Steps have identified some compulsion that causes problems for us and others. Usually, we try to control the compulsive behavior, but never attain more than short-term success. We use our will power against it, we pray for help, but nothing seems to work!

Feeling "hopeless and helpless" we enter a treatment program or join a Twelve Step group. We learn that our will alone cannot control our chronic addictions. We ask ourselves, "If reason and will power can't change things, what can?"

The answer is where reason and will power fail, surrender succeeds. The spirit of Step One says, "We can't control our compulsions, so why don't we stop trying? How many ways have we tried and failed? We need to quit pretending things aren't that bad, that somehow we can make them better. We must be completely honest about what has happened in our lives as a result of our compulsions – only then can we create a space
within where the Spirit can work."

Step One presents a paradox, it says the way we regain control of our life is to give up trying to control it. This doesn't make sense at first, but later it will be seen as the beginning of wisdom.

Strengthened with all might, according to His glorious power, unto all patience and long-suffering with joyfulness. (Colossians 1:11)

TODAY'S STEP: I acknowledge my wants and needs, then turn them over to my Higher Power.

"For me alcoholism has proven to be a bitter-sweet legacy – bitter, because of the pain I have suffered, and sweet, because if it weren't for that pain, I wouldn't have searched for and found a better way for living." --Al-Anon Faces Alcoholism

Overcoming Shame

A sense of shame is one of the most toxic emotions we can experience. Modern medical understanding of addictions and compulsivity tells us our "driven-ness" is often an effort to escape from or compensate for a profound sense of shame.

What is this shame that can envelop and paralyze us? We may feel shame about our estrangement from God. We may harbor shameful feelings about our inability to pull in the reins on addictive or compulsive behaviors. We may regret and feel ashamed for the damage we have inflicted on others through our life-styles. We may carry memories of false shame about the dysfunction of our childhood families.

At Step One, we face a turning point. Will we allow this flood of guilt to overwhelm us and drive us back into the practice of our dependencies? Or will we yield this colossal unmanageability over to the care of God? The choice is ours.

Although we may associate brokenness, or powerlessness, with defeat, in reality this admission is the first building block toward lasting victory over all our addictions and dependencies. A paradox of our recovery is that we must give up control of our life in order to gain control.

Usually the admission of powerlessness cannot be achieved unless we have first assessed the magnitude and the gravity of what our addiction has cost us. We may want to compile a list of the losses that have resulted from the practice of our dependencies. These losses may include such things as diminished vocational achievement, impaired intimacy in our most important relationships, and even a ruptured spiritual relationship with God. Only as we appreciate the full grief of our losses can we approach the surrender required in Step One.

Have mercy on me, O Lord, for I am in trouble; My eye wastes away with grief . . . For my life is spent with grief, And my years with sighing; My strength fails because of my iniquity, And my bones waste away. (Psalm 31:9-11)

TODAY'S STEP: I accept who I am, where I am, and I continue to push forward one day at a time.

"A life spent in making mistakes is not only more honorable but more useful than a life spent in doing nothing." -- George Bernard Shaw

Admitted We Were Powerless

Step One is the gateway to the Recovery process. Without it, there is very little hope that we can effectively achieve our goal.

In this critical step we are called upon to admit our personal powerlessness over the dilemma in which we find ourselves. We are called upon to admit our life has reached a stage of such despair that we see no possibility of ever setting it right again.

Despite all we have been taught about never giving up, never yelling "uncle", never admitting defeat, we now find ourselves facing the unrelenting fact that all of our old beliefs have withered and blown away in the reality of our present situation.

We shall learn, as we pursue Step One, that we are facing some puzzling paradoxes:

    (1) "We have to surrender to win."
    (2) "To keep what we have, we have to give it away."
    (3) "Failure is not final – it is actually a stepping stone to success."

Our minds cry out against the idea of personal powerlessness and resist acknowledging that, in reality, we are not in charge. We are accustomed to accepting full responsibility for the events in our lives, as well as in the lives of others. This supports our need to deny we are powerless. We live in the delusion that we are in control. Until we discover how we can be responsible persons and also be powerless, we cannot take the first step toward liberating ourselves from the bondage of our past. The degree to which we are able to surrender is the degree to which we acknowledge our powerlessness.

Although working Step One can be painful, the road to Recovery can only begin with honest self-confrontation and surrender. Admitting our human limitations forms the foundation for working each of the Twelve Steps.

The spirit of the Lord God is upon me; because the Lord hath anointed me to preach good tidings unto the meek; he hath sent me to bind up the broken-hearted, to proclaim liberty to the captives, and the opening of the prison to them that are bound (Isaiah 61:1)

TODAY'S STEP: Day by day, I entrust my problems to a power greater than myself. I am not in control. I'm not God.

"Some people imagine that hope is the highest degree of optimism, a kind of super-optimism. I get the image of someone climbing higher and higher to the most fanciful pinnacle of optimism, there to wave the little flag of hope. A far more accurate picture would be that hope happens when the bottom drops out of our pessimism. We have nowhere to fall but into the ultimate reality of God's motherly caring." -- David Steindl-Rast, **Gratefulness, The Heart of Prayer**

Hope and Surrender

The ordeals we suffer purge us of unfounded optimism. When the "bottom drops out of our pessimism" we are forced to let go of the idea that we are "doers" who can conquer life by the application of our individual will.

The First Step of **all** Twelve Step programs addresses just this issue of the bottom dropping out. In the case of Adult Children of Alcoholics (**ACoA**), the First Step reads, "<u>We admitted we were powerless over the effects of addiction – that our lives had become unmanageable.</u>" We might apply this attitude of surrender to **all** areas of life in which we have struggled fruitlessly to change.

At first glance, hope and surrender may seem to be strange partners. But when, as Steindl-Rast says, we "fall into the ultimate reality of God's motherly caring," we find we have landed in the lap of hope itself. Steindl-Rast asserts that hope is a patient waiting for God, a stillness that allows us to hear the inner voice of guidance. In **Gratefulness, The Heart of Prayer,** he says,

"As long as we wait for an improvement of the situation of our desires

Be still, and know I am God. (Psalm 46:10)

TODAY'S STEP: I am beginning to understand that surrender is not defeat and I welcome powerlessness.

"He who gives himself up to vanity, and does not give himself up to meditation, forgetting the real aim of life and grasping at pleasure, will in time envy him who has exerted himself in meditation." -- The Buddha

The Power of Meditation

In his book, **As A Man Thinketh,** James Allen describes meditation as the acquirement of a knowledge of eternal principles, which results in our ability to become one with the Eternal. The end of meditation is, according to Allen, the direct knowledge of Truth, God, and the realization of divine and profound peace. He further believes that:

"He who earnestly meditates first perceives a truth, as it were, afar off, and then realizes it by daily practice. It is only the doer of the Word of Truth that can know of the doctrine of Truth, for though by pure thought the Truth is perceived, it is only actualized by practice."

"In our meditations, therefore, let your heart grow and expand with ever-broadening love, until, freed from hatred, and passion, and condemnation, it embraces the whole universe with thoughtful tenderness. As the flower opens its petals to receive the morning light, so open your soul more and more to the glorious light of Truth. Soar upward upon the wings of aspiration; be fearless, and believe in the loftiest possibilities. Believe that a life of absolute meekness is possible; believe that a life of stainless purity is possible; believe that a life of perfect holiness is possible; believe that the realization of the highest truth is possible. He who so believes, climbs rapidly the heavenly hills, whilst the unbelievers continue to grope darkly and painfully in the fog-bound valleys."

"So believing, so aspiring, so meditating, divinely sweet and beautiful will be your spiritual experiences, and glorious the revelations that will enrapture your inward division. As you realize the divine Love, the divine Justice, the divine Purity, the Perfect Law of Good, or God, great will be your bliss and deep your peace. The veil of the material universe, so dense and impenetrable to the eye of error, so thin and gauzy to the eye of Truth, will be lifted and the spiritual will be revealed."

Acquaint now thyself with Him, and be at peace. (Job 22:21)

TODAY'S STEP: My life is brightened, my burdens lifted and my hopes become realities whenever I look to my Higher Power for inspiration.

"As we learn to depend upon our Higher Power through applying the Al-Anon program to our lives, fear and uncertainty are replaced by faith and confidence." -- *One Day At A Time In Al-Anon*

"Easy Does It"

One of the wonderful benefits we receive by going to meetings is we always find new ways to work our program. At one of my regular Al-Anon meetings an attendee was celebrating her fourth year. She shared her story and then, as she opened the meeting for discussion, she passed around a basket full of slips of paper with Al-Anon slogans printed on them. She suggested we each take one and try to apply it to our day. It was remarkable how many of us seemed to get the perfect slogan!

The very next day I found myself in a stressful situation. I was struggling to solve a tough problem, growing frustrated and upset, but no closer to a solution. I asked my Higher Power for guidance and suddenly remembered the basket. In my mind, I imagined myself reaching into a basket full of slogans. Again, I got exactly what I needed. The slogan I visualized was "Easy Does It." It reminded me to stop trying to force a solution and wait until I could approach the problem more gently. I felt much better, my thinking was clearer, and in time a solution appeared.

I have heard that the time to be especially gentle with ourselves is <u>not</u> when we're doing well, but when we're doing poorly. We may be able to push ourselves hard when things are going our way, but we invite trouble if we try this when we're already struggling to manage the basic activities of life. We tend to be very hard on ourselves, so hard at times that we make our own lives unmanageable. As a result, we often accomplish less than we would if we took a more gentle approach. "Easy Does It", suggests not only that we learn to slow down, but also that we learn to lighten up.

Knowing which Al-Anon tool to apply is not always easy, especially in the middle of a crisis. But we can be grateful for a Higher Power who knows our needs, and for meetings that help us to find new ways to use these tools in our lives.

See how the farmer waits for the precious fruit of the earth, waiting patiently for it until it receives the early and the latter rain. (James 5:7-8)

TODAY'S STEP: God will strengthen me when life gets hard.

"We should have much peace if we would not busy ourselves with the sayings and doings of others."   -- Thomas a Kempis

<u>*Tradition One*</u>

Our common welfare should come first; personal progress for the greatest number depends upon unity.

1. Am I in my group a healing, mending, integrating person, or am I a divisive? What about gossip and taking other member's inventories?

2. Am I a peacemaker? Or do I, with pious preludes such as "just for the sake of discussion," plunge into argument?

3. Am I gentle with those who rub me the wrong way, or am I abrasive?

4. Do I make competitive AA remarks, such as comparing one group with another or contrasting AA in one place with AA in another?

5. Do I put down some AA activities as if I were superior for not participating in this or that aspect of AA?

6. Am I informed about AA as a whole? Do I support, in every way I can, AA as a whole, or just the parts I understand and approve of?

7. Am I as considerate of AA members as I want them to be of me?

8. Do I spout platitudes about love while indulging in and secretly justifying behavior that bristles with hostility?

9. Do I go through AA meetings or read just enough AA literature to really keep in touch?

10. Do I share with AA all of me, the bad and the good, accepting as well as giving the help of fellowship?

Repent therefore and be converted, that your sins may be blotted out, so that times of refreshing may come from the presence of God. (Acts 3:19)

TODAY'S STEP: I move confidently toward my ideal, knowing my steps are guided by my Higher Power.

"Suffering isn't ennobling, recovery is." -- Christian N. Barnard

Suggested Welcome for Al-Anon Meetings

We welcome you to the (*Group Name*) Al-Anon Family Group and hope you will find in this fellowship the help and friendship we have been privileged to enjoy.

We who live, or have lived, with the problem of alcoholism understand as perhaps few others can. We, too, were lonely and frustrated, but in Al-Anon we discover that no situation is really hopeless, and that it is possible for us to find contentment, and even happiness, whether the alcoholic is still drinking or not.

We urge you to try our program. It has helped many of us find solutions that lead to serenity. So much depends on our own attitudes, and as we learn to place our problem in its true perspective, we find it loses its power to dominate our thoughts and our lives.

The family situation is bound to improve as we apply the Al-Anon ideas. Without such spiritual help, living with an alcoholic is too much for most of us. Our thinking becomes distorted by trying to force solutions and we become irritable and unreasonable without knowing it.

The Al-Anon program is based on the Twelve Steps (adapted from Alcoholics Anonymous), which we try, little by little, one day at a time, to apply to our lives along with our slogans and the Serenity Prayer. The loving interchange of help among members and daily reading of Al-Anon literature thus make us ready to receive the priceless gift of serenity.

Al-Anon is an anonymous fellowship. Everything that is said here, in the group meeting and member-to-member, must be held in confidence. Only in this way can we feel free to say what is in our minds and hearts, for this is how we help one another in Al-Anon.

Blessed be the . . . Father of Our Lord Jesus Christ, the . . . God of all comfort, who comforts us in all our tribulation that we may be able to comfort those who are in any trouble. (2 Corinthians 1:3-4)

TODAY'S STEP: I am willing to turn my will and my life over to my Higher Power, to let go of willfulness and to surrender myself to Recovery.

"The coming to consciousness is not a discovery of some new thing; it is a long and painful return to that which has always been. It is when we admit our powerlessness that the guide appears" – Helen M. Luke

Smokers Anonymous

Smokers Anonymous is a self-help program based on the 12 Steps of Alcoholics Anonymous. Smokers Anonymous is a fellowship of men and women who gather together to obtain freedom form nicotine addiction and smoking obsession. Any person with a sincere desire to stop smoking is welcome. We have learned to admit we were powerless over smoking, for us no amount of willpower would work and that by helping other smokers we will help ourselves stay <u>ex-smokers.</u>

Nicotine is the most addicting drug that human beings put into their systems. 99 out of 100 people who smoke one cigarette become addicted. What does addiction mean? The dictionary says, "a slave to someone or something." <u>Are you a slave?</u> Do you:

- (a) Walk into meetings and look to see where the ashtrays are before you look for your friends;
- (b) Wait for a table in the smoking section rather than be seated immediately in the non-smoking section;
- (c) Leave a movie in the middle to have a few quick puffs in the theater lobby;
- (d) Search frantically through pockets, drawers, under chair cushions, car seats, etc. for a cigarette; and,
- (e) Leave the safety and comfort of your home late at night because you're out of cigarettes?

Some of us "slaves" have even gone through the garbage can for cigarette butts or picked up someone's discard from the street or public ashtrays. Some of us have even gone so far as to "hide" our smoking from loved ones (as do many addicts of other substances) and engaged in "secretive" smoking.

Once you know you are powerless, you can stop wasting your energy trying to control your smoking. You can stop blaming yourself for being a weak person. Instead, you can say, "I am addicted to nicotine. My body is physically dependent on nicotine. My life is unmanageable!"

Carry each others burdens, and in this way you will fulfill the law of Christ. (Galatians 6:2)

TODAY'S STEP: Day by day, I entrust my problems to a power greater than myself.

"The only prison we have to escape from is the prison of our own minds." --
Anonymous

<u>*Maturity*</u>

MATURITY is the ability to control anger and settle differences without violence or destruction.

MATURITY is patience. The willingness to pass up immediate pleasure in favor of the long-term gain.

MATURITY is perseverance. The ability to sweat out a project or situation in spite of opposition and discouraging setbacks.

MATURITY is the capacity to face unpleasantness and frustration, discomfort and defeat, without complaint or collapse.

MATURITY is the ability to make a decision and stand by it. The immature spend their lives exploring endless possibilities, then do nothing.

MATURITY means dependability, keeping one's word, and coming through a crisis. The immature are masters of the alibi – confused and disorganized. Their lives are a maze of broken promises, former friends, unfinished business and good intentions, which never materialize.

MATURITY is the art of living in peace with that which we cannot change.

MATURITY is accepting yourself and not having to make excuses for your behavior.

MATURITY IS ADMITTING YOU ARE POWERLESS!!!

In **Quit Smoking with the 12 Steps of Smokers Anonymous**

When wisdom enters your heart, And knowledge is pleasant to your soul, Discretion will preserve you; Understanding will keep you. (Proverbs 2:10-11)

TODAY'S STEP: I pray that my Higher Power will give me the courage and strength to recognize the Truth about myself, and to help me accept that I am powerless.

"There are things about ourselves that we need to get rid of; there are things we need to change. But at the same time, we do not need to be too desperate, too ruthless, and too combative. Along the way to usefulness and happiness, many of those things will change themselves, and the others can be worked on as we go. The first thing we need to do is recognize and trust our own Inner Nature, and not lose sight of it. For within the Ugly Duckling is the Swan, inside the Bouncy Tigger is the Rescuer who knows the Way, and in each of us is something Special, and that we need to keep." -- Benjamin Hoff, *The Tao of Pooh*

Finding the Right Group

There are several ways to find a good group – one that is right for you.

- Read over the **Self-Help Resources** in Appendix B. Write or call the national headquarters and inquire about meetings in your area, i.e., Al-Anon, Alcoholics Anonymous, Alateen, Narcotics Anonymous, Over-Eaters Anonymous, etc.

- Check the phone book, both the white and yellow pages. Some listings use the full name of the group (CoDependents Anonymous); others list by initials (CoDA).

- Check with your local community agencies, treatment centers, hospitals, mental-
health units, social-service agencies, or churches. They may have information about groups in your area.

- Check with the primary addiction recovery groups in your area, such as Alcoholics Anonymous. They may have information about other Twelve Step meetings and codependency groups related to that addiction. For instance, Alcoholics Anonymous will probably be able to point you to Al-Anon; Cocaine Anonymous will probably be able to tell you where the Co-Anon groups meet.

- Another good way to find a group is by contacting the National Self-Help Clearinghouse, 365 5th Avenue, Suite 3300, New York, New York 10016, (212) 817-1822, www.selfhelpweb.org/. This organization is connected to seventy clearinghouses across the country and responds promptly to requests.

. . . but with God all things are possible. (Matthew 19:26)

TODAY'S STEP: As I work the Steps, I grow in my capacity to be happy.

"What is it that every man seeks? To be secure, to be happy, to do what he pleases without restraint and without compulsion." -- Epictetus

Levels of Twelve Step Involvement

No one is forced to do anything in a 12 Step Program. It is one of the few organizations that support the inherent constitutional right to do what we want. There is no coercion to participate on any level. If you want to belong, that's fine. You are welcome to attend meetings and work the Steps. If you don't want to belong, that's fine also!

For most members, however, their involvement progresses through a number of levels. At the first level, they attend meetings. At the second, they get a sponsor who can show them how the program works. At the third level, they read Twelve Step literature and discuss it with other members of the Program. At the fourth level, they start working the Twelve Steps.

As members start to grow and change – as a result of attending meetings and working the Steps – they are ready to move to a fifth level of involvement and begin sponsoring others. After they gain experience as sponsors, they are then ready for the sixth level of involvement, general service work, guided by AA's Twelve Traditions, the set principles that act as bylaws. General Service work is designed to benefit Twelve Step Programs as a whole.

Notice the progression: (a) Individuals help themselves first, then they (b) help other people in the program, then they (c) help the program as a whole. In summary, the levels of involvement are as follows:

1.   Attending meetings;
2.   Getting a sponsor;
3.   Reading and discussing Program literature;
4.   Working the Twelve Steps;
5.   Sponsoring others; and,
6.   Doing service work.

That your love will overflow more and more, and that you will keep on growing in knowledge and understanding. I want you to understand what really matters, so that you may live pure and blameless lives. . . (Philippians 1:9-10)

TODAY'S STEP: If I want to become skillful at applying the Program to my life, I need to do more than go to an occasional meeting. I must make a commitment and practice, practice, practice.

"Oh, I've been a victim all my life", he said. "No, Joe," she said. "Your whole life is ahead of you." -- **Joe and the Volcano**

The Detachment Step

The First Step is the Step that helps us begin detaching – a Recovery concept that means we release and detach from others – lovingly, whenever possible.

This Step helps us begin to identify the proper use and abuse of willpower. We begin feeling instead of running from our emotions. We identify how we have neglected ourselves, so we may better love ourselves in any circumstance.

It is the first step toward removing ourselves as victims – of others, of us, and of life. This is the <u>Detachment Step</u>. Detachment means to detach from *the emotion* of the situation/conflict.

This Step is about boundaries. We learn the limits and extent of our responsibilities and ourselves. We learn to identify when we're trying to do the impossible or trying to do that which is not our job.

Then, we stop doing the impossible and focus our attentions on the possible – living our lives, taking care of ourselves, feeling and responding appropriately. We can love ourselves and others without feeling the overwhelming need to control and manipulate them and their situations to our liking.

When you focus on others, before you decide to "help" others ask yourself 2 questions:

1)   Is he/she capable to doing this for him/herself?
2)   If I do this, will it give rise to resentment?

Often, this Step puts us in touch with our feelings – feelings of fear, hurt, or shame. It puts us in touch with grief. At first, this Step can feel dark and frightening. It doesn't have to, not for long. It renders us powerless over what we cannot control, so we can become empowered. Once we accept whatever loss or area of powerlessness we're facing, we're free to feel and deal with our feelings, then move forward with life.

I am learning to be content in whatever circumstances I am. (Philippians 4:11)

TODAY'S STEP: I avoid making excuses for my own or someone else's behavior.

"Everything has its wonders, even darkness and silence, and I learn, whatever state I may be in, therein to be content." -- **Helen Keller**

"HOW = Honesty, Open-Mindedness, and Willingness"

In order to work Step One effectively, we need three ingredients: Honesty, Open-Mindedness, and Willingness. These are the crucial components of the "HOW" of success, and they are essential to Recovery. Without them, our chances of succeeding are negligible. So it is necessary to admit that the unmanageability of our lives is directly related to our actions.

We have cultivated self-delusion because the pain of seeing ourselves as solely responsible for our sorry state of affairs is almost too much to bear. This is the time to remind ourselves that, in the past, we didn't have the knowledge or experience to acknowledge or manage our worsening situation. Once we're able to acknowledge this inability, we open the door to information that helps us eliminate our feelings of guilt and shame. It's by admitting and owning these feelings that it becomes possible to rid ourselves of them.

Our pride has kept us from seeking help from others. We were afraid of being viewed as stupid or uninformed. But now we're willing to ask for help. We're willing to begin to relinquish our old ideas and attitudes so that we can accept the guidance now being offered to us.

We can't control our Recovery. We can't force ourselves to let go any faster, nor insist upon serenity. But we can take small actions to remind ourselves that we are willing participants in this process. We have every reason to be hopeful, for each step we take is a step toward living life more fully. We have been affected by a disease of attitudes and values. When we treat ourselves with love and approval, that's when we will know we are recovering.

Where shall I go from your Spirit? Or where shall I flee from your presence? If I ascend up into heaven, you are there: If I make my bed in hell, behold, you are there. If I take the wings of the morning, and dwell in the uppermost parts of the sea; even there shall your hand lead me, and your right hand shall hold me. (Psalm 139:7-10)

TODAY'S STEP: How do I feel today? How am I doing? If I can answer those questions truthfully, I am more likely to pursue the help I need and to share the happy times with others as well.

"True freedom lies in the realization and calm acceptance of the fact that there may very well be no perfect answer." -- Allen Reid McGinnis

What is Acceptance?

By Bill W.

"On entering AA, we become the beneficiaries of a very different experience. Our new way of staying sober is literally founded upon the proposition that 'Of ourselves, we are nothing, the Father doeth the works.' In Steps One and Two of our recovery program these ideas are specifically spelled out: 'We admitted that we were powerless over alcohol . . . that our lives had become unmanageable' – 'Came to believe that a power greater than ourselves could restore us to sanity.' We couldn't lick alcohol with our remaining resources and so we accepted the further fact that dependence upon a Higher Power (if only our AA group) could do this hitherto impossible job. The moment we were able to fully accept these facts, our release from the alcohol compulsion had begun.
For most of us this pair of acceptances had required a lot of exertion to achieve. Our whole treasured philosophy of self-sufficiency had to be cast aside. This had not been done with old-fashioned will power; it was instead a matter of developing the willingness to accept these new facts of living. We neither ran nor fought. But accept we did. And then we were free. There had been no irretrievable disaster."

"This kind of acceptance and faith is capable of producing 100 percent sobriety. In fact it usually does; and it must, else we could have no life at all. But the moment we carry these attitudes into our emotional problems, we find that only relative results are possible. Nobody can, for example, become completely free from fear, anger, and pride. Hence in this life we shall attain nothing like perfect humility and love. So we shall have to settle, respecting most of our problems, for a very gradual progress, punctuated sometimes by heavy setbacks. Our old-time attitudes of 'all or nothing' will have to be abandoned." Everyone has an "as is" sign. No one is perfect.

Do not love the world or anything in the world. If anyone loves the world, the love of the Father is not in him. For everything in the world – the cravings of sinful man, the lust of his eyes and the boasting of what he has and does – comes not from the Father but from the world. The world and its desires pass away, but the man who does the will of God lives forever. (1 John 2:15-18)

TODAY'S STEP: I let go of old ideas about myself and discover a new self through Recovery.

"True words are not beautiful;
Beautiful words are not true.
A good man does not argue;
He who argues is not a good man.
A wise man has no extensive knowledge;
He who has extensive knowledge is not a wise man.
The sage does not accumulate for himself.
The more he does for others, the more he has himself.
The more he gives to others, the more he possesses of his own.
The Way of Heaven is to benefit others and not to injure.
The Way of the sage is to act but not to compete. --*The Way of Lao-Tzu*

"Acting As If"

The behavior we call "Acting As If" can be a powerful Recovery tool. Acting as if is a way to practice being positive. It's a positive form of pretending. It's a tool we use to get ourselves unstuck. It's a tool we make a conscious decision to use.

There are many areas where acting as if – combined with our other Recovery principles – will set the stage for the reality we desire. We can act as if we love ourselves, until we actually do begin to care for ourselves. We can act as if we have a right to say no, until we believe we do.

When a problem plagues us, acting as if can help us get unstuck. We act as if the problem will be or already is solved, so we can go on with our life. Often, acting as if we are detached will set the stage for detachment to come in and take over. Acting as if can be helpful when a feeling begins to control us. We make a conscious decision to act as if we feel fine and are going to be fine.

Acting as if is a positive way to overcome doubts, fear and anxiety. We do not have to lie; we do not have to be dishonest with ourselves. We open up the positive possibilities of the future, instead of limiting the future by today's feelings and circumstances.

Verily, I say unto you, If ye have faith, and doubt not, ye shall not only do this which is done to the fig tree, but also if ye shall say unto this mountain, be thou removed, and be thou cast into the sea; it shall be done. (Matthew 21:21)

TODAY'S STEP: My sense of humor helps me to carry – and to get – the message of the Twelve Steps.

"I was thirty-five years old the first time I spoke up to my mother and refused to buy into her games and manipulation. I was terribly frightened and almost couldn't believe I was doing this. I found I didn't have to be mean. I didn't have to start an argument. But I could say what I wanted and needed to say to take care of myself. I learned I could love and honor myself, and still care about my mother – the way I wanted to – not the way she wanted me to." -- Anonymous, ***The Language of Letting Go***

<u>*Welcome to Al-Anon*</u>

As a newcomer you may feel you are here tonight for the alcoholic . . . that your presence here may teach you how to stop his or her drinking. The truth is you are here
because of the alcoholic and not **for** the alcoholic. You will soon learn that you did not cause the alcoholic to drink, nor can you cure the alcoholic. You are here for **yourself**. You and only you are responsible for dealing with your recovery from the effects of the disease of alcoholism.

You will find love, understanding, and a lot of hope from the Al-Anon Family Group. The people around you tonight are experiencing in varying degrees the hurt, the anger, and the anxiety you are experiencing. We in Al-Anon share our experiences because it helps us to focus on ourselves and our recovery. We do this with the use of the Al-Anon tools of the Program (Steps, Traditions, slogans, meetings, sponsorship, service, literature), which will be provided to you.

Al-Anon will work for you if you allow it to – it's as effective as you make it. It's the safe place, the right place to be. Feel free to ask any questions or you may feel more comfortable just listening. That's fine too. There are no "musts" in Al-Anon.

We all have dark times in our lives, but the journey to better times is often what makes us happier, stronger people. When we stop expecting instant relief, we may come to believe that where we are today is exactly where our Higher Power would have us to be. Finally, what you say or hear here and who you see here tonight stays in this room. Your anonymity is protected at all times.

Let my speech always be filled with grace... so that I will know how to respond to each person. (Colossians 4:6)

TODAY'S STEP: I avoid making excuses for my own or someone else's behavior.

"What another would have done as well as you, do not do it. What another would have said as well as you, do not say it; written as well, do not write it. Be faithful to that which exists nowhere but in yourself – and thus make yourself indispensable." -- Andre Gide, **Les Nourritures Terrestres** (Fruits of the Earth)

<u>*What Really Counts*</u>

Jesus talked about money and possessions in at least one third of his parables. He usually concluded that money couldn't buy what really counts. In fact, the most important elements in life have no price tags.

It is interesting that Twelve-Step Recovery charges no fee. A person's wealth, possessions, or station in life are irrelevant. There is a cost, however. We must invest ourselves. Our possessions are not important. We are. As playwright Henrik Ibsen said, "Money may buy the husk of things, not the kernel. It brings you food not appetite, not faithfulness, days of pleasure but not peace or happiness."

Jesus and the Twelve Steps can supply the kernel. Where our hearts/desires lie, our money follows. **"Do not store up for yourselves treasures on earth, where moth and rust destroy, and where thieves break in and steal. But store up for yourselves treasures in heaven, where moth and rust do not destroy, and where thieves do not break in and steal. For where your treasure is, there your heart will be also." (Matthew 6:19-22)**

Jesus also directed us to look within for our treasures. **"Command those who are rich in this present world not to be arrogant nor to put their hope in wealth, which is so uncertain, but to put their hope in God, who richly provides us with everything for our enjoyment. Command them to do good, to be rich in good deeds, and to be generous and willing to share." (1 Timothy 6:17-20)**

"People who want to get rich fall into temptation and a trap and into many foolish and harmful desires that plunge men into ruin and destruction. For the love of money is a root of all kinds of evil. Some people, eager for money have wandered from the faith and pierced themselves with many grief's." (1 Timothy 6:9-11)

TODAY'S STEP: I practice the discipline of H.O.W. – Honesty, Open-mindedness and willingness everyday with my feelings, attitudes and actions.

"There is a life force, an energy that is translated through you into action. And because there is only one of you in all time, this expression is unique ... it is not your business to determine how good it is, nor how valuable, nor how it compares with other expressions. It is your business to keep it yours clearly and directly, to keep the channel open." -- Martha Graham

"An Attitude of Gratitude"

Say thank you until you mean it. Thank God for everyone and everything sent your way.

"An attitude of gratitude" unlocks the fullness of life. It turns what we have into enough, and more. It turns denial into acceptance, chaos to order, confusion to clarity. It can turn a meal into a feast, a house into a home, a stranger into a friend. It turns problems into gifts, failures into successes, the unexpected into perfect timing, and mistakes into important events. It can turn an existence into a real life, and disconnected situations into important and beneficial lessons. Gratitude makes sense of our past, brings peace for today, and creates a vision of tomorrow.

Your attitude reflects your thought life. What are you thinking now? "An attitude of gratitude" makes things right. It turns negative energy into positive energy. There is no situation or circumstance so small or large that it is not susceptible to gratitude's power. We can start with who we are and what we have today, apply an attitude of gratitude, and then let it work its magic.

Say thank you, until you mean it. If you say it long enough, you will believe it.

Taken from Melody Beattie, *The Language of Letting Go*

PRAYER: God, help me to shine the transforming light of gratitude on all the circumstances of my life.

We always thank God for all of you, making mention of you in our prayers. We continually remember before our God and Father your work produced by faith, your labor promoted by love, and your endurance inspired by hope in our Lord Jesus Christ. (1 Thessalonians 1:2-4)

TODAY'S STEP: Thankfulness today will help me see the miracles at work in my life and in the lives of others on the road to recovery.

"Man will only become better when you make him see what he is like." -- Anton Pavlovich Chekhov

Types and Prevalence of Addiction

Any substance that we ingest, or any activity or behavior that we engage in, can become an addictive habit or disorder.

> *Addiction refers to a relationship with a substance or activity that is excessive or compulsive, causes problems in one or more areas of our lives, causes distress when we are not engaging in it, and often exerts a good deal of control over our lives, even when we are not engaging in the addictive behaviors.*

Addiction is better seen as a "disorder" with a characteristic set of symptoms rather than something that is easily or simplistically defined. The more common substance-related addictions involve abuse of alcohol, tobacco, or other drugs; compulsive overeating; and compulsive dieting. The most commonly seen addictions related to activities or behaviors include compulsive sex (pornography, multiple affairs, etc), compulsive gambling, workaholism, making money and accumulating wealth, spending money (shopping), seeking power, and stealing or committing crimes. Recently, attention has also been given to love and relationship addiction, as well as to the so-called positive addictions such as exercising, running, and meditation.

The personal pain – whether it is physical, emotional, or spiritual suffering – that goes along with any type of addiction is hard to quantify. Such pain certainly does not stand out when one looks at statistics. Nonetheless, let us look at some statistics for several of the addictions, keeping in mind that numbers in no way tell us anything about the specific people represented in these numbers.

- A recent report to the U.S. Congress entitled **Alcohol and Health** estimates that 18 million adults eighteen years of age and older are addicted to alcohol.
- The National Institute of Mental Health reported that 13.7% of adults have experienced problems with alcohol.
- 5.9% of the adults studied had a problem with drug abuse and drug addiction.
- 2% to 3% of adults have serious gambling problems.
- Millions of people suffer from compulsive overeating, anorexia and/or bulimia.

I will go in the strength of the Lord God. (Psalm 71:16)

TODAY'S STEP: God will strengthen me when life gets hard

"There is a guidance for each of us, and by lowly listening we shall hear the right word – Place yourself in the middle of the stream of power and wisdom, which flows into your life. Then, without effort, you are impelled to truth and to perfect contentment."
– Ralph Waldo Emerson

<u>*But Is It A "Disease"?*</u>

Is codependency a disease? As psychiatrist Timmen Cermak in *Diagnosing and Treating Codependence* (1986) points out, "Therapists in traditional mental health approaches have attempted to treat (separately) the symptoms of codependence, diagnosing clients as having anxiety disorders, depression, hysterical personality disorders, or dependent personality disorders, to name a few."

Cermak also says, "Once we accept that codependence exists on a par with other personality disorders such as borderline, narcissistic, and dependent personalities, it should be clear that it deserves to be treated with the same level of sophistication."

But since neither the language nor the criteria used to describe codependence are consistent or organized into a generally accepted substantive framework by those who work with the disorder, it has been impossible to do the research required to establish scientific validity for viewing it as a legitimate personality "disease." Until this research is done, the psychological community's own rules forbid including codependence in the nomenclature as a disease.

In the meantime, those who deal with people in the grips of the compulsive symptoms of codependence are not waiting for the official labeling of the disease. Whatever codependence is, it certainly **acts** like a disease. And as Cermak notes, "According to what we have learned it would seem at least to fit the usual descriptions of a disease (with discernable symptoms that are predictable, progressive, and debilitating)." As any contemporary bibliography on codependence suggests, many therapists are struggling to give form and structure to the river of data about codependence and its symptoms that is overflowing the banks of chemical dependency treatment centers into the other mental health fields.

Don't copy the behavior and customs of this world, but be a new and different person with a fresh newness in all you do and think . . . (Romans 12:2)

TODAY'S STEP: God help me to believe in myself and help me to let go of old beliefs and feelings that are hurting me.

<h1 style="text-align:center"><u>Step Two</u></h1>

<u>Came to believe that a power greater than ourselves could restore us to wholeness.</u>

Accepting our powerlessness leads us naturally into Step Two. By this time, we have discovered the impact that being raised in a dysfunctional family had on our lives. Our present condition is a result of the many decisions we made to survive in that chaotic environment. We are now faced with behavior that produces unmanageable situations over which we are powerless. For some of us, belief in the strength of self-will was all we thought we needed until, in Step One, we realized the true state of our ineffective behavior. As we accept the idea of a Power greater than ourselves, we begin to function in a healthier way, and our lives become more manageable. We recognize that we are just human beings, learning to live within our human limitations.

Step Two is referred to as the Hope Step. It is the starting point from which we begin our journey toward a more spiritual view of life. In Step One, when we recognize our condition, we felt hopeless and helpless. Step Two instills new hope, as we see help is available if we simply take the risk to believe and trust in a Power greater than ourselves. If we follow the guidance of that Power, we no longer need to struggle. We now have a chance to dramatically decrease our old patterns of behavior and gradually become the persons we were meant to be. Step Two provides a foundation for the spiritual development that will help us achieve a greater sense of personal fulfillment.

As Newcomers, we often encounter stumbling blocks when working this Step. One obstacle is the difficulty we have in believing a Power greater than ourselves exists. We may find it impossible to imagine, through 'believing," the intensity of our obsessions and compulsions could decrease.

Another problem posed by Step Two is the implication that disorder and ineffective behavior permeates our lives. Having recognized that our lives are unmanageable, we now know we need new direction. These are powerful issues for us; they can be frightening when we face them for the first time. For many of us, they are definite contradictions of our former beliefs about ourselves and our lives.

The discovery and acceptance of a Power greater than ourselves is the beginning of our turning away from our self-will. Through working the Steps, we can experience a growing trust in our Higher Power.

<u>***SECOND STEP PRAYERS***</u>

<u>"Came to believe that a Power greater than ourselves could restore us to wholeness."</u>

I pray for an open mind so I may come to believe in a Power greater than myself. I pray for humility and the continued opportunity to increase my faith. I don't want to be crazy any more.

In this moment, I can believe I am never alone; I can experience the sense of freedom that having a Higher Power offers me. I can remind myself that believing is also an action, and if I am willing to practice it, one moment at a time, I will develop faith.

<u>*MEDITATIONS*</u>

Bless me, dear Father, and let me understand all that is happening in my life today. I ask for the Christ Light to shine on all my dark corners so I may look upon the problems that will confront me. I pray for the gentleness of saints and to learn that no matter how much I feel right, there is always another side to consider. Teach me humility, which is true strength, and let my thoughts and actions today be constructive and helpful. Grant me the ability to help someone in need and lighten a shadow in his life as I ask Thee for the same gift. Teach me consideration and help me to shift the concern I have for myself to others more in need. Take from me the fear of losing my image in the eyes of others. In Thy sweet mercy, let those who love me know me as I really am. All this, dear Father, I ask in Thy Holy Name.

<u>*AFFIRMATIONS*</u>

Each day I become stronger in my faith and in the outcome of my own future.

My faith lives in every part of my life. It is always there and always with me, creating even more strength, confidence, and belief within me.

I take full responsibility for my thoughts. I use the capability of my mind in the best possible way.

I allow no thought that is harmful to me to dwell in my mind at anytime.

"I do not ask to walk smooth paths nor bear an easy load, I pray for strength and fortitude to climb the rock strewn road. Give me such courage I can scale the hardest peaks alone, and transform every stumbling block into a stepping stone." – G.B. Burket

When you were born, you didn't come with an owner's manual; these guidelines make life work better.

The Rules for Being Human

1. You will receive a body. You may like it or hate it, but it's the only thing you are sure to keep for the rest of your life.
2. You will learn lessons. You are enrolled in a full-time informal school called "Life on Planet Earth". Every person or incident is the Universal Teacher.
3. There are no mistakes, only lessons. Growth is a process of experimentation. "Failures" are as much a part of the process as "success."
4. A lesson is repeated until learned. It is presented to you in various forms until you learn it – then you can go on to the next lesson.
5. If you don't learn easy lessons, they get harder. External problems are a precise reflection of your internal state. When you clear inner obstructions, your outside world changes. Pain is how the universe gets your attention.
6. You will know you've learned a lesson when your actions change. Wisdom is practice. A little of something is better than a lot of nothing.
7. "There" is no better than "here". When your "there" becomes a "here" you will simply obtain another "there" that again looks better than "here."
8. Others are only mirrors of you. You cannot love or hate something about another unless it reflects something you love or hate in yourself.
9. Your life is up to you. Life provides the canvas; you do the painting. Take charge of your life – or someone else will.
10. You always get what you want. Your subconscious rightfully determines what energies, experiences, and people you attract – therefore, the only foolproof way to know what you want is to see what you have. There are no victims, only students.
11. There is no right or wrong, but there are consequences. Moralizing doesn't help. Judgments only hold the patterns in place. Just do your best.
12. Your answers lie inside you. Children need guidance from others; as we mature, we trust our hearts, where the Laws of Spirit are written. You know more than you have heard or read or been told. All you need to do is to look, listen, and trust.
13. You will forget all of this. 14. You can remember any time you wish.

(From the book *"If Life is a Game, These are the Rules"* by Cherie Carter-Scott)
Cast your cares on the Lord and he will sustain you. (Psalm 55:22)

TODAY'S STEP: I avoid making excuses for my own or someone else's behavior.

"The Lord works from the inside out. The world works from the outside in. The world would take people out of the slums. Christ takes the slums out of people, and then they take themselves out of the slums. The world would mold men by changing their environment. Christ changes men, who then change their environment. The world would shape human behavior, but Christ can change human nature."   -- Ezra Taft Benson

Every Day A New Beginning

Friends came to clean the desk of a Cardinal who had died. Inscribed on a small placard was the following prayer:

Tire not of new beginnings;

Build thy life, never on regret

Always on resolve!

Shed no tear on the blotted page of the past,

But turn the leaf – and smile –

To see the clean white page before thee.

Tire not of new beginnings! The life of sobriety is a new beginning. Build your life on the resolve to follow the AA 12 Step program in its entirety. Many cities have been completely destroyed and then rebuilt by willing hands. The alcoholic also has a rock bottom and by the time it is reached, his/her life is a shambles. The Twelve Steps are excellent for rebuilding our lives. To make the building ready for occupancy, the first three steps are the foundation. The other nine are the maintenance steps and without constant attention to these, decay can set in. The Bible tells us that *"Unless the* L*ord* *builds the house, the builders labor in vain. Unless the* L*ord* *watches over the city, the guards stand watch in vain" (Psalm 127:1).*

You didn't know you were in the building business, did you? You are not building a house, but you are building a life. Check your foundation from time to time. Remember that constant maintenance makes for a good building.

Search me, O God, and know my heart: try me, and know my thoughts. (Psalm 139:23)

TODAY'S STEP: I let consequences and responsibility fall where they belong.

"Life is a self-fulfilling prophecy; you won't necessarily get what you want in life, but in the long run you will usually get what you expect." -- Dennis Waitley

Before I entered into a Program I didn't know what Faith or Trust was, but now I know these two concepts only work when we recognize and accept that they are based on the following principles:

1. I am **"A child of God"**;

2. My inheritance is **"the Kingdom of Heaven"**; and,

3. **"I can do all things through Christ, who strengthens me"** (Philippians 4:13).

The Acceptance Prayer

God grant me the serenity to accept my addiction (or those of others) gracefully and humbly. Grant me also the ability to absorb the teachings of the Program, which by its past experience is trying to help me. Teach me to be grateful for the help I receive.

Guide me, Higher Power, in the path of tolerance and understanding of my fellow members and fellow man, guide me away from the path of criticism, intolerance, jealousy and envy of my friends. Let me not prejudge, let me not become a moralist, keep my tongue and thoughts from malicious idle gossip.

Help me to grow in stature spiritually, mentally and morally. Grant me that greatest of all rewards, of being able to help my fellow sufferers in their search out of the addiction that has encompassed them.

Above all, help me to be less critical and impatient with myself.

For he satisfied the longing soul, and fills the hungry soul with goodness (Psalm 107:9)

TODAY'S STEP: Faith is the recognizing that the longer I suffer under trying circumstances, the more certain I am to appreciate my deliverance

"Wrong, wrong thou art doing to thyself, O my soul; and all too soon thou shalt have no more time to do thyself right. Man has but one life; already thine is nearing its close, yet still has thou no eye to thine own honor, but art staking thy happiness on the souls of other men." -- Marcus Aurelius, **Meditations**

On Being Codependent

To many, codependency is the current buzz word to use when discussing addictive behavior. But for millions it's more than a classification . . . it's a painful reality. The term codependency finds it roots in alcohol treatment. Specialists in this field realized that family members and friends played a significant role in perpetuating or enabling the disease process by adopting dysfunctional behavior patterns in an attempt to adapt to the alcoholic in their life.

In the book **Love is a Choice**, codependency is defined as an addiction to people (by assuming the role of rescuer or victim), behavior (such as work, anger, sex, perfectionism), and things (including alcohol/drugs, money, food). Codependency arises from the fallacy of trying to control inner feelings by manipulating other people and circumstances. The following 10 points can identify a codependent:

1. A codependent is driven by one or more compulsions.
2. The codependent is bound and tormented by the way things were in the dysfunctional family of origin.
3. The codependent's self-esteem is very low.
4. A codependent is certain his or her happiness hinges on others.
5. Conversely, a codependent feels inordinately <u>responsible</u> for others.
6. The codependent's relationship with a spouse or significant other is marred by a damaging, unstable lack of balance between dependence and independence.
7. The codependent is a master of denial and repression.
8. The codependent worries about things he or she can't change and may well try to change them.
9. A codependent's life is punctuated by extremes.
10. A codependent is continually looking for the something that is lacking or missing in life.

The way of a fool is right in his own eyes, but he who heeds counsel is wise. (Proverbs 12:15)

TODAY'S STEP: God help me to believe in myself and help me to let go of old beliefs and feelings that are hurting me.

"It is granted only to the heart that abounds with integrity, trust, generosity and love to realize true prosperity; for prosperity, like happiness, is not an outward possession, but an inward realization." -- James Allen, **As a Man Thinketh**

EPITAPH

I drank for happiness, and became unhappy.

I drank for joy, and became miserable.

I drank for sociability, and became argumentative.

I drank for sophistication, and became obnoxious.

I drank for friendship, and made enemies.

I drank for sleep, and awoke without rest.

I drank for strength, and became weak.

I drank "medically", and acquired health problems.

I drank for relaxation, and got the shakes.

I drank for bravery, and became afraid.

I drank for confidence, and became doubtful.

I drank to converse easily, and slurred my speech.

I drank to feel heavenly, and ended up feeling like hell.

I drank to forget, and became a slave.

I drank to erase my problems and saw them multiply.

I drank to cope with life and I died.

I pray that I may not expect too much from the world and that I may be content with the rewards that come from serving God.

. . . No eye has seen, no ear has heard, and no mind has imagined what God has prepared for those who love him. (1 Corinthians 2:9)

TODAY'S STEP: I trust Truth, my instincts, and my ability to ground myself in reality.

"Our fault lies, not in our lack of talent or potential, but in our refusal to believe that it exists. Only after we can accept such a belief and have thus gained enough confidence to look within ourselves can our development go full steam ahead." -- Jan Dunlap, **Exploring Inner Space**

<u>A Power Greater Than Ourselves</u>

Before we can welcome in a Higher Power to restore us to wholeness, we will probably have to engage in some emotional and spiritual "housecleaning":

1. We must bring into abstinence or balance all the addictive agents through which we have sought to meet our deepest needs. Chemicals, money, sex, career, anything and everything about which we may have become excessive, must be put into proper perspective – not lifted up to be worshipped.
2. We must transcend the god of reason if we have been worshipping God through an exclusively intellectual approach.
3. We must renounce the tendency to play God ourselves. We must grow beyond selfishness, narcissism, and grandiosity.
4. We must also renounce putting other people or human institutions in the role of gods.

Not only must we be rid of "false gods", but we may need to overcome old sources of bitterness toward God:

1. We may have identified God with an abusive parent.
2. We may have had negative experiences with a church (hypocrisy, bigotry, condemnation).
3. We may be struggling with a sense that God has failed us – that He has allowed us to become codependent.
4. We may be angry that God has not instantaneously healed us of our addictive illnesses.

Do not judge according to appearance, but judge righteous judgment. (John 7:24)

TODAY'S STEP: I accept who I am, where I am, and I continue to reach forward one day at a time.

"Self-reverence, self-knowledge, self-control, these three alone lead life to sovereign power." -- Lord Alfred Tennyson, **Oenone** *1829 poem*

Brave men and women (as well as cowardly men and women) are not born that way; they become that way through their acts. Acts like these make us not just grow up, but grow up well.

IF (Rudyard Kipling)

If you can keep your head when all about you are losing theirs and blaming it on you; If you can trust yourself when all men doubt you, but make allowance for their doubting too;

If you can wait and not be tired by waiting, or, being lied about, don't deal in lies,

Or, being hated, don't give way to hating, and yet don't look too good, nor talk too wise; If you can dream – and not make dreams your master; If you can think – and not make thoughts your aim;

If you can meet with triumph and disaster and treat those two imposters just the same; If you can bear to hear the truth you've spoken twisted by knaves to make a trap for fools,

Or watch the things you gave your life to broken, and stoop and build'em up with worn-out tools; If you can make one heap of all your winnings and risk it on one turn of pitch-and-toss,

And lose, and start again at your beginnings and never breather a word about your loss; If you can force your heart and nerve and sinew to serve your turn long after they are gone,

And so hold on when there is nothing in you except the Will, which says to them: "Hold on!"

If you can talk with crowds and keep your virtue, or walk with Kings – nor lose the common touch; If neither foes nor loving friends can hurt you; if all men count with you, but none too much;

If you can fill the unforgiving minute with sixty seconds' worth of distance run –

Yours is the Earth and everything that's in it,

     And – which is more – you'll be a Man, my son!

Above all else, guard your heart, for everything you do flows from it. (Proverbs 4:23)

TODAY'S STEP: When I rely on my Higher Power's help I can achieve.

"There is an instinct for newness, for renewal, for a liberation of creative power. We seek to awaken in ourselves a force, which changes our lives from within. And yet the same instinct tells us that this change is a recovery of that which is deepest, most original, and most personal in ourselves. To be born again is not to be somebody else, but to become ourselves. -- Thomas Merton, **Love and Living**

<u>*"Came . . . Came To . . . Came To Believe"*</u>

Having completed Step One, we're starting to feel a little more familiar with how the process of Recovery works. But now that we're facing Step Two, we've begun to have second thoughts about whether we're willing to proceed. We're nervous about doing an in-depth analysis of our own mental health. And we're equally fearful and reluctant about relinquishing our own self-reliance to a power we may feel we don't have even a nodding acquaintance with.

This is where we have to experiment a little with faith in ourselves, and in the process. By the time we have successfully worked through Step Two, we have developed a deeper understanding of why self-will and self-determination – no matter how we struggle to apply them – are simply not powerful enough to affect our Recovery.

Also, by the end of Step Two it should be increasingly clear how our compulsion/addiction has compelled us to act in ways that are not healthy. Many of us acquired behavior patterns and personality traits we thought would protect us from the painful realities of life. Some of the common behavior patterns are victimization, defiance, self-centeredness and indifference. The presence of these behaviors and attitudes indicates that we suffer from some form of emotional, mental and behavioral disability.

Step Two helps us see that our lives can be restored to wholeness. In the context of the Program, wholeness is defined as "being in sound health, not diseased or injured, not broken, damaged or defective." As we attend meetings and work the Steps, we discover the peace and serenity possible only through surrendering our self-will and humbly seeking to improve the quality of our lives.

Though you have not seen him, you love him; and even though you do not see him now, you believe in him and are filled with an inexpressible and glorious joy (1 Peter 1:8)

TODAY'S STEP: I trust that God will bring out the best in me and others.

"Send me the right thought, word, or action. Show me what my next step should be. In times of doubt and indecision, please send Your inspiration and guidance."
-- Alcoholics Anonymous

<u>One Step at a Time</u>

Though alcoholics enter AA to stop drinking, they quickly learn that Recovery involves more than just giving up alcohol and drugs. The secret is to learn to live differently by: (a) Principles rather than personality; (b) Self-knowledge instead of denial; and, (c) Faith rather than ambition. Success comes from sticking with the Program and working the Steps as follows:

- **Admit powerlessness over addiction:** Acknowledging that you have lost control over chemicals and your life has become unmanageable sets the stage for the entrance of the Higher Power, who can help you do what you haven't been able to accomplish on your own.
- **Assume faith in a Higher Power:** You accept the need for outside assistance in Recovery, forsaking further attempts to beat your addiction through willpower.
- **Abandon insistence on personal control:** You turn your will and life over to whatever outside power you believe in.
- **Examine yourself:** You study your own behavior (often quite a change from an earlier preoccupation with criticizing others) in terms of right and wrong.
- **Make personal changes:** You become willing to have your Higher Power remedy these character defects.
- **Make amends to those you harmed:** You seek to atone for the wrongs of the past where possible.
- **Pray and Meditate:** You ask your Higher Power for guidance (prayer) and promise to listen to and reflect on the answers (meditation).
- **Carry the message:** You share your "experience, strength and hope" with those who still suffer, as a way of reinforcing the message in your own thinking.

God will guide me continually . . . . (Isaiah 58:11)

TODAY'S STEP: I may move forward in confidence, knowing my steps are guided by my Higher Power.

"We are what and where we are because we have first imagined it." -- Donald Curtis

The Things That Haven't Been Done Before   (Edgar Guest)

The things that haven't been done before, those are the things to try;

Columbus dreamed of an unknown shore at the rim of the far-flung sky,

And his heart was bold and his faith was strong as he ventured in dangers new,

And he paid no heed to the jeering throng or the fears of the doubting crew.

The many will follow the beaten track with guideposts on the way.

They live and have lived for ages back with a chart for every day.

Someone has told them it's safe to go on the road he has traveled o'er

And all that they ever strive to know are the things that were known before.

A few strike out, without map or chart, where never a man has seen.

From beaten paths they draw apart to see what no man has seen.

There are deeds they hunger alone to do; though battered and bruised and sore,

They blaze the path for the many, who do nothing not done before.

The things that haven't been done before are the tasks worthwhile today?

Are you one of the flock that follows, or are you one that shall lead the way?

Are you one of the timid souls that quail at the jeers of a doubting crew,

Or dare you, whether you win or fail, strike out for a goal that's new?

Behold, I show you a mystery; We shall not all sleep, but we shall all be changed, in a moment, in the twinkling of an eye . . . . (1 Corinthians 15:51)

TODAY'S STEP: I my move confidently toward wholeness, knowing my steps are guided by my Higher Power.

"Unless a man has courage, he has no security for preserving any other virtue." -- Samuel Johnson

The Courage to Change

Courage is the basic virtue. Of what use is wisdom if you don't have the courage to act wisely? Of what value is love if you don't have the courage to love? Of what importance is truth if you don't have the courage to speak out? Of what consequence is faith without the courage to seek it? Courage activates all other goodness.

It also requires honesty. It takes courage to confront the truth of our unmanageable lives and then admit it, it takes courage to surrender our lives and wills to God. It takes courage to make our Fourth and Fifth Steps. It takes courage to face our moral life and honestly take our inventory; and then admit our findings to another human being. To make our best efforts to make amends, continue our inventory, maintain our conscious contact with God, and share our program with others – all our Steps take courage. If you have no fear or vulnerability, courage is irrelevant. If you have no fear you may be hiding in denial or arrogance.

The Twelve Steps are for the brave. We walk the way of Recovery facing fearful truths – with every person who walks along with us. We can be courageous because we do not walk alone. We are with one another and God. It is knowing we have the support and friendship of our companions that supplies the courage we often lack. God is with us – and for us, even though we can't see him – giving us the courage and the strength to persevere. More than this, He helps us see that our trials serve a purpose: to move us down the path toward greater faith. Fear and faith cannot co-exist.

The LORD is my shepherd I shall not want. He makes me lie down in green pastures; He leads me beside [quiet waters. He restores my soul; He guides me in the paths of righteousness For His name's sake. Even though I walk through the valley of the shadow of death, I fear no evil, for You are with me; Your rod and Your staff, they comfort me. You prepare a table before me in the presence of my enemies; You have anointed my head with oil; my cup overflows. Surely goodness and loving kindness will follow me all the days of my life, and I will dwell in the house of the LORD forever. (Psalm 23:1-6)

TODAY'S STEP: I have courage to go forward; to meet the new day, to handle whatever confronts me. Peace is coupled with courage, now and forever.

"Sow a thought, and you reap an act;

Sow an act, and you reap a habit;

Sow a habit, and you reap a character;

Sow a character, and you reap a destiny."
                Quoted by Samuel Smiles in **Life and Labor**

<u>As Ye Sow, So Shall Ye Reap</u>

The hardest part of Recovery is it requires us to change. We may be intrigued by the idea of Recovery. We may be inspired by the stories about Recovery. We may be convinced of our need for Recovery. These and many other cognitive processes are relatively easy for us. But the *doing* of Recovery is hard because it means change. And change is difficult. We understandably resist change. We are angry that we have to change. We feel shame that we need to change. And we are afraid we will not be able to change. We know there will be moments when we'll find ourselves saying, "I can't do it. It's too hard." "Can't" and "hard" are words to remove from our vocabulary.

But change is also the most exhilarating part of Recovery. We don't have to live in bondage to our addictions. We don't have to run in fear from relationships. We don't have to live as if we were responsible for the world. We can learn serenity. We can find freedom. We can experience love.

Change is the most difficult and the most wonderful part of the Recovery process. It engages us in an internal battle. It is not a comfortable battle. But our capacity to change is the key to our hope. Change is scary, especially at the emotional and spiritual level. But Recovery can never occur in others, or continue in us, without the willingness to let God bring about change.

God has given us the ability to change and grow. He calls us to change. He gives us the perspectives and disciplines and encouragements we need. And, as we allow and invite him, God himself works within us to strengthen us, heal us and make us new.

In all things showing yourself to be a pattern of good works. (Titus 2:7)

TODAY'S STEP: I can strengthen my assets, first by knowing them, and then by emphasizing them repeatedly. I am willing to change.

"Take away the cause, and the effect ceases." -- Miguel de Cervantes, **Don Quixote de la Mancha**

Is it possible to have great values, to have all our rules aligned to support them and not be living our values in the moment? If we are honest with ourselves, we know the answer is yes. All of us at one time or another have let events control us, instead of controlling our decisions as to what those events mean. We need a clear-cut way to ensure that we consistently live the values to which we've committed ourselves on a daily basis. We need to follow a Code of Conduct similar to the **OPTIMISTS' CLUB CREED.**

<u>Promise Yourself . . . .</u>

To be strong that nothing can disturb your peace of mind.

To talk health, happiness, prosperity to every person you meet.

To make all your friends feel there is something of value in them.

To look at the sunny side of everything and make your optimism come true.

To think only the best, to work only for the best, and to expect the best.

To be just as enthusiastic about the success of others as you are about your own.

To forget the mistakes of the past and press on to the greater achievements of the future.

To wear a cheerful countenance at all times and give every living creature you meet a smile.

To give so much time to the improvement of yourself that you have no time to criticize others.

To be too large for worry, too noble for anger, too strong for fear, and too happy to permit the presence of trouble.

Do you not know that you are the temple of God and that the Spirit of God dwells in you? (I Corinthians 3:16)

TODAY'S STEP: I practice the discipline of H.O.W. – Honesty, Open-mindedness and Willingness every day.

"In a full heart there is room for everything, and in an empty heart there is room for nothing." -- Antonio Pochia

Committed to Commitment

There is a lot of fear involved with commitment. In the first place, you may be frightened about commitment because of your past experiences. But do you really want that to be an excuse for the rest of your life? If so, you had better be prepared to be an emotional cripple, because that's what you are setting yourself up to be.

You'll never find the right person, because you will never feel safe. Commitment means safety – it means that you don't have to worry, wonder, and fret about whether your partner is going to be there in the morning. Commitment means you and your partner pledge to accept your couple status and concentrate on practicing and improving the skills necessary to make your relationship work. Love is a commitment, not a feeling.

The following acronym (with specific words italicized) may help to reinforce the essential ideas of commitment:

C : I **care** about this partner.

O : I can be totally **open** with him/her.

M : I can **make** amends in my relationship

M : I feel that we **matter** to each other

I : I feel the **intrigue** of our relationship.

T : I can **trust** my partner and he/she can **trust** me.

M : I feel our **minds** blending.

E : I feel **energy** when I'm with him/her.

N : I feel **non-threatened** by my partner.

T : I enjoy spending **time** with my partner.

.... God is Love; and he that dwells in love dwells in God, and God in him. (1 John 4:16)

TODAY'S STEP: I am open to the love in my life and to the love of my Higher Power.

"Deep within man dwell those slumbering powers; powers that would astonish him, that he never dreamed of possessing; forces that would revolutionize his life if aroused and put into action." -- Orison Swett Marden

You Can If You Think You Can

In his inspirational book ***You Can If You Think You Can,*** Dr. Norman Vincent Peale shows us that health, vitality, and aliveness can be a way of life. All we need to do to experience these remarkable benefits in our lives is to **Think, Practice,** and **Pray** about each of these basic principles:

1. Realize you can by yourself do much to make yourself a healthy, vital, and alive individual.

2. Affirm and keep on affirming that the powerful life force is flowing through your mind, your spirit, and your body.

3. Rid yourself of all sick thoughts – hate, resentment, inferiority, and the like.

4. Every day practice emptying your mind of all unhealthy attitudes.

5. Keep your mind tuned up to keep your body in tone.

6. Hold the thought of all elements of the body working together in perfect rhythm.

7. Help the doctor by thinking healthy thoughts. Remember that while the doctor treats you, God heals you.

8. Think health, practice health, and pray health.

9. See yourself as a whole person.

10. Visualize God, who created you, as constantly recreating you in every element of being.

But they that hope in the Lord shall renew their strength; they shall mount up with wings as eagles. They shall run, and not get tired; and they shall walk and not become weary. (Isaiah 40:31)

TODAY'S STEP: Emotional health is from within; not without.

"A consistent man believes in destiny, a capricious man in chance."
"Man is not the creature of circumstances; circumstances are the creatures of men."

"Nothing can resist the human will that will stake even its existence on its stated purpose." - Benjamin Disraeli, **Vivian Grey**

The Need for Turbulence – A. Philip Parham

On the Boeing 707 jet aircraft, a line of small blades is placed halfway down the upper wing. These little blades sticking up from the otherwise smooth wings are called "vortex generators." They are put on the plane for the purpose of creating turbulence in the airflow passing over the wing. The plane designers had discovered that the Boeing 707 would not steer accurately when the air current was too smooth.

For whatever reason, our Recovery does not steer accurately when everything is too smooth either. We seem to need a little roughness and turbulence in our program to make progress. Many recovering persons experienced their worst relapse or "slip" when everything was going smoothly. If we don't encounter rough seas of difficulties, we get cocky and complacent and can easily get off course and crash. Without struggle and strain we become lazy and vulnerable prey to foolish errors. We need to stay alert. Paul said, "We rejoice in our sufferings" (Romans 5:3), because our problems and rough times produce endurance and toughness that sees reality as a struggle, not an easy highway.

So often, however, we feel afraid that we don't have the resources to handle a certain person, problem or situation – much less the power to let go of our addictions. Nothing can calm our fears like the knowledge that we are being taken care of and provided for by God.

The fear won't vanish immediately, but as we work the Steps and draw closer to God, serenity and confidence will grow, and our fears will fade.

And let the beauty of the Lord our God be upon us, and establish the work of our hands for us. (Psalm 90:17)

TODAY'S STEP: There are many things I can do to improve my life and to further my Recovery, but I cannot heal myself. I need to continually ask God's help in becoming free of all that blocks me from my true self.

"I know of no more encouraging fact than the unquestionable ability of man to elevate his life by a conscious endeavor." - Henry David Thoreau, ***Where I Lived, and What I Lived For***

<u>Ten Seeds of Greatness*</u>

1. **SELF-ESTEEM.** We must feel love inside ourselves before we can give it to others.

2. **CREATIVITY.** Our minds can't tell the difference between real experience and one that is vividly and repeated imagined.

3. **RESPONSIBILITY.** Our rewards in life depend on the quality and amount of the contribution we make.

4. **WISDOM.** A large vocabulary which implies broad, general knowledge – characterizes the more successful persons, regardless of their occupations.

5. **PURPOSE.** The reason so many individuals fail to achieve their goals in life is that they never really set them in the first place.

6. **COMMUNICATION.** A touch is worth a thousand words.

7. **FAITH.** Life is a self-fulfilling prophecy; you won't necessarily get what you want in life, but in the long run you will usually get what you expect.

8. **ADAPTABILITY.** The good days are here and now!

9. **PERSEVERANCE.** Winners work at doing things that the majority of the population are not willing to do.

10. **PERSPECTIVE.** Seeing life from within – how we see life makes all the difference. Happiness is the spiritual experience of living every minute with love, grace, and gratitude. You cannot look for success. The treasure is within you. *Taken from Dennis Waitley's, ***Seeds of Greatness***

Delight yourself also in the Lord, and He shall give you the desires of your heart. (Psalm 37:4)

TODAY'S STEP: I need to believe in myself and my dreams. I am created to fulfill my destiny

"I am not discouraged, because every wrong attempt discarded is another step forward." - Thomas A. Edison, *Life*

Overcoming Failure

Dr. Maxwell Maltz, in his book ***Creative Living for Today,*** believes that the secret of successful living is to rise above our failures. According to Dr. Maltz, the elements of failure are: Frustration, Aggressiveness, Insecurity, Loneliness, Uncertainty, Resentment, and Emptiness – (**F-A-I-L-U-R-E**). Let's consider each of them:

1. **Frustration.** We feel frustration when we fail to achieve important goals or to satisfy basic desires. A morbid concentration on one's grievances with life will only make one's problems more severe. Far better to focus on one's successes and gain confidence from seeing oneself winning.

2. **Aggressiveness.** Frustration produces aggressiveness (misdirected). It is usually linked up with the setting of inappropriate goals, which cannot be achieved. This leads to frustrated rage, which leads to failure.

3. **Insecurity.** This is another unpleasant feeling; it is based on a feeling of inner inadequacy and living with impossible expectations.

4. **Loneliness.** We are all lonely now and then, but this is the extreme feeling of being separated from other people, from yourself, from life and from a Higher Power.

5. **Uncertainty.** This failure-type symptom is characterized by indecisiveness. The uncertain person usually sees himself as perfect; therefore, he cannot afford to be wrong because he doesn't want to be criticized.

6. **Resentment.** This is the excuse-making reaction of the failure-type personality to his/her status in life. Unable to bear the pain of his/her failure he/she seeks scapegoats.

7. **Emptiness.** Emptiness is symptomatic of a weak self-image and the lack of the capacity for creative living.

Strengthen those with tired hands, encourage those with weak knees. Say to those who are fearful hearted, Be strong. . . . (Isaiah 35:3-4)

TODAY'S STEP: By calling on my Higher Power for help daily I can learn from every situation

"A man, who suffers before it is necessary, suffers more than is necessary." -- Lucius Annaeus Seneca

When Life Gets Hard

There comes a time in everyone's life when trouble and difficulties seem to gang up. When this happens – *When Life Gets Hard* – Dr. Norman Vincent Peale suggests we:

FIRST - Don't try to do it all yourself. Do not struggle and fret. Do not strain and complain. Do all you can about things and then put everything into God's hands, trusting Him to bring it out right. **"Let Go and Let God".**

SECOND - Pray for guidance and believe that direction is now being given you. Believe this guidance can be trusted. Depend on it. For it won't fail you.

THIRD - Pray for and practice a calm attitude. Disturbing things will remain disturbing as long as you are disturbed.

FOURTH - Saturate your consciousness with faith, the creative faith that things will turn out right. Say aloud every day, "Thou wilt keep him in perfect peace whose mind is stayed on thee."

FIFTH – Remind yourself of one great truth; hard experiences **will** pass away. They **will** yield. They **can** be changed.

SIXTH – There is always light in the darkness. Believe that. Look for the light. The light is the love of God.

SEVENTH – Ask the Lord to release your own creative ingenuity, your own strength and wisdom, which taken together can handle any problem successfully.

EIGHTH – Never forget that God cares for you, He loves you. He wants to help you. Turn to Him. Accept His help.

NINTH – Remember that all human beings experience troubles similar to your own.

TENTH – Finally, hold on to this great promise: "God is our refuge and strength, a very pleasant help in trouble." God will see you through and a brighter day will dawn for you.

In all things, don't grumble or complain. (Philippians 2:14)

TODAY'S STEP: God will strengthen me when life gets rough.

"The secret of success is learning how to use pain and pleasure instead of having pain and pleasure use you. If you do that, you're in control of your life. If you don't, life controls you." - Anthony Robbins, ***Awaken the Giant Within***

<u>*Change "Want" to "Need"*</u>

"To the degree you give others what they want (need), they will give you what you want (need)." This is the major principle of Robert Conklin's book, ***How to Get People to Do Things.*** It is the key to persuading, leading, motivating, selling, supervising, influencing, guiding others – getting people to do things for you.

It seems incredibly simple. Perhaps it is, if you really understand it. But few do. There are some implications of the rule you must know and apply before you can make it work for you. Otherwise, the principle seems to work in reverse: people resist you, act against you, do the things you do not want them to do.

The way the law works is you must **first** give others what they want; then they will give you what you want. Most people have this twisted around. Of course, it takes patience -- and a few other things. Like knowing **what** it is people want. And knowing **how** to give them the things they want. Knowing what it is **you** want and what you're willing to give in order to get it.

Wants and needs are separate substances. Wants are frivolous, itchy, plundering, often greedy forces that are never satisfied. Meet one want, and there are two more to replace it. But needs are the deeper currents of one's existence. They are meaningful, worthy, and not as capricious as wants.

- People want sympathy; they need empathy.
- People want riches; they need fulfillment.
- People want big cars and expensive homes; they need transportation and shelter.
- People want fame; they need recognition.
- People want power; they need support and cooperation.
- People want prestige; they need respect.
- People want adoration; they need love.

Do not be overcome by evil, but overcome evil with good. (Romans 12:21)

TODAY'S STEP: I acknowledge my wants and needs, then turn them over to my Higher Power.

"If you are distressed by anything external, the pain is not due to the thing itself, but to your own estimate of it; and this you have the power to revoke at any moment . . . . Do not suppose you are hurt and your complaint ceases and you are not hurt."
Marcus Aurelius, ***Meditations***

<u>Letting Go of Negative Thinking</u>

Undoubtedly every human life has its quota of suffering, but the only purpose and service of suffering is to awaken understanding. With each increase of understanding, the quota of suffering lessens.

We fall into trouble in two ways: (1) Either by consciously thinking limiting thoughts, or (2) By allowing thoughts of limitation to be thought in us on an involuntary level. We need to learn how to:

1.   Face trouble;
2.   Look at it; and,
3.   Establish a transcendent relationship to it.

Exaggerating the negative element in our lives is familiar behavior for all too many of us. But this obsession is our choice. We can stop at any moment. We can decide to let go of a situation we can't control, turn it over to God, and be free to look ahead at the possibilities for happiness.

If we can learn to accept a serious situation in our lives as a special opportunity for growth and as an opportunity to let God work in our lives; then crises will lessen in number and in gravity in direct proportion to the partnership we develop with our Higher Power.

The stronger our dependence on that power, for all answers and all directions, the greater will our comfort be. No crises need worry us. Serenity is the gift promised when we let God handle our lives. The solution is to ask for help!!!

If you diligently heed the voice of the LORD **your God and do what is right in His sight, give ear to His commandments and keep all His statutes, I will put none of the diseases on you…. for I am the L**ORD **who heals you. (Exodus 15:26)**

TODAY'S STEP: I let go of old ideas about myself and discover a new self through Recovery.

"I conceive that pleasures are to be avoided if greater pains be the consequence, and pains to be coveted that will terminate in greater pleasure." - Michel Eygeun de Montaigue, *Essays*

Detachment

The following statement, based on Al-Anon's Conference Approved Literature, is written with the hope that it will help us to understand the concept of detachment within Al-Anon and Alateen. Detachment helps families look at their situations realistically and objectively, thereby making intelligent decisions possible.

Alcoholism is a family disease. Living with the effects of someone else's drinking is too devastating for most people to bear without help. In Al-Anon we learn individuals are not responsible for another person's disease or recovery from it. Detachment helps us to help ourselves.

We let go of our obsession with another's behavior and begin to lead happier and more manageable lives, lives with dignity and rights; lives guided by a Power greater than ourselves. In Al-Anon we learn:

- Not to suffer because of the actions or reactions of other people;
- Not allow ourselves to be used or abused in the interest of another's Recovery;
- Not to do for others what they can do for themselves;
- Not to manipulate situations so others will eat, go to bed, get up, pay bills, etc.
- Not to cover up for another's mistakes or misdeeds;
- Not to create a crisis; and,
- Not to prevent a crisis if it is in the natural course of events.

Detachment is neither kind nor unkind. It does not imply evaluation of the person or situation from which we are detaching. It is simply a means for us to recover from the adverse effects of the disease of alcoholism upon our lives.

Watch and pray that ye enter not into temptation: The spirit indeed is willing, but the flesh is weak. (Matthew 26:41)

TODAY'S STEP: I know I need the help of a power greater than myself.

"It is the mind that maketh good or ill, that maketh wretch or happy, rich or poor."
Edmund Spenser, *Paradise Lost*

Relationship Depression Quiz*

Answer the following questions YES or NO. (If a parent or parents were not your
primary caregivers when you were a child, substitute the person(s) most like parents
to you.)

1. My parents were divorced before I was 20.   _____
2. One or both of my parents died before I was 20.   _____
3. One or both of my parents were very sick with a life-threatening
    Illness or chronically ill for more than a year during my childhood. _____
4. I was physically or sexually abused as a child.   _____
5. One or both of my parents were alcoholic or seriously addicted to
    drugs, gambling, shopping, eating, etc.   _____

6. I have been shunned or badly treated at school or work because of my
    gender, age, race, creed, sexual orientation, or other personal qualities

    I can't or won't change.   _____

7. I've been divorced one or more times.   _____

8. My intimate partner had an affair or affairs.   _____

9. My friends and family are often unavailable to give me what I need
    when I'm stressed.   _____

10. I'm uncomfortable with intimacy; I seem to choose the "wrong"
     people or sabotage relationships that may be "right".   _____

Total Number of Questions Answered YES:

(0-2)   You possess excellent social skills and had a healthy family background.

(3-5)   You probably experience a moderate degree of Relationship Depression.

(6-7)   Beware! You're experiencing a significant degree of unhealthy Relationship

         Depression.

(8-10)   Danger! Your Relationship Depression is unhealthy and destructive.
         Without help, your relationships will continue to be unsuccessful and
         debilitating. *Taken from Ellen McGrath, *When Feeling Bad is Good*, Henry
         Holt & Co.: New York, NY, 1992 (p.123-124).

**Be of good courage . . . let the Lord do that which is good in His sight. (1 Chronicles
19:13)**

TODAY'S STEP: I let go of denial and accept responsibility for myself and my life.

"We are what we think. All that we are arises with our thoughts. With our thoughts, we make our world." -- The Buddha

How to Acquire a "Success-Type Personality"

Dr. Maxwell Maltz, in his best-seller *Psycho-Cybernetics,* gives us a prescription for the development of a "Success-Type Personality", which is composed of the letters of the word **"SUCCESS"** itself:

S – ense of direction. Get yourself a goal worth working for. Always have

something ahead of you to look forward to – to work for and hope for.

U – nderstanding. Look for and seek out true information concerning yourself, your problems, other people, or situations. Admit your mistakes and errors, correct them and go forward.

C – ourage. Be willing to make a few mistakes, to suffer a little pain to get what you want.

C – harity. Act as if other people are important and treat them accordingly. Respect others' problems and needs.

E – steem. Begin to appreciate other people more; practice treating them as if they had some value – and surprisingly enough your own self-esteem will go up.

S – elf Confidence. Use errors and mistakes as a way of learning – then dismiss them from your mind. Remember and picture to yourself past successes.

S – elf Acceptance. Accept yourself as you are – and start from there. You cannot realize the potentialities inherent in that unique and special something, which is "You" if you keep turning your back upon it, feeling ashamed of it, hating it, and refusing to recognize it.

For I know the thoughts that I think toward you, says the Lord, thoughts of peace and not of evil, to give you a future and a hope. (Jeremiah 29:11)

TODAY'S STEP: There are so many ways in which I can improve the quality of my life. Instead of fretting about what I can't have or can't do, I'll take action to create something positive in my life today.

"The beginning of a habit is like an invisible thread, but every time we repeat the act we strengthen the strand, and add to it another filament, until it becomes a great cable and binds us irrevocably, thought and act."   -- Orison Swett Marden

Tradition Two

For our group purpose there is but one authority – a loving God as He may express Himself in our group conscience. Our leaders are but trusted servants; they do not govern.

In Al-Anon, a group conscience is reached after thorough discussion of group concerns – guided by members' own experiences and a loving God as He expresses Himself in that conscience. He is the ultimate authority in all group decisions. Through Al-Anon, we have learned we can have discussions and that it is okay for members to have different points of view. No individual imposes his/her will on the group, or keeps silent when they have a burning desire to speak out. There are no dictators. No one is in charge. There is no one to fear. Therefore, whenever there is controversy over any subject, a group conscience meeting is called.

The second part of Tradition Two deals with leadership roles in Al-Anon. Our Group Reps, District Reps and Delegates have volunteered to serve as leaders. They have been entrusted with the authority to vote on our behalf, but never blindly. They act according to the best information available, their own conscience and the welfare of Al-Anon as a whole. We entrust them to do that. The same idea applies to leaders at the group level. However, whenever anyone feels these individuals do not have Al-Anon's welfare at heart, we discuss the incident, we reason things out and we rely on a loving God to express Himself in our group conscience.

Applying Tradition Two in our family lives is another way of letting God work through us. As we talk to each other, listen to what the other person is saying, and then reason things out with one another, we find the good of the family as a whole prevails. That's what Tradition Two is all about.

Let no one seek his own, but each one the other's well-being. (1 Corinthians 10:24)

TODAY'S STEP: With the help of a Higher Power, decision-making can be one of life's great adventures. Each crossroad brings a new challenge, and I am capable of dealing with whatever comes my way.

"Good and evil, reward and punishment, are the only motives to a rational creature: these are the spur and reins whereby all mankind are set on work, and guided." - John Locke, *Some Thoughts Concerning Education*

<u>Discipline</u>

Children need discipline to feel secure; so do adults. Discipline means understanding there are logical consequences to our behavior. Discipline means taking responsibility for our behavior and the consequences.

Discipline means:

1. **Learning to wait for what we want.**

2. **Being willing to work for and toward what we want.**

3. **Being where we need to be when we need to be there, despite our feelings.**

4. **Performing the day-to-day tasks, whether these be Recovery behavior or washing the dishes.**

5. **Trusting that our goals will be reached though we cannot see them.**

Discipline can be grueling. We may feel afraid, confused, and uncertain. Later, we will see the purpose. But this clarity of sight usually does not come during the time of discipline. We may not even believe we're moving forward. But we are.

The task at hand during times of discipline is simple:

Listen, Trust and Obey.

Take up the whole armor of God put on the belt of truth, the breastplate of righteousness, the shoes of peace . . . above all, the shield of faith . . . the helmet of salvation and the sword of the Spirit . . . . (Ephesians 6:13-17)

TODAY'S STEP: I allow myself to recognize and accept whatever feelings pass through me.

"Experience is not what happens to a man; it is what a man does with what happens to him." -- Aldous Huxley

<u>*Overcoming Guilt and Resentment*</u>

In the book, ***You Can't Afford the Luxury of a Negative Thought,*** John Roger & Peter McWilliams suggest a few techniques to help us get back on track whenever we're caught in the cycle of guilt or resentment.

1. **Change the Image.** Ask yourself, "What am I upset about?" and let whatever it is be OK. Accept it. Give yourself and others permission to do what you or they have already done. Allow your image to adjust to reality. You don't have to like it, but you don't have to hate it either.
2. **Forgive.** Forgive the others and forgive yourself. Forgive yourself for whatever you did. Forgive the others for whatever they did. Then forgive yourself for judging yourself or others.
3. **What's the Payoff?** Are you enjoying the intensity of it all? Are you feeling "right"? What are you getting from this?
4. **Move.** Do something physical. Run around the block. Do aerobics. If you're in bed, move your arms a lot. Get the energy moving.
5. **Refocus.** Focus on something positive.
6. **Is It Worth Dying For?** If you had a choice – defending that inaccurate image or your life – which would it be?
7. **Be Grateful.** Find something to be grateful for.
8. **Observe.** Observe the anger or resentment. Observe the feeling. Don't do anything to it or with it. Don't pay attention to the thoughts feeding the feeling. Pay attention to the feeling itself.
9. **Surrender.** Let go of the struggle. Don't try to get rid of the feeling. Just surrender. Flow with it.
10. **Sacrifice.** Give it up. You thought sacrifice meant giving up the good things? It can also mean giving up the not-so-good things. Sacrifice your guilt and resentment. Give them up.

When you pass through the waters, I will be with you; And through the rivers, they shall not overflow you . . . Thus says the Lord, who makes a way in the sea and a path through the mighty waters. (Isaiah 43:2-16)

TODAY'S STEP: I avoid making excuses for my own or someone else's behavior.

"Some men see things as they are, and say, 'Why?' I dream of things that never were, and say, 'Why not?'" – George Bernard Shaw

*Dreaming God's Dream**

What's the purpose of life anyway? Only to eat, drink, work, play, make love?

Or do we have a brain designed to dream dreams?

Isn't our mind created to be an architect, drawing plans?

Can't we imagine beautiful accomplishments?

Think of this: The human being is the only creature in the universe

that has the capacity for exercising creative imagination!

This divine quality of dreaming what you want to be,

where you want to go, what you'd love to do,

projects you hope to achieve, goals you'd like to reach –

all of this makes us human and the most unique creature in all of creation!

We really are "made in the image" of the Creator – God!

So you are fulfilling your destiny as a child of God in human flesh

when you start dreaming the beautiful dreams God Himself is inspiring in your mind.

A radio is designed to pick up the sounds that are here in this room now.

A television is engineered to pick up the moving pictures that are in the air waves around you now.

Your mind was invented and created by God to pick up the messages and mental pictures He is sending your way. That's exciting! Faith is dreaming God's dreams for us! *Taken from Robert H. Schuller, ***Tough Minded Faith For Tender Hearted People***

Tomorrow the Lord will do wonders among you. (Joshua 3:5)

TODAY'S STEP: I move confidently toward wholeness knowing my steps are guided by my Higher Power.

"Half measures availed us nothing. We stood at the turning point. We asked His protection and care with complete abandon." – **Alcoholics Anonymous**

<u>*Sanity/Insanity*</u>

Our minds, our bodies, our emotions and our spirits are all affected by illness, stress and crises. When one part of our-self is out of sync, the totality of our being is also adversely affected. We have discovered one of the kindest things we can do for ourselves in Recovery is nourish our entire being. We find this particularly helpful in Step Two. This is because the more we do healing things for ourselves; the more clearly we come to recognize the lifestyle we were living was less than sane.

How long has it been since you paid attention to your physical health? Took a walk along the beach, or in the country? Visited an art gallery? Enjoyed a sunset? Heard a symphony? Watched a ballet? Cheered at a sports event? Attended the theater? Had a massage? Participated in a sport? Took a trip? Or just set aside a day for yourself to read or do nothing? Good nutrition, adequate exercise and restful sleep are important elements that help us nourish and replenish our minds and bodies.

Many of us experienced severe sleep problems. Worry, fear and guilt are thieves that enter our consciousness and rob us of our needed rest. One interesting note about the Recovery process comes from those who have been working the Steps for some time. They've discovered that once they were able to confront and amend their lifestyle, their night worries, anxiety and insomnia tended to disappear.

Know God;

Know peace.

No God;

No peace.

I will give you peace in the land, and you will be able to sleep without fear. (Leviticus 26:6)

TODAY'S STEP: I am beginning to understand surrender is not defeat and I welcome my powerlessness.

Step Three

Made a decision to turn our will and our lives over to the care of God as we understood God.

Step Three requires that we take affirmative action as a result of the developing awareness we have gained from working the first two Steps. In Step One, we admitted we were powerless, that our lives had become unmanageable. In Step Two, we came to believe that a Power greater than our-selves could restore us to wholeness. In Step Three we make a decision to turn our will and our lives over.

Step Three commands more of us than the first two Steps, because we are now asked to trust in a Higher Power. If we have accepted our behavior and are ready to turn our lives over to a new manager, we see that allowing a Higher Power to guide our lives will reduce our fears and resentments to a manageable level.

The slogan "Let Go and Let God" expresses the central theme of Step Three. The idea of "letting go" and trusting the outcome can be especially helpful when we realize that surrendering our burdens actually frees us to experience healing and growth. As long as we do the appropriate "footwork" and do not expect God to do everything, we will see that our Higher Power takes good care of us.

The Twelve Steps is a spiritual program – a tool for healing. Step Three is an opportunity to let a spiritual Power greater than ourselves take charge of the rest of our lives. This liberates us from the pressure of feeling responsible for everything and everyone, or expecting someone else to take responsibility for us. As we surrender to our Higher Power and allow others to experience their own Higher Power, we develop a feeling of peace and serenity in our lives. **NOTE**: There is a paradox in the way this Program works. The less we try to manage our lives, the more effective we become. When we give up managing our own lives and trust in our Higher Power's plan for us, we find we are calmer and more accepting of things around us.

Most of us start this Program in an effort to stop repeating painful cycles of ineffective and damaging behavior. We are usually in search of answers to the complex questions of life. In the past, some of us may have experimented with lifestyles and beliefs that appeared to offer solutions. We may have been looking for a personal relationship with a Higher Power that transcended things of this world. This life-giving experience is available through the Twelve Step Program.

THIRD STEP PRAYERS

"Made a decision to turn our will and our lives over to the care of God as we understood God."

"God, I offer myself to Thee, to build with me and to do with me as Thou wilt. Relieve me of the bondage of self, that I may better do Thy will. Take away my difficulties, that victory over them may bear witness to those I would help of Thy Power, Thy Love, and Thy Way of Life. May I do Thy will always!" (*Alcoholics Anonymous,* p. 63)

In this moment I can choose my own Higher Power. I can set aside all the old beliefs about who I am not and be who I am – a child of God. I can remind myself that a faith in a Higher Power becomes a faith in me, and my Recovery lies in being true to myself and to my Higher Power. I am now willing to enter into partnership with my Higher Power.

"Higher Power, I trust your guidance will free me from my ineffective behavior so I may better do your will. Free me from the personal struggles and difficulties rooted in my dysfunctional family life. Show me how to love and care for the precious child within me. I seek wholeness so my life may bear witness to those I would help of Your Power, Your Love and Your Way of Life. I seek to do Your Will always."

MEDITATIONS

Release me, dear Father, from the bonds of pride. Help me to understand that others, too, have a point of view. Teach me to listen and not to be critical of the thoughts and actions of my fellow men. Expand my tolerance so I may help those who may be searching. My vision of life often becomes focused only on my personal needs and desires. With Thy almighty blessing I pray that this day I can truly give myself and not be concerned about my own welfare and feelings. Relieve me of my narrow scope of thinking, release me from my ego, and in Thy love let my actions be a worthwhile acknowledgement that Thou, dear Father, live in me this day forevermore.

AFFIRMATIONS

I am at peace with myself. And I find myself thinking only those thoughts which give me even more peace and serenity.

My view of life gives me a perspective of balance – and I see things as they really are – in their proper place of importance in my life.

"Dream lofty dreams, and as you dream, so shall you become. Your vision is the promise of what you shall at last unveil." - James Allen, ***As a Man Thinketh***

<u>*Milestones in Recovery*</u>

Through working in partnership with our Higher Power and participating in a Twelve Step Program, we can look forward to achieving the following milestones:

- We feel comfortable with people, including authority figures.

- We have a strong identity and generally approve of ourselves.

- We accept and use personal criticism in a positive way.

- As we face our own life situation, we find we are attracted by strengths and understand the weakness in ourselves; we accept responsibility for our own thoughts and actions.

- We feel comfortable standing up for ourselves when it is appropriate.

- We are enjoying peace and serenity, trusting in God is guiding our Recovery.

- We love people who love and take care of themselves.

- We are free to feel and express our feelings even when they cause us pain.

- We have a healthy sense of self-esteem.

- We take prudent action and consider the consequences.

- We rely more and more on our Higher Power.

But as for me, I trust in You, O Lord. I say "You are my God". (Psalm 31:4)

TODAY'S STEP: I move confidently toward wholeness, knowing my steps are guided by my Higher Power.

"Go confidently in the direction of your dreams! Live the life you've imagined. Our truest life is when we are in dreams awake" – Henry David Thoreau

*The Ten Cognitive Distortions**

1. **All-or-nothing thinking:** You see things in absolute categories. If your performance isn't perfect, you feel you're a total failure.
2. **Over-generalization:** You view a single negative event as a never-ending pattern of defeat.
3. **Mental filter:** You pick out a single negative detail and dwell on it so exclusively that it colors your whole vision of reality – like the drop of ink that discolors the entire beaker of water.
4. **Disqualifying the positive:** By rejecting positive experience (it "doesn't count"), you nurture a negative belief that is contradicted by everyday experience.
5. **Jumping to conclusions:** You interpret events negatively, even though there is no evidence to support your conclusions, by . . . (a) Mind-reading. You simply assume that people are reacting negatively to you. (b) Fortune-telling. You anticipate that things will turn out badly, then convince yourself the prediction is established fact.
6. **Catastrophizing or minimization:** You exaggerate the importance of, for example, your goof-up or someone else's achievement; or, you minimize into insignificance your own desirable qualities or the other fellow's imperfections.
7. **Emotional reasoning:** You assume that your emotions necessarily reflect reality: "I feel like an idiot, so I must be one."
8. **Labeling:** Instead of describing your error, you attach a negative label to yourself, e.g., "I'm a loser."
9. **"Should" statements:** You try to motivate yourself with shoulds and shouldn'ts (or musts and oughts). The emotional consequence is guilt. When you direct these statements toward others, telling them what they "should" do, you reap anger and resentment.
10. **Personalization:** You see yourself as the cause of some negative external event for which, in fact, you were not responsible.

Taken from: **Feeling Good: The New Mood Therapy.* David D. Burns, MD, William Morrow & Co., Inc.: New York, NY, 1980.

If you can believe, all things are possible to him who believes. (Mark 9:23)

TODAY'S STEP: I need to believe in myself and my dreams.

"Pain makes man think. Thought makes man wise. Wisdom makes life endurable." -- John Patrick

<u>*Tradition Three*</u>

The relatives of alcoholics, when gathered together for mutual aid, may call themselves an Al-Anon Family Group, provided that, as a group, they have no other affiliation. The only requirement for membership is that there be a problem of alcoholism in a relative or friend.

Tradition Three is about membership in Al-Anon. The first part tells us that we gather together for mutual aid, provided we have no other affiliation. With the increasing number of Twelve Step programs for food, sex, gambling, etc., there is a concern that members of those programs will bring their literature and their program to our groups. This shows affiliation – precisely what Tradition Three cautions against.

Once, when a member at an Al-Anon group requested they use literature he had picked up at another Twelve Step program, a long-timer protested, saying it was the identifying and copyrighted statements of another self-help fellowship. She felt the spirit of our principle of non-affiliation would, therefore, be violated if it were used. The group agreed whole-heartedly.

The second part of Tradition Three deals with our only requirement for membership, " . . . .

that there be a problem of alcoholism in a relative or friend." When a Newcomer shared that her therapist had suggested she go to Al-Anon because of her low self-esteem and her inability to confront her husband, she was told very bluntly Al-Anon was not for her, she had to have an alcoholic in her life to be a member of Al-Anon. She left the group in tears. Several years later she came back to Al-Anon after recognizing her father had indeed had a problem with alcohol. She had every right to be in Al-Anon after all. Membership in Al-Anon is truly a personal decision. Only we can decide whether or not we belong. Shouldn't others have the same opportunity?

How much better it is to get wisdom than gold! And to get understanding is to be chosen rather than silver. (Proverbs 16:16)

TODAY'S STEP: As I work the Steps, I grow in wisdom and my capacity to be happy.

"Self is the only prison that can ever bind the soul; Truth is the only angel that can bid the gates unroll; And when he comes to call thee, arise and follow fast; His way may lie through darkness, but it leads to light at last." - James Allen, *As a Man Thinketh*

The Promises

"I'm sick and tired of being sick and tired," is a lament often heard at AA meetings. It represents that point in time when we finally make up our minds we are tired of being strangled in the grips of doubt and fear. Finally we begin to recognize that we are "powerless over alcohol" (substances, behaviors or people) and the devastating effects of "self-destructive" behavior which have caused us to hit "bottom" (**Step 1).**

As an alcoholic, we may frequently say we want to "change", but until we are willing to "go to any lengths" to experience a new level of living and spirituality we will usually continue to drink and ultimately self-destruct. Once we are willing to change and "come to believe that a power greater than ourselves can return us to sanity" (**Step 2)**; is when we "can expect a miracle". The miracle is we **will** change and we **will** experience "The Promises" (of Recovery) described in *"The Big Book":*

"We are going to know a new freedom and a new happiness. We will not regret the past nor wish to shut the door on it. We will comprehend the word serenity and we

will know peace. No matter how far down the scale we have gone, we will see how our experiences can benefit others. That feeling of uselessness and self-pity will disappear. We will lose interest in selfish things and gain interest in our fellows. Self-seeking will slip away. Our whole attitude and outlook upon life will change.

Fear of people and economic security will leave. We will intuitively know how to handle situations which used to baffle us. We will suddenly realize that God is doing for us what we could not do for ourselves." (pages 83 and 84 of *Alcoholics Anonymous)*

When we finally make up our minds that we have "had it," and we turn our life and will over to God (**Step 3),** God turns toward us.

Draw near to God, and He will draw near to you. (James 4:8)

TODAY'S STEP: God will strengthen me when life gets tough.

"God, I offer myself to Thee — to build with me and to do with me as Thou wilt. Relieve me of the bondage of self, that I may better so Thy will. Take away my difficulties, that victory over them may bear witness to those I would help of Thy power, Thy love, and Thy way of life. May I do Thy will always!" ***Alcoholics Anonymous,*** p.63

"Let Go and Let God"

What happens when we physically hold on tightly to something? Our knuckles ache as our fists clench. Fingernails bite into our palms. We exhaust ourselves. We hurt! We lose balance. On the other hand, when we trust God to give us what we need, we let go. We face forward. Our hands are free for healthy, loving, and enjoyable activities. We find unexpected reserves of energy.

Before we complain about our suffering, we might do well to examine ourselves. We may be surprised by the amount of pain we can release by simply letting go.

When we let go of a situation, we allow life to unfold according to God's will, not ours. We open our minds and let other ways of thinking or behaving enter in. When we let go of another person, we are affirming their right to live their own life, to make their own choices, and to grow as they experience the results of their actions. A Higher Power exists for others, as well. Our obsessive interference disrupts not only our connection with them but also our connection with our own spiritual selves.

By keeping the focus on ourselves, we let go of other people's problems and can better cope with our own. What can we do for ourselves today? How much can God give us if we are not open to receive? When we hold onto a problem, a fear, or resentment, we shut ourselves off to the help that is available to us. All we have to do is become the least bit willing to loosen our clutched fists a tiny, grudging bit, and miracles will happen. Struggling and worrying won't help solve our problems — doing our part and trusting our Higher Power with the rest will!

The way of peace I have not known. There is no justice in my ways. I have made myself crooked paths. (Psalm 59:8)

TODAY'S STEP: I acknowledge my wants and needs, then turn them over to my Higher Power.

"A condition of complete simplicity
(Costing not less than everything)." - T.S. Eliot, **Little Gidding**

<u>Turning Our Will and Our Lives Over</u>

In the words of Socrates, "Life contains but two tragedies. One is not to get our heart's desire; the other is to get it." Translation: Our will gets us into trouble. We aim for some goal or other, but even when we get it, we are rarely satisfied. It doesn't make our life complete, so we raise the ante, set a new goal, and push even harder. Or we don't get what we want and feel inadequate or deprived. Maybe that's why none of the Twelve Steps talks about carrying out our will.

The only time we can experience lasting satisfaction is when we let go of self-will and commit ourselves to seeking the will of our Higher Power. Prayer and meditation are two means by which we seek to discover what God's will holds for us, and they help us gain access to the power to carry it out.

Sometimes our hopes and desires are forms of guidance. When we are willing to place God's will above our own, those dreams can become a wonderful reality. The path to our true heart's desire is to surrender to the will of our Higher Power.

Is there an area in your life you treat as though it were too important to turn over to a Higher Power? Are your efforts to control that area making your life better and more manageable? We can hold on to our will until things become so painful that we are forced to submit, or we can put our energy where it can do some good now, and surrender to our Higher Power's care.

"I have held many things in my hands, and I have lost them all; but whatever I have placed in God's hands, that I still possess." – Martin Luther

And Jesus said unto him, No man, having put his hand to the plough, and looking back, is fit for the Kingdom of God. (Luke 9:62)

TODAY'S STEP: I am beginning to understand that surrender is not defeat and I welcome powerlessness.

"Emotion is the chief source of all becoming conscious. There can be no transforming of darkness into light and of apathy into movement without emotion." - Carl Gustav Jung, *From Psychological Reflections: A Jung Anthology*

The Path to Recovery from Addiction

Even though the Recovery movement has burgeoned in the last decade, addiction is a frequently overlooked source of anxiety and/or depression, both for the addict and for his or her loved ones. One in ten Americans are alcoholics, and significantly more people are directly affected by the alcoholism of a close friend or loved one. Psychotherapy has a poor track record in the treatment of addictions, as C. G. Jung himself found out when he treated Bill W., one of the cofounders of the Alcoholics Anonymous self-help fellowship.

Jung wrote a now-famous letter to Bill W., stating that alcoholism was too deeply seated to be cured by psychological means and that Bill W's hopes lay in a spiritual conversion. He had that conversion, of course, and out of it came the Twelve Step programs that have been called the greatest spiritual force in America today.

The power of Twelve Step programs is multifaceted. Hearing the stories of other recovering alcoholics is inspiring, and a body of simple wisdom and profound truths have emerged from those in Recovery. The slogans "One Day At A Time," "Live And Let Live" and "Let Go And Let God" are solid principles for anyone seeking to live a happy, well-balanced life.

The integral parts of The Program are:

1.   Admitting powerlessness over our addiction and others;
2.   Asking a Higher Power for help;
3.   Taking responsibility for our actions; and,
4.   Learning to forgive.

The last and most important commitment is helping others gain and maintain their sobriety. According to Bill W. "We recovered alcoholics are not so much brothers in virtue as we are brothers in our defects, and in our common strivings to overcome them" – **As Bill Sees It.**

If anyone desires to come after Me, let him deny himself, and take up his cross daily, and follow me. (Luke 9:23)

TODAY'S STEP: I let consequences and responsibility fall where they belong.

"Habit is either the best of servants or the worst of masters." -- Nathaniel Emmons

<u>Obsessions and Stinking Thinking</u>

Obsessions are recurrent ideas, thoughts, images or impulses that invade our consciousness. We usually do not feel like we have much control over these things. They may be a constant preoccupation with the object of our addiction (food, sex, alcohol, drugs, gambling), or they may pop in and out of our consciousness, the result is often the same – feeling overwhelmed, uncomfortable, and controlled. Obsessions go hand in hand with addiction and for some people are a tremendous source of worry and torment because they can be hard to get rid of.

Faulty thinking, referred to as "stinking thinking" in self-help programs, is our inaccurate beliefs or specific thoughts that may support our addiction by letting us talk ourselves into engaging in this addictive habit again. Some examples of these "worrisome" ideas include:

- I feel bad, so why not use drugs (eat, gamble, have sex) to feel good?

- I'm worthless. I just want to relax.

- Gambling (drugs, alcohol, sex, food) is the only thing that gives me a lift and makes me feel good.

- Sex (drugs, alcohol, gambling, food) works for me.

- I can't have fun unless I get some sex (drugs, alcohol, gambling, food).

- Relapse can't happen to me. I'll just have one.

- I'm in control now. I'll never go back to where I was.

- Recovery is such a drag. It's going so slow and it isn't what it's cracked up to be.

Teach me to do Thy will, for Thou art my God: Thy spirit is good . . . . *(Psalm 143:10)*

TODAY'S STEP: I ask my Higher Power to help me let go of fear, doubt, and anxiety and to fill me with faith, trust and serenity.

"Men are wise in proportion, not to their experience, but to their capacity for experience." -- George Bernard Shaw

"Keep Coming Back . . . . It Works, If You Work It"

Chapter 5 of *Alcoholics Anonymous* is a faithful guide for those of us who want to practice The Program. The following Ten Points represent an <u>epitome</u> of the life-saving directions in this chapter. We commit ourselves to work toward Recovery and spiritual awakening by sincerely and responsibly trying to do what "The Big Book" suggests:

1.   **Completely giving ourselves** to this simple Program;

2.   Practicing **rigorous honesty;**

3.   Being **willing to go to any lengths** to recover;

4.   Being **fearless and thorough** in our practice of the 12 Step principles;

5.   Realizing that for us there is **no easier, softer way;**

6.   **Letting go of our old ideas** absolutely;

7.   Recognizing that **half measures will not work;**

8.   **Asking God's protection and care** with complete abandon;

9.   Being **willing to grow** along spiritual lines;

10. Accepting the following pertinent ideas as proved by 12 Step experience:
     (a) that **we cannot manage our own lives;**

     (b) that probably **no human power can restore us to sanity;**

     (c) that **God can and will,** if sought.

If you have the willingness to go to "any lengths" in order to adopt these principles as a way of life; you will attain spiritual awakening, self-control, sanity, peace and joy.

When I am weak, then I am strong. *(2 Corinthians 12:10)*

TODAY'S STEP: I am willing to turn my life over to my Higher Power, to let go of willfulness and to surrender myself to Recovery.

"Nothing splendid has ever been achieved except by those who dared believe that something inside of them was superior to circumstance." -- Bruce Barton

The Secret of Abounding Happiness

James Allen in his book *From Poverty to Power* affirms that if we have not yet realized unbounded happiness in our lives we may begin to actualize it by holding before us the lofty ideal of unselfish love, and aspiring towards it. As we rise above the sordid self, as we break the chains that bind us, as we begin to realize the joys of giving, as distinguished from the misery of grasping – giving of our substance; giving of our intellect; giving of the love and light that is growing within us – then we will understand that it is indeed "more blessed to give than to receive."But the giving must be **of the heart** without the taint of self, without desire for reward. Allen exhorts us to **"Lose yourself in the welfare of others; forget yourself in all that you do; this is the secret of abounding happiness."**

I followed happiness to make her mine,

Past towering oak and swinging ivy vine.

She fled, I chased, o'er slanting hill and dale,

O'er fields and meadows, in the purpling vale;

Pursuing rapidly o'er dashing stream,

I scaled the dizzy cliffs where eagles scream;

I traversed swiftly every land and sea,

But always happiness eluded me.

Exhausted, fainting, I pursued no more,

But sank to rest upon a barren shore,

One came and asked for food, and one for alms;

I placed the bread and gold in bony palms.

One came for sympathy, and one for rest;

I shared with every needy one my best;

When, lo! Sweet happiness, with form divine,

Stoop by me, whispering softly, "I am thine."

"Taking the First Step with a good thought, the second with a good word, and the third with a good dead, I entered Paradise."

May the Lord make you increase and abound in love to one another and to all. *(1 Thessalonians 3:12)*

TODAY'S STEP: I trust Truth, my instincts, and my ability to ground myself in reality.

"Be more concerned with your character than your reputation, because character is what you really are, while your reputation is merely what others think you are." -- John Wooden

What Al-Anon Is, And What It Is Not

Al-Anon is not a therapy, nor does it duplicate a counselor/client relationship. It is a worldwide, self-help organization where each autonomous group adheres to a set of guidelines for the purpose of promoting Recovery for each of its members. Membership is entirely voluntary. Each group endorses basic precepts to ensure effective operation. A simple explanation of group functioning based on Al-Anon's Twelve Traditions follows:

1. Individual Recovery depends on group unity. While each member is free to express his own opinion, group conscience is formed by the majority determining the group's direction.
2. Common suffering promotes spiritual growth. No one member is different from, or more important than another.
3. Al-Anon's role is to provide a program of spiritual recovery.
4. Individual Al-Anon groups have complete freedom to choose their own meeting programs.
5. The ultimate success of Al-Anon and the recovery of its members depends on limiting the program to one purpose – helping families and friends of alcoholics.
6. Al-Anon focuses on personal growth for the family member.
7. Support for Al-Anon's world-wide services comes from the membership itself.
8. No one person is an expert on alcoholism at an Al-Anon meeting.
9. The equality of members requires only spiritual principles and logical procedures agreed upon the majority.
10. Al-Anon as a fellowship has no opinion on outside issues.
11. The Al-Anon program is based on attraction rather than promotion.
12. Anonymity is the spiritual foundation of these Traditions. It is a common problem that brings Al-Anon members together, and subordinating the individual will to a source of spiritual strength adds to the healing process.

Choose for yourselves this day whom you serve . . . But as for me and my house, we will serve the Lord. (Joshua 21:15)

TODAY'S STEP: I take responsibility for my own behavior, not for someone else's.

"We have made thee neither of heaven nor of earth, neither mortal nor immortal, so that with freedom of choice and with honor, as though the maker and molder of thy self, thou mayest fashion thyself in whatever shape thou shalt prefer, thou shalt have the power out of thy soul's judgment, to be reborn into the higher forms, which are divine." --God's speech to Adam from Pico della Mirandola's, ***Oration on the Dignity of Man***

Learning How to Pray

Many of us had to learn how to pray. We're told that trying to pray is praying. We began with very simple prayers: "God, help me know your will for me." "Thank you, God, for helping me today."

We learn prayer helps us with our overdependence on people, places, and things by giving us the insight and strength to rearrange our priorities. Prayer doesn't change God, but it changes those who pray.

Today in our prayers, we seek our Higher Power's will for us. We no longer bargain with God.

Prayer is seeking answers and direction in life. Meditation is listening for answers from a Higher Power and developing the faith within us to accept those answers. Reflection is finding ways to change the answers we get from prayer and meditation into action.

Reflection is understanding how to use the Twelve Steps. It is not snap judgment. It asks us to think of the pros and cons of our possible choices and to understand what directions we will take to give us the best results.

The process of spiritual connection from prayer to meditation to reflection is active, not passive. It is taking our part in the process and marveling at God's.

We have learned through times of quiet reflection to work into our lives the answers our Higher Power has given us as a result of our prayer and meditation.

For thou hast made him a little lower than the angels, and hast crowned him with glory and honor. (Psalm 8:5)

TODAY'S STEP: I connect with my Higher Power daily through prayer and meditation in the morning and at night, and anytime in-between.

"Give me beauty in the inward soul; may the outward and the inward man be at one. Having the fewest wants, I am nearest to the gods." -- Socrates, From *Diogenes Laeretius, Lives of Eminent Philosophers,* bk. II, sec. 25

The Magic of Gratitude and Acceptance*

Gratitude and acceptance are two magic tricks available to us in Recovery. No matter whom we are, or what we have, gratitude and acceptance work.

We may eventually become so happy that we realize our present circumstances are good. Or we master our present circumstances and then move forward into the next set of circumstances.

If we become stuck, miserable, feeling trapped and hopeless, try gratitude and acceptance. If we have tried unsuccessfully to alter our present circumstances and have begun to feel like we're beating our heads against a brick wall, try gratitude and acceptance.

If we feel like all is dark and the night will never end, try gratitude and acceptance.

If we've tried everything else and nothing seems to work, try gratitude and acceptance.

If we've been fighting something, try gratitude and acceptance.

When all else fails, go back to the basics.

Gratitude and acceptance work.

Today, God, help me let go of my resistance. Help me know the part of a circumstance will stop hurting so much if I accept it. I will practice the basics of gratitude and acceptance in my life, and for all my present circumstances.

*Taken from Melody Beattie, *The Language of Letting Go*

Rejoice in the Lord always. Again I will say, rejoice! (Philippians 4:4)

TODAY'S STEP: Thankfulness today will help me see the miracles at work in my life and in the lives of others on the road to Recovery.

"We are what we repeatedly do." -- Aristotle

"We are all invited to be who we are." -- Henry David Thoreau

Circles of Learning

I love the circles in the program. I love our tradition of reading through the Steps in Step meetings, and when we finish, reading through the Steps again. Same with *The Big Book*.

When we finish the stories, we start in with the forewords. We never let up on learning who we are and what we need. We never graduate; we just begin again.

We need these circles of learning. We need always to regard ourselves as perpetual beginners in The Program. After all, we're no further away from our next drink than anybody else. Insanity could strike at any moment, and we've got to be prepared. We've got to know enough about ourselves and the defenses we have learned in The Program to deal with any emotional fit that could make us drink/act out again.

For us, the four most dangerous fits are:

- **Rage** – those furious gusts of ego justification that tell us we are absolutely right, absolutely wronged, absolutely deserving of justice. (But since life never provides justice the way we think it should, we will provide our own justice. Glug, glug, glug.)

- **Glee** – those giddy gusts of ego fulfillment that tell us it will always be all right, we will always be on top. (And just to make sure we stay up there, we'll get stoned.)

- **Lust** – that high stepping lowlife who tells us our satisfaction will never end. (If we just pop that pill, or joint, or jug.)

- **Self-pity** – the sob sister of rage, who tells us we have suffered much too much, much too long. (Poor me, poor me, pour me a drink.)

I have set before you life and death, blessing and cursing; therefore choose life, that . . . you . . . may live. (Deuteronomy 30:19)

TODAY'S STEP: I am seeking a saner approach to everything I encounter. The slogans are a valuable source of sanity in chaotic situations. If I am tempted to act out of anger or frustration, I will remember "Easy Does It."

"Hold yourself responsible for a higher standard than anybody else expects of you." -- Henry Ward Beecher

The Habit of Happiness

Habitually, we put on either our right shoe first or our left shoe. Tomorrow morning determine which shoe you put on first. Now, consciously decide that for the next 21 days you are going to form a new habit by putting on the other shoe first. Now each morning as you decide to put on your shoes in a certain manner, let this simple act serve as a reminder to change other habitual ways of thinking, acting and feeling throughout the day. Say to yourself as you put on your shoes, *"I am beginning the day in a new and better way."* Then, consciously decide that you will:

1. Be as cheerful as possible.

2. Feel and act a little friendlier, smiling often.

3. Be a little less critical and a little more tolerant of other people, their faults, failings and mistakes. Place the best possible interpretation upon their actions.

4. Act as if success is inevitable, and you already are the sort of person you want to be. Practice "acting like" and "feeling like" this new person.

5. Practice not allowing your own opinions to color facts in a pessimistic or negative way.

6. Hand out praise three times during the day.

7. React as calmly and as intelligently as possible, regardless of what happens.

8. Ignore completely and close your mind to all those pessimistic and negative "facts" which you can do nothing to change.

Be steadfast, immovable, always abounding in the work of the Lord, knowing that your labor is not in vain. (1 Corinthians 15:58)

TODAY'S STEP: I have courage to go forward; to meet the new day, to handle whatever confronts me. Peace is coupled with courage, now and forever.

"We lift ourselves by our thought; we climb upon our vision of ourselves." -- Orison Swett Marden

Feel Your Feelings

Coping with emotions begins with awareness of what we are feeling. As simple as this sounds, many people have trouble knowing what they feel. Many mislabel what they are feeling. For example, when we say to ourselves, "I'm feeling upset," what do we really mean? Are we really saying we feel afraid, angry, disappointed, ashamed, or depressed?

When we first stop our addictive habit it is common to be flooded with many feelings that seem rather foreign. Often we feel uncomfortable with these emotions, especially if our addiction covered them up. Being aware of when we feel sad, afraid, happy, angry, and so on is a good way to begin the process of handling emotions in a constructive way. We need not deny nor minimize our true emotions. Here are some suggestions for understanding and handling feelings:

STEP 1. Recognize and label your feelings.

STEP 2. Be aware of how your feelings show in body language, physical symptoms, and behaviors.

STEP 3. Look for the causes of uncomfortable feelings (events, situations, and perceptions).

STEP 4. Evaluate the effects of your emotions on yourself and other people.

STEP 5. Learn new coping strategies to help you deal with emotions.

STEP 6. Rehearse new coping strategies.

STEP 7. Put your new coping strategies into action.

STEP 8. Change your strategies as needed, based on an evaluation of whether or not they were effective.

Peace I leave with you, My peace I give to you; not as the world gives do I give to you. Let not your heart be troubled, neither let it be afraid. (John 14:27)

TODAY'S STEP: My reward for practicing the principles of The Program in all my affairs is the priceless gift of serenity.

"It is only with the heart that one can see rightly; what is essential is invisible to the eye." -- Antoine de Saint-Exupery

Characteristics of Addiction

Regardless of the addiction, a generic formula that helps explain the cause is:

Body + thinking + emotions + personality + environment

+ coping skills + [alcohol, drugs, food, sex, gambling] = **ADDICTION**

Why and how a person becomes addicted may not particularly matter at first. What is more important than finding the possible causes is to stop the addiction. Think of a burning building. Flames have engulfed it entirely. Firefighters are not going to try to figure out what caused the fire; instead, they will work to put it out. Later, when the fire has been extinguished, they will search for possible causes. The same is true for an addicted person. The fire of addiction first needs to be put out, then the person is in better shape to search for what may have caused the problem.

Negative effects on various areas of functioning characterize addiction. Medical, family, job, relationship, financial, and spiritual problems are common among addicts. Addiction also tends to be progressive. It usually gets worse if not stopped or if the person doesn't enter some type of recovery program. Certain types of addictions are potentially fatal. For example, premature deaths from accidents, suicides, and medical diseases occur with greater frequency among tobacco addicts, alcoholics, drug addicts, and compulsive overeaters.

Now the good news! **Addictive illnesses are treatable.** Hundreds of thousands of people have stopped their addictive habits and put their lives back together. Many have not only stopped the addiction, but have developed into healthier, happier, and better people as a result of being in recovery. Trusting in the help and guidance of professionals and other recovering addicts in self-help programs such as Alcoholics Anonymous, Narcotics Anonymous, Overeaters Anonymous and Al-Anon has enabled many people to enjoy the immense rewards offered by Recovery. Today "we" have a choice.

In You, O Lord, I put my trust; Let me never be put to shame. (Psalm 71:1)

TODAY'S STEP: I trust that God will bring out the best in me and others.

"The only way to discover the limits of the possible is to go beyond them into the impossible." Arthur C. Clarke

Spiritual vs. Religious

People who are recovering from alcoholism or other addictions through Twelve Step programs hear phrases such as "the spiritual part of the program" or "this is a spiritual program." Twelve Step programs clearly separate themselves from religions and, yet, are equally clear in claiming to be spiritual programs. What does it mean to be "spiritual rather than religious?"

One simple way of understanding spirituality is to see that it is concerned with our ability, through our attitudes and actions, to relate to others, to ourselves, and to God as we understand Him. All of us, addicted or not, have a way of relating to our own lives, other people, and God, which tends toward the negative, self-defeating, and destructive. The question is not whether we will be spiritual, but whether we are moving in the direction of a negative or positive spirituality.

Spirituality is a simple way of living. There are four basic movements that recovering people need to make to put their lives on a positive spiritual basis – the first of these is a movement from fear to trust; the second, from self-pity to gratitude; the third, from resentment to acceptance; and, the fourth, from dishonesty to honesty.

Many of us had trouble believing that a God existed when we began our recovery program, because for years we thought we were the master of our affairs. When we realized how much help we needed, we first looked to other members and our group for support. By rejecting at first the idea of a Power **higher** than ourselves, many of us did accept the idea of a Power **other** than ourselves. It is important to our recovery to rely on God, as our belief in a Higher Power is what can and does save us from our addiction (only two of the Steps talk about addiction; the other ten talk about spiritual growth).

As we made spiritual progress, most of us now have a clear and ongoing belief in a Higher Power we call God.

Trust in the Lord with all my heart; and lean not unto my own understanding. In all my ways acknowledge him, and he shall direct my paths. (Proverbs 3:5-6)

TODAY'S STEP: I trust that God will direct me in the right way to go.

"To be disciplined within, where all is permissible, where all is concealed --- that's the point." -- Michel Eygeun de Montaigne

Overeaters need to understand the dynamics that cause their eating compulsion before they can begin to change this addiction. Let's look at twelve common reasons for compulsive overeating identified by Drs. Frank Minirith, Paul Meier, Robert Hemfelt, Sharon Sneed and Don Hawkins, in *Love Hunger: Recovery From Food Addiction.*

<u>12 Common Reasons for Compulsive Eating</u>

1. Overeaters may respond compulsively to cultural pressures.
2. Overeaters may subconsciously desire added pounds to protect themselves from love and intimacy.
3. Overeaters may use food to satisfy their need for immediate gratification.
4. Overeaters may use food as a tranquilizer.
5. Overeaters may concentrate on their desire for food to avoid facing their problems.
6. Overeaters may eat to punish themselves or others.
7. Overeaters may eat to relieve depression or stress.
8. Overeaters may eat to rebel against themselves or others.
9. Overeaters may eat to express their need to control their circumstances.
10. Overeaters may have a faulty perception of their body image.
11. Overeaters may have emotional feelings about food, which were developed at their parent's dinner table.
12. Overeaters may use food as a nurturer to satisfy their love hunger.

. . . add to your faith virtue, to virtue knowledge, to knowledge self-control, to self-control perseverance. (2 Peter 1:5-6)

TODAY'S STEP: There are many things I can do to improve my life and to further my Recovery, but I cannot heal myself. I need to continually ask God's help in becoming free of all that blocks me from my true self.

"The blossom vanishes of itself as the fruit grows. So will your lower self vanish as the Divine grows within you." -- Vivekenanda

The key to effectively working Step Three lies in our willingness to turn as much of our lives as we can over to the care of God. This is difficult for many of us because we are accustomed to functioning by self-will alone. Our mistrust may have prevented God from having a meaningful place in our lives, and the idea of letting an unrecognized Power be our guide is too unfamiliar to us. We may have learned to pray to God as we would to a celestial Santa Claus, asking for things we wanted and always expecting to receive them. We may have asked for guidance in achieving our worldly goals, but this is vastly different from turning our whole being over to a Higher Power and trusting that we will be safely guided.

The Twelve Steps is a spiritual program and Step Three is an opportunity to let our Higher Power take charge of the rest of our lives. This liberates us from the pressure of feeling responsible for everything and everyone, or expecting someone else to take responsibility for us. As we become willing to surrender we also become open to receiving His gifts.

Step Three Gift

Striving for recognition . . . Wanting to look good . . .

Accomplishment . . . A relationship that fits my pictures.

All a mirage, relentless . . .Thirsting to fill the emptiness within . . .

Incessantly demanding more and more.

Yet – ever-present, within, Serene and uncritical . . .

Poised in the gentle stillness of infinite patience . . .

Spirit . . . My Higher Power . . .

Comforting Love . . .And Healing

Awaits.

Into Thy hand I commit my spirit. (Psalm 31:5)

TODAY'S STEP: I am willing to turn my will and my life over to my Higher Power, to let go of willfulness and to surrender myself to Recovery.

"The tragedy of life is not so much what men suffer, but rather what they miss." -- Thomas Carlyle

"Success, Without Joy of Living, Is a Game of Fools"

Charles Lamb once declared, "Our spirits grow gray before our hairs." One starts out in youth with anticipation. Excitedly he looks down the approaching years with the spirit of adventure, but before he has traveled far, life starts blowing its cold winds upon him. He tries his wings, perhaps they fail him; and some, sadly enough, having been disillusioned a time or two, give over the dreams and plod wearily on over a pathway from which the romance has fled. This is one of the saddest things that can happen to anyone, to lose the thrill and zest of living.

Perhaps William Wordsworth gave us the best description of the sad process that takes place in many:

Heaven lies about us in our infancy!

Shades of the prison-house begin to close upon the growing boy.

But he beholds the light, and whence it flows, he sees it in his joy;

The youth, who daily farther from the east must travel, still is Nature's priest,

And by the vision splendid is on his way attended;

At length the man perceives it die away, And fade into the light of common day.

(Ode. Intimations of Immortality from Recollections of Early Childhood)

There is one certain way to decide whether you are old – namely, what is your attitude of mind when you arise in the morning? The person who is young awakes with a strange feeling of excitement; the individual who is old, regardless of age, arises with an unresponsive spirit, not expecting any great things to happen. The one real measure of age is how well we retain the romance of life.

The romance of life is so priceless a possession that it is a supreme tragedy to lose it. Though one may acquire much in wealth, fame, or honor, the real joy of life does not lie there but, rather, in keeping the romance of living going. Nothing gives such complete and profound happiness as the perpetually fresh wonder and mystery of exciting life.

O Lord, You are my God . . . a strength to the needy in . . . distress, A refuge from the storm. (Isaiah 25:1-4)

TODAY'S STEP: God will shelter me from the cold winds and strengthen me when I ask for His help.

"You can hold back from the suffering of the world, but perhaps this very holding back is the one suffering you could have avoided." -- Kafka

Original Pain Work

"Original pain work" is a term that helps us describe and heal a particularly acute and deep part of our aggrieved hurts. Like grieving and recovery in general, this process cannot be forced or rushed, or our *Child Within* will likely go deeper into hiding. While there are many approaches to facilitating original pain work, the following **eight** actions can help in this process and are examples of some of its components in an effective healing sequence.

1. I tell my story of any current upset, as it may occur, to safe and supportive people, for example, in my therapy group, individual therapy, or to my sponsor.
2. I cognitively and experientially connect my current upset, conflict and feelings around them to my past. To help with this process I can ask myself, "What does any of this current experience remind me of?," ,"What age was I" and then begin to answer.
3. I may write about it in my journal or in an unmailed letter. Or I may work through this conflict and its emotional pain by any of several other possible experiential techniques.
4. I bring in and read my unmailed letter (or describe whatever else I've done experientially) to my therapy group or therapist. I may also enact parts of the resolution of my original pain with these safe people, such as by using further experiential techniques (for example, gestalt or psychodrama techniques facilitated by my therapist).
5. In the company of these safe people, I then discharge the stored toxic energy until I feel as complete with it as I can.
6. Then I listen to feedback from the therapy group or therapist.
7. After listening to each person's feedback, I describe how my doing all of the above feels now.
8. I connect any future upsets and conflicts with what I have learned above.

My sheep hear my voice, and I know them, and they follow me. And I give them eternal life, and they shall never perish; neither shall anyone snatch them out of my hand. (John 10:27-28)

TODAY'S STEP: God will hear my prayers and comfort me when I am grieving.

"The greatest weapon against stress is our ability to choose one thought over another. When you have to make a choice and don't make it, that is in itself a choice. The art of being wise is the art of knowing what to overlook. If you want a quality, act as if you already had it." Common sense and a sense of humor are the same thing, moving at different speeds. A sense of humor is just common sense, dancing. -- William James

<u>Count That Day Lost</u>

Each day is an opportunity to build a supply of positive spiritual experiences. If we get into the habit of taking an inventory of the day's events in the evening before we go to sleep we can better judge whether it was lost or well spent. Mary Ann Evans, better known as George Eliot (1819-1880), shows us how to tell the difference, and that is worth a day's expense.

If you sit down at set of sun and count the acts that you have done,

And, counting find one self-denying deed, one word

That eased the heart of him who heard, one glance most kind

That fell like sunshine where it went – Then you may count that day well spent.

But if, through all the livelong day, You've cheered no heart, by yea or nay –

If, through it all

You've nothing done that you can trace

That brought the sunshine to one face –

No act most small

That helped some soul and nothing cost –

Then count that day as worse than lost.

Give, and you will receive. Your gift will return to you in full—pressed down, shaken together to make room for more, running over, and poured into your lap. The amount you give will determine the amount you get back. (Luke 6:38)

TODAY'S STEP: I remind myself each morning that God cares for me. I am in His care and safe. It's easy to turn my will and my life over to a Higher Power I can trust.

"We lie loudest when we lie to ourselves." -- Eric Hoffer

Language of Denial

If you grew up in an alcoholic or dysfunctional family, you can safely assume that the habit of denial is a basic aspect of your personality. To find out, listen carefully to yourself. See if you may be speaking the language of denial without even knowing it. Do any of these phrases sound familiar?

- If I can just get through the next month (six months, year, five years), I'll be okay.

- I'll never end up like my mother (or father).

- I don't have negative feelings. I'm not angry.

- I can't start taking care of myself until I start feeling better.

- All I need to do is lose ten pounds.
-
- I know it didn't work before, but this time will be different.

- All I need is a little time to myself. I'm ok.

- Don't worry. I'm fine! It's just a bad habit, I can handle it.

- There's nothing really wrong with me, except I can't seem to shake this virus.

- I didn't do anything wrong. " Not me".

If your language and thoughts are peppered with these kinds of statements, you have surrounded yourself with a wall of denial. If you consistently deny feelings of anger, fear, frustration, stress, worry or inadequacy, you can be sure that the physical and emotional strain is taking its toll on your vitality and creativity. Denial keeps us imprisoned – awareness and acceptance break the bonds – and knowing the Truth about ourselves sets us free.

I have chosen the way of truth . . . (Psalm 119:30)

TODAY'S STEP: I'm awakening. I ask God to reveal areas in my self I can't see.

"The man who lies to himself and listens to his own lie comes to such a pass that he cannot distinguish the truth within him, or around him, and so loses all respect for himself and for others. And having no respect he ceases to love, and in order to occupy and distract himself without love he gives way to passions and coarse pleasures, and sinks to bestiality in his vices, all from continually lying to himself and to others." -- Fedor Mikhailovich Dostoevswky

DENIAL = "Don't Even Know I Am Lying"

Inherent in the words "had become unmanageable," is the recognition that we got to this stuck place over an extended period of time. There was a point in our lives where we managed very well indeed. However, the euphoric memory of those past successes may now be crowding out our ability to surrender; to admit we are no longer capable of controlling our destiny.

The Big Book of Alcoholics Anonymous tells us they have rarely seen a person fail who has thoroughly followed the path. They further state that those men and women who do not recover have not been able to be completely honest with themselves. They also say that those who succeed seem to have the ability to grasp and develop a program that demands rigorous honesty.

The fact we've decided to try this program implies we've chosen to attempt to develop rigorous honesty. We may well find, though, the search for such honesty is much more difficult than we had anticipated.

Both honest self-deception and self-delusion have been pervasive stumbling blocks on our path to Recovery, because they have been so hard to identify. But, as we progress, we will be better able to recognize them and they'll become valuable tools to help unravel the tangled web of our lives.

Only by understanding the elaborate defense system that our addictive behavior has set up are we able to concede our powerlessness and find the way out of the maze of our honest self-deception. In fact, we will find that "honest self-deception," "failure is not final," and "surrendering to win," will be recurring themes as we pursue our goal of serenity.

For You will light my lamp; the Lord my God will enlighten my darkness. (Psalm 18:28)

TODAY'S STEP: I awaken from denial and accept responsibility for myself and my life.

"If we would only stop lying, if we would only testify to the truth as we see it, it would turn out at once that there are hundreds, thousands, even millions of men just as we are, who see the truth as we do, are afraid as we are of seeming to be singular by confessing it, and are only waiting, again as we are, for someone to proclaim it."
Tolstoy

Alcoholism: The Disease of Denial

Alcoholism touches each of us in some way. Practically everyone has been affected by the alcoholism of a friend, a loved one, or a colleague. Unfortunately, many people do not understand the concept of alcoholism as a disease, the stages of illness and the dynamics of its progression, or how it affects the lives of the people around the alcoholic.

Alcoholism can be called the disease of denial and self-delusion. The alcoholic knows his or her drinking problem creates major problems, knows how unhappy he or she is making others, and is aware that he or she is the source of great anger and the cause of pain. But the alcoholic denies and minimizes the drinking and family and friends share the denial, deluding themselves into believing the person is not an alcoholic. The label "alcoholic" is seen by many to be worse than the drunkenness, the hurt inflicted, the loss of livelihood, and the physical deterioration.

In general, our understanding of alcoholism is steeped in misinformation and fear. If the reality of treatment and Recovery were understood, alcoholics and their families might have less difficulty with the term itself. An increasing number of Americans now accept the disease concept of alcoholism, but many still grope to understand it. A few reject the disease concept outright and argue against it. Still, the intellectual acceptance by the public is significant in how it affects public policy, government programs, industry, community agencies, and treatment efforts. Acceptance of alcoholism as a disease also offers hope of Recovery.

The National Council on Alcoholism (NCA) describes alcoholism as a chronic and progressive disease with the following physiological criteria:

- Continued drinking despite medical advice to stop;
- The presence of serious social problems; and,
- The apparent loss of control.

For there is nothing covered that will not be revealed, nor hidden that will not be known. (Luke 12:2)

TODAY'S STEP: I let go of denial and accept responsibility for myself and my life.

"Death is psychologically just as important as birth. As the arrow flies to the target, so life ends in death. Shrinking away from it is something unhealthy and abnormal, which robs the second half of life of its purpose." -- Carl Jung

The A-B-C Method

Dr. Albert Ellis developed "rational emotive therapy," an approach that helps people learn to think differently about themselves and their difficulties. Many people assume that events cause emotional reactions. Dr. Ellis's approach assumes that your self-talk or beliefs about the events determine the emotional consequences. He suggests following the A-B-C method to help you change your viewpoints.

The first step in the A-B-C method is to identify the events activating your feelings (A). The next step is to identify your beliefs or self-talk about these events (B). Next identify the emotional consequences of your thinking and pay attention to how strong your feelings are (C). For example:

A -- **activating event:** Chuck turns in a written report to his boss, who returns it a few days later with a lot of corrections made in red ink.

B -- **belief:** Chuck thinks it is terrible that his boss did not like his report, he wonders if he is incompetent, and he believes his boss dislikes him.

C -- **consequences:** Chuck feels anxious and upset.

Counterstatements: Chuck could dispute his self-defeating thoughts (B) by countering with statements like these:

1. My boss made a lot of changes. Next time I'll make sure I know what he wants in the report before I write it.

2. The boss is tough, but he makes a lot of good suggestions. I've learned something from his critical comments and can use it in the future.

3. Everyone in the office gets corrections from the boss, so it's really nothing personal. He's very particular, but usually correct in his suggestions or criticisms.

My son was dead and has come to life again; he was lost and now is found. (Luke 15:24)

TODAY'S STEP: I let go of old ideas about myself and discover a new self through Recovery.

"A complete life may be one ending in so full an identification with the not-self that there is no self left to die." -- Bernard Benson

The Tools of Recovery: Abstinence

The Twelve Steps of Overeaters Anonymous are a program of Recovery. The tools are some methods through which we work and live the 12 Steps. A tool is a means to an end. It can never be an end in itself. In order for a tool to work, it must be used. So, too, with our tools of Recovery for if we do not act upon them, there can be no Recovery.

In Overeaters Anonymous, abstinence means to abstain from compulsive overeating. There are no absolutes for abstinence. It is both a _tool_ that facilitates working the Twelve Steps and a _result_ of living the Steps.

As a tool, abstinence brings the symptom of compulsive overeating to an immediate halt. We willingly adopt a disciplined, well-balanced eating plan. From this vantage point, we can begin to follow the Twelve Step Recovery program a day at a time. Now, we are able to move beyond the food to a fuller living experience.

As a result of practicing the Twelve Steps, the symptom of compulsive overeating is removed on a daily basis. Thus, abstinence is also a change in attitude directly due to the program.

For many OA's abstinence means:

- Freedom from the bondage of compulsive eating.

- Planning and developing a manner of living that puts food in its proper perspective.

- That state of being in which a Power greater than ourselves has removed the compulsion to overeat, or at such times when it is experienced, we need not act it out because we have the power to resist.

- The process of surrendering to something greater than ourselves; the more total our surrender, the more fully realized our freedom from food and negative thinking.

Do not withhold good from those to whom it is due, when it is in your power to do it (Proverbs 3:27)

TODAY'S STEP: I am beginning to understand that surrender is not defeat and I welcome my powerlessness.

"Love does not dominate; it cultivates." -- Johann Wolfgang von Goethe

It takes a lot of faith to love. The fear of having your love rejected, the anxiety of "getting involved," the worry about not being appreciated, are only a few of the negative thoughts that keep people from loving others.

Faith Is Love in Action

Love is finding a need and filling it;

I believe I can help someone in need.

Love is finding a hurt and healing it;

I believe I can comfort someone in pain.

Love is finding a problem and solving it;

I believe I can come up with solutions.

Love is feeling someone's grief and consoling them;

I believe I can soothe the troubled mind.

Love is seeing the chasm and bridging it;

I believe I can be reconciling, unifying spirit!

The whole purpose behind the walk of faith is that through personal commitment and self-development, we are able to fulfill the plan that God has for our lives! Therefore, the central aspect of our walk of faith must be to center our lives on the will of God.

How can we keep from being distracted form this goal? We need to daily concentrate on the following realities:

1. Real faith always leads to commitment.
2. Commitment always demands and results in conversion.
3. Conversion is the process of radical change.
4. The ultimate experience of faith is the process of making a commitment to believe in God and devoting our life to serving Him as He leads,
5. Real love is my deciding to make your problem my problem.

If I give all my possessions to feed the poor... but do not have love, I have gained nothing (1 Corinthians 13:3)

TODAY'S STEP: Faith is recognizing that the longer I suffer under trying circumstances, the more certain I am to appreciate my deliverance.

"This life therefore, is not righteousness, but growth in righteousness, not health but healing, not being but becoming, not rest but exercise. We are not what we shall be, but we are growing toward it, the process is not yet finished, but it is going on, this is not the end, but it is the road. All does not yet gleam in glory, but all is being purified." -- Martin Luther

Dealing with Stress

The Twenty-third Psalm has doubtless been of help in subduing stress for many. A modernized version of the Psalm by Toki Miyashina (from ***Psalm 23: Several Versions Collected*** by K. H. Strange) is a translation of the Japanese, which seems to have a healing effect on today's fast-paced and stressful society.

This poem is not only beautiful, but it is therapeutic as well. Anyone who will commit it to memory and say it over and over again until it sinks into his deep unconscious can, in due course, find effective healing of any-stressful condition. With this certain cure available, it is little less than pathetic to permit ourselves to be dominated by tension; to be victimized by anxiety.

The Lord is my Pace-setter, I shall not rush;

He makes me stop and rest for quiet intervals,

He provides me with images of stillness, which restore my serenity.

He leads me in the ways of efficiency through calmness of mind,

And His guidance is peace.

Even though I have a great many things   to accomplish each day,

I will not fret for His presence is here,

His timelessness, His all importance, will keep me in balance,

He prepares refreshment and renewal in the midst of my activity,

By anointing my mind with His oils of tranquility.

My cup of joyous energy overflows,

Surely harmony and effectiveness shall be the fruits of my hours,

For I shall walk, in the pace of my Lord

And dwell in His house forever.

You are my rock and my fortress...You will lead me and guide me. (Psalms 31:3)

TODAY'S STEP: Wh**en *I exert my will I am leaving no room for God to work His Plan. It is freeing to not be in control. A miracle of the program is gaining hope and trust.***

"No one has ever loved anyone the way everyone wants to be loved." -- Mignon McLaughlin

Love and Freedom

Addiction finds its way into all our loves. We can discern how much by asking ourselves two questions. First, how free are we to give up the persons or things we love? As we become more addicted, letting go seems increasingly impossible. Our most addicted loving is our most desperate loving: "I cannot live without you," "If I don't get that promotion, my life is over," "Everything depends on buying that house," or "I can't think of anything, but that mistake I made."

Second, how free are we within our love? How much space is there for us to be ourselves? To say No? To what extent can we play? How much is our freedom confined, restricted, perhaps even imprisoned, by our attachment to the person or thing we love? Our most addicted loving is also our most choice less loving: "I cannot tell her how I feel because she would leave me," or worse, "I cannot tell him because he would beat me." In one way or another, we all know what it is to relinquish our freedom for love.

It is critical to understand what freedom means here. Because love is giving of ourselves, it always involves some choice to direct and restrain our behavior. When we love, we do not follow every impulse that comes along. We have self control, a higher concern, a deeper desire; we value our beloved more than we value our passing whims. The freedom question, then, is not whether we can do whatever we want, but whether we can do what we most deeply want, respecting those we are in relationship with.

It is a critical distinction, the difference between attachment-binding desire, and commitment-honoring desire. It is the difference between codependence and compassion, between neediness and mutuality, between shame and dignity.

Love is patient; love is kind and envies no one. Love is never boastful, nor conceited, nor rude; never selfish, not quick to take offense. Love keeps no score of wrongs; does not gloat over other men's sins, but delights in the truth. There is nothing love cannot face; there is no limit to its faith, its hope, and its endurance. (Corinthians 13:4-7)

TODAY'S STEP: I create a healthy atmosphere of love and nurturing around and within me. I accept the love and support of my sponsor and my group.

Step Four

<u>"Made a searching and fearless moral inventory of ourselves."</u>

Our entrance into the Twelve Step Program often occurs after a series of painful events resulting from reality pushing aside our fantasy world. Our resultant fears and anxieties may have weakened the defenses of our denial system and forced us to look at ourselves and acknowledge the consequences of our behavior. The shock, disbelief and acceptance of the problems in our lives form the foundation for a life-changing adventure that involves self-discovery, healing and Recovery.

During the first three Steps, we initiated many changes that have far-reaching effects on our lives. In Step Four, we must look at ourselves and our lives honestly, possibly for the first time. If we do this carefully, a new awareness of ourselves will begin. Our increased sensitivity may help us discover some aspects of our character that are alarming or overwhelming to us. If we carefully worked Steps One through Three, this discovery should be rewarding.

As we begin to discover the origins of our behavior, we start to develop an enlightened and mature perspective about being Adult Children. Much of our early trauma was caused by things over which we had no control. We can see how our wounded inner child continues to influence much of our current adult behavior. We can stop engaging in hurtful childish behavior and feeling frustrated when the wounded inner child appears. Step Four uncovers many childhood traumas that can be transformed and healed with the help of our Higher Power.

As we prepare our <u>Fourth Step Inventory</u>, we look at our character traits and review both our limitations and our strengths. Our inability to accept our limitations often produces behavior that is destructive to us and exploits the limitations of others. Before we can seriously work on our problem areas, we need to acknowledge and examine our limitations. Our self-understanding will be accelerated as we discover how we talk to ourselves and others -- the ideas, beliefs and attitudes that govern the ways in which we see our world and how we relate to it.

The <u>Inventory</u> we are preparing is for our benefit. It will be the tool for making a major breakthrough in our Recovery and setting us on the road to freedom. The negative, unwanted and excess emotional baggage we have been carrying can be gradually put aside in light of our new understanding. As we abandon old, useless attitudes, we must remember that our Higher Power is always with us, offering the support and guidance we need to continue this work.

FOURTH STEP PRAYERS

"Made a searching and fearless moral inventory of ourselves."

Dear God,

It is I who have made my life a mess. I have done it, but I cannot undo it alone. My mistakes are mine, and I will begin a searching and fearless moral inventory. I will write down my wrongs, and I will also include that which is good. I pray for the strength to complete the task.

In this moment, I am willing to see myself as I truly am, a growing, unfolding spiritual being resting in the hands of a loving God. I can separate who I am from what I've done, knowing the real me is emerging – loving, joyful and whole.

MEDITATIONS

Today I must be in control of all my emotions, they must not injure anyone or lead me to injure myself. Dear Lord, my life is so full of problems. So often I go from day to day trying to ignore their many consequences. I pray for heavenly forces to rejuvenate me and fill my whole being with divine strength so I may be in control of everything I say and do. Insecurity clouds my vision, the love and respect I yearn for from others is spoiled by my childish demand for unnecessary attention. I think and say things I am truly sorry for, I hesitate to make apologies, because I do not feel capable of doing so correctly. I am too concerned with myself and ask Thee, dear Father, to release me from the prison of false ego that I have built around myself. Fortify me with strength of character and let me direct my energies into making others happy. I ask this in all my humility.

AFFIRMATIONS

I know that greatness begins in the minds of the great. I know what I believe about my self is what I will become -- so I believe in the best for my self!

I am practical and realistic, and I keep my feet on solid ground. I also give my self the freedom to live up to my fullest expectations.

I never limit my self by the short-sighted beliefs of others. Instead, I open my self up to the broad horizons of unlimited possibilities.

The three great essentials to achieve anything are, first, hard work, second, stick-to-itiveness, third, common sense." Thomas Edison

A Survival and Serenity Checklist

[ ]   I make attitude changes within myself to begin and continue growing and recovering.

[ ]   I am powerless over people, places and things – the only one I can change is myself.

[ ]   I have choices; I don't have to stay stuck unless I choose to.

[ ]   I keep the focus on me and stay in the now.

[ ]   My spirituality is restored; I believe in a Power greater than myself; I ask for God's help and His will to be done.

[ ]   I'm responsible for both my happiness and my unhappiness.

[ ]   I deserve and have self-esteem and self-confidence.

[ ]   I don't have to accept unacceptable behavior.

[ ]   I feel and deal with my feelings, not stuff them as I did before.

[ ]   I strive for continued growth and recovery through service work.

[ ]   I do not place unreasonable expectations on people.

[ ]   I celebrate what I do have and do not complain about what I don't have.

[ ]   I detach with love.

[ ]   I work on self-honesty.

[ ]   I work to achieve balance in my life, not extremes.

The eternal God is my refuge, and underneath are the everlasting arms . . . . (Deuteronomy 33:27)

TODAY'S STEP: When I rely on my Higher Power's help I can achieve anything.

"The important thing is this: To be able at any moment to sacrifice what we are for what we could become." -- Charles Du Bois

<u>Ten Commandments for Human Relations</u>

(Recovery from Isolation)

As we begin to feel better about ourselves, we become more willing to take risks and expose ourselves to new people and surroundings. We seek friends and relationships that are more nurturing, safe and supportive. It becomes easier to express our feelings when we recognize people will accept us for who we really are if we are willing to:

- **Speak to people.** There is nothing as nice as a big cheerful word of greeting.

- **Smile at people.** It takes 72 muscles to frown and only 14 to smile.

- **Call people by name.** The sweetest music to anyone's ear is the sound of their own name.

- **Be friendly and helpful.** If you would have friends, be friendly.

- **Be cordial.** Speak and act as if everything you do is a genuine pleasure.

- **Be generous with praise and cautious with criticism.**

- **Be thoughtful of the opinions of others.** There are three sides to a controversy; yours, the other person's and the right one.

- **Be alert to give service.** What counts most in life is what we do for others.

- **Be genuinely interested in people.** You can like almost everyone if you try.

- **Be considerate of the feelings of others.**

Teach me the way in which I should walk; For to You I lift up my soul (Psalm 143:8)

TODAY'S STEP: I visualize myself achieving my goal of changing for the better.

"Learn to forgive. With bitterness in your soul you can never be happy." -- Anonymous

Fear and Resentment

The Big Book of Alcoholics Anonymous has some excellent guidelines on how to do an inventory. Their experience of taking stock identifies resentment as the "number one" offender. "It destroys more alcoholics than anything else. From it stem all forms of spiritual disease, for we have been not only mentally and physically ill, we have been spiritually sick. When the spiritual malady is overcome, we straighten out mentally and physically."

The word "resentment" has its root in the Latin word "sentire" – to feel. Resentment actually means re-feeling in its most negative sense.

A useful way of dealing with resentment is to make a list of those persons toward whom we hold resentments and then take a look at "why" we feel that way. Have those people affected our self-esteem, our security, our personal relationships, our sexual relationships or our ambitions? In what manner have these people behaved to cause this reaction from us? Are they patronizing? Do they threaten our professional standing or careers? Have they bested us in competition, either socially or through their superior business tactics? Have they turned others away from us? Are they unresponsive to our seductiveness?

More often than not, we find that the underlying cause of these resentments is fear: Fear of being discounted; fear of losing our stature in the community; fear of financial failure, fear of being deserted by our friends, fear of losing our ability to attract the opposite sex. There are also many other fears underlying resentment that we could add to our list.

Resentments are, without a doubt, the most dangerous threat to our continuing recovery. Time after time, people have reported that their inability to let go of resentments led to a relapse into their former addictive/compulsive lives. If I haven't forgiven someone, I am *holding* resentment.

You open Your hand and satisfy the desire of every living thing. (Psalm 145:16)

TODAY'S STEP: I am not afraid because God is my courage and my strength.

"Today I have got myself out of all my perplexities; or rather, I have got the perplexities out of myself – for they were not without, but within; they lay in my own outlook." Marcus Aurelius, **Meditations**

<u>Tradition Four</u>

Tradition Four says each group is autonomous, free to conduct meetings in a way that suits its members as long as it abides by the Traditions and doesn't harm the overall unity of Al-Anon.

Why should we get our noses bent out of shape because another Al-Anon group chooses to follow a meeting format different from one familiar to us? Why should we assume **our** way is the **right** way?

In Al-Anon we learn to "Think" before we react to angry outbursts and accusations. We learn to hold our tongues when tempted to interfere in something that is clearly none of our business. We learn the value of silence.

But silence can be more damaging than cruel words when it's used to punish. Deliberately ignoring someone's attempts to communicate is no better than engaging in a battle of words. Rage expressed non-verbally through cold looks is still rage. When we seek to hurt someone else with silence or any other weapon at our disposal, we always hurt ourselves. When we remember to "Keep An Open Mind," we find the principles of the Al-Anon program remain exactly the same, no matter which group or which city or which state we visit.

Each of us plays an essential part in this remarkable fellowship, supporting one another as we recover from the effects of alcoholism. With this solid foundation of love and support, our individual differences can only make us richer as a whole. Today, try to make choices that support this goal.

Be quick to hear, slow to speak, slow to anger. **(James 1:19)**

TODAY'S STEP: I am seeking a saner approach to everything I encounter. The slogans are a valuable source of sanity in chaotic situations. If I am tempted to act out of anger or frustration, I will remember "Easy Does It."

"What we call the beginning is often the end, and to make an end is to make a beginning. The end is where we start from." -- T. S. Eliot

Am I An Addict?

Only you can answer this question. We lived to use and used to live. Very simply, an addict is a person whose life is controlled by drugs.

1. Do you ever use alone? YES [ ] NO [ ]

2. Have you ever substituted one drug for another, thinking that one particular drug was the problem? YES [ ] NO [ ]

3. Have you ever manipulated or lied to a doctor to obtain prescription drugs? YES [ ] NO [ ]

4. Have you ever stolen drugs or stolen to obtain drugs? YES [ ] NO [ ]

5. Do you regularly use a drug when you wake up or when you go to bed? YES [ ] NO [ ]

6. Have you ever taken one drug to overcome the effects of another? YES [ ] NO [ ]

7. Do you avoid people or places that do not approve of you using drugs? YES [ ] NO [ ]

8. Have you ever used a drug without knowing what it was or what it would do to you? YES [ ] NO [ ]

9. Has your job or school performance ever suffered because of your drug use? YES [ ] NO [ ]

10. Have you ever been arrested as a result of using drugs? YES [ ] NO [ ]

11. Have you ever lied about what or how much you use? YES [ ] NO [ ]

12. Do you put the purchase of drugs ahead of your financial responsibilities? YES [ ] NO [ ]

13. Have you ever tried to stop or control your using? YES [ ] NO [ ]

14. Have you ever been in a jail, hospital or drug rehabilitation center because of your using? YES [ ] NO [ ]

15. Does using interfere with your sleeping or eating? YES [ ] NO [ ]

My grace is sufficient for you . . . (2 Corinthians 12:9)

TODAY'S STEP: Day by day, I entrust my problems to a power greater than myself.

"Failure is, in a sense, the highway to success, inasmuch as every discovery of what is false leads us to seek earnestly after what is true, and every fresh experience points out some form of error, which we shall afterward carefully avoid." -- John Keats

How to Conquer the Ten Most Common Causes of Failure

From his widely acclaimed book, ***The Road to Successful Living,*** Louis Binstock introduces us to the major stumbling blocks we may have unknowingly erected in our lives, errors we may be making, again and again, that are hurting us every day. The ten most common causes of failure are:

1. **Blaming others.** The practice of blaming others accounts not only for perhaps half of our failures, but also for our failure to cash in on failures. We do not recognize failure for what it is, and consequently, we cannot deal with it.
2. **Blaming ourselves.** Instead of wrestling with the problem behind the failure and struggling to resolve it – to prevent its recurrence – we blame ourselves.
3. **Having no goals.** A person must know where he wants to go and what he wants, if he is going to get anywhere.
4. **Choosing the wrong goals.** Setting our sights upon one goal and allowing it to represent self-fulfillment, we sometimes discover after many years of struggle that attaining the object of our efforts does not always bring happiness.
5. **Taking short cuts.** Most of us instinctively choose the shortest, easiest, quickest way to success, only to discover that the success was illusory.
6. **Taking the long road.** Too often if you wait or travel too long, you never reach home.
7. **Neglecting little things.** The good executive keeps his finger on the little things: he knows they may, if mishandled, become big problems. We must appreciate and care for the details.
8. **Quitting too soon.** Often it is not the wrong start, but the wrong stop that makes the difference between success and failure – "Don't stop trying in trying times."
9. **Hanging on to the past.** Memories of the past can infuse us with courage and confidence and creative power; or they can bind us in a dark shroud of dejection and defeat.
10. **Recognizing the illusion of success.** The achievement of success is most precarious when it appears to be permanent. Success, being fickle, must be continuously wooed; she can never be won forever and ever.

Oh Lord, I pray, send now prosperity. (Psalm 118:25)

TODAY'S STEP: By calling on my Higher Power for help daily I can learn from every situation.

"We can't form our children on our own concepts; we must take them and love them as God gives them to us." -- Johann Wolfgang von Goethe, ***Hermann and Dorothea***

Children Learn What They Live

If children live with criticism, they learn to condemn.

If children live with hostility, they learn to fight.

If children live with fear, they learn to be apprehensive.

If children live with pity, they learn to feel sorry for themselves.

If children live with ridicule, they learn to be shy.

If children live with jealousy, they learn what envy is.

If children live with shame, they learn to feel guilty.

If children live with tolerance, they learn to be patient.

If children live with encouragement, they learn to be confident.

If children live with praise, they learn to appreciate.

If children live with approval, they learn to like themselves.

If children live with acceptance, they learn to find love in the world.

If children live with recognition, they learn to have a goal.

If children live with sharing, they learn to be generous.

If children live with honesty and fairness, they learn what truth and justice are.

If children live with security, they learn to have faith in themselves and in those around them.

If children live with friendliness, they learn that the world is a nice place in which to live.

If children live with serenity, they learn to have peace of mind.

With what are your children living? -- Dorothy L. Nolte

. . . live as children of light. (Ephesians 5:8)

TODAY'S STEP: If I touch someone else, God touches me too.

"Love is not consolation, it is light." -- Simone Weil

"Recovery Is a Journey, Not a Destination"

Recovery is learning to function in relationships. And we learn to function in relationships by participating in relationships.

Certain behaviors and attitudes nurture relationships and help them grow. Healthy detachment, honestly, self-love, love for each other, tackling problems, negotiating differences, and being flexible help nurture relationships. We can enhance relationships with acceptance, forgiveness, a sense of humor, an empowering, but realistic attitude, open communication, respect, tolerance, patience, and faith in a Higher Power.

- Caring about our own and each other's feelings helps.
- Asking instead of ordering helps.
- Not caring, when caring too much hurts, helps too.
- Being there when we need each other helps.
- Having and setting boundaries and respecting other people's boundaries improves relationships.

On the other hand, certain behaviors and attitudes harm relationships. Low self-esteem, taking responsibility for others, neglecting ourselves, unfinished business, and trying to control other people or the relationship can cause damage. Certain attitudes such as hopelessness, resentment, perpetual criticism, naiveté, unreliability, hard heartedness, negativity, or cynicism can ruin relationships.

- Being too selfish, or not selfish enough, can hurt relationships.
- Too little or too much tolerance can harm relationships.
- Looking for all our good feelings, excitement, or stimulation from our relationships can damage them.
- Having expectations too high or too low can hurt relationships.
- Not learning from our mistakes can cause us to repeat the same mistakes.

Let everything you say be good and helpful, so that your words will be an encouragement to those who hear them. (Ephesians 4:29)

TODAY'S STEP: I create a healthy atmosphere of love and nurturing around and within me. I accept the love and support of my sponsor and my group.

"There is no security on this earth; there is only opportunity." -- Gen. Douglas MacArthur

<u>Anxiety</u>

Anxious feelings are common in Recovery. When you give up an addictive habit, you are likely to feel anxious for a while. You may wonder if you can handle the demands of Recovery and worry about whether or not you will relapse. Anxiety may stem from the typical challenges of Recovery, such as how to handle a craving for an addictive substance.

A strong desire for cocaine will cause a drug addict to feel anxious. A strong desire for gambling will make a compulsive gambler experience anxiety. Increased fantasies and thoughts about sex can cause anxiety in a sex addict. Eating in moderation in front of other people can cause a compulsive overeater to feel anxious. Each addiction creates its own challenges for the person who attempts to recover from it.

In cases of alcoholism and drug addiction, anxiety can result from your body's adjustment to being without chemicals. Anxiety, depression, and cravings are just a few of the common symptoms of sobriety experienced by alcoholics and drug addicts, particularly in the first several months of Recovery.

The list below presents some methods you can use to handle anxiety:

- Practice challenging and changing your anxious thoughts and beliefs.

- Find out specific problems or things that cause you to feel anxious and work on changing these when possible.

- Evaluate your diet. Is your use of caffeine, tobacco, sugar, or other foods contributing to anxiety?

- Learn to meditate and to use relaxation techniques.

- If your anxiety level continues to cause you significant distress, consult a mental health professional.

The Lord is my rock and my fortress and my deliverer. (Psalm 18:2)

TODAY'S STEP: I ask my Higher Power to help me let go of fear, doubt, and anxiety and to fill me with faith, trust and serenity.

"No one is alone if they've come to believe in a Power greater than themselves."

"But For the Grace Of God"

The Higher Power's role is to assist in adopting the principles outlined in the Twelve Steps. Though alcoholics enter AA to stop drinking, they quickly learn that Recovery involves more than just giving up alcohol and drugs. The secret is to learn to live differently: by principles rather than personality, self-knowledge instead of denial, faith rather than ambition. Broadly stated, the Steps suggest we:

- **Admit powerlessness over addiction:** Acknowledging we have lost control over chemicals and our lives have become unmanageable sets the stage for the entrance of our Higher Power, who can help us do what we haven't been able to accomplish on our own.

- **Assume faith in a Higher Power:** We accept the need for outside assistance in Recovery, forsaking further attempts to beat our addiction through willpower.

- **Abandon insistence on personal control:** We turn our will and lives over to whatever outside power we believe in.

- **Examine ourselves:** We study our own behavior (often quite a change from an earlier preoccupation with criticizing others) in terms of right and wrong.

- **Make personal changes:** We become willing to have our Higher Power remedy our character defects.

- **Make amends to those we harmed:** We seek to atone for the wrongs of the past where possible.

- **Pray and meditate:** We ask our Higher Power for guidance (prayer) and promise to listen to and reflect on the answers (meditation).

- **Carry the message:** We share our experience with those who still suffer, as a way of reinforcing the message in our own thinking.

Do not be conformed to this world, but be transformed by the renewing of your mind, that you may prove what is that good and acceptable and perfect will of God. (Romans 12:2)

TODAY'S STEP: When faced with difficult or painful situations, I remember a loving God is always here for me.

"Life is like the trumpet. If you don't put anything in, you don't get anything out."
-- W. C. Handy

Owning Our Feelings

Melody Beattie, author of **Codependent No More, Beyond Codependency, The Language of Letting Go,** and **Codependent's Guide to the Twelve Steps,** writes about the problem of codependency and talks about the importance of (1) Owning our feelings, (2) Not blaming our problems on other people, and (3) Asking God for help to deal with our pain and frustration.

In **The Language of Letting Go**, she demonstrates how easy it is for us to blame our problems on others. "Look at what he's doing." "Look how long I've waited." "Why doesn't she call?" "If only he'd change – then I'd be happy." Often, we feel our accusations are justified and we believe the solution to our pain and frustration is getting the other person to do what we want. But these self-defeating illusions put the power and control of our life in other people's hands. (This is called **Codependency.**)

The solution to our pain and frustration is to acknowledge our own feelings. We feel the anger, the grief; then we let go of the feelings and find peace – within ourselves. We know our happiness isn't controlled by another person, even though we may have convinced ourselves it is. (This is called **Acceptance.**)

Then we decide that although we'd like our situation to be different, maybe our life is happening this way for a reason. Maybe there is a higher purpose and plan in play, one that's better than we could have orchestrated. (This is called **Faith.**)

Then we decide what we need to do, what is within our power to take care of ourselves and move toward health. (This is called **Recovery.**)

Examine me, O Lord, and prove me; Try my mind and my heart. (Psalm 26:2)

TODAY'S STEP: I face my problems squarely and without blame.

<u>Addiction's Ten Commandments</u>

Addiction bears many of the trappings of religious sects: ritualistic behavior, ecstatic experience, strict codes of conduct, even martyrdom. R. Rogers & C. McMillin in ***Under Your Own Power: A Secular Approach to 12-Step Programs*** offer us their view of the "Ten Commandments" for the faithful followers of the imaginary *Church of the Exalted Chemical.*

The First Commandment: **THOU SHALT HAVE NO OTHER GODS BEFORE THE DRUG.** Think of all the alcoholics who have sacrificed career, family, and even life itself to the God of Alcohol.

The Second Commandment: **THOU SHALT HONOR THE DRUG THY FATHER AND MOTHER.** Devotion to the drug supersedes family loyalties – husbands leave their wives, wives forsake their husbands, parents abandon their kids – all to use drugs.

The Third Commandment: **THOU SHALT KILL ANY WHO THREATEN THE DRUG.** Armed kids roam poor neighborhoods, dealers use Uzis, and random violence claims as many victims as homicides.

The Fourth Commandment: **THOU SHALT SACRIFICE THY CHILDREN TO ME.** How many children are born with Fetal Alcohol Syndrome or how many must be detoxified from heroin or cocaine?

The Fifth Commandment: **THOU SHALT SET ASIDE TIME TO WORSHIP ME.** How many alcoholics limit or swear off drinking during the week, only to binge on the weekends?

The Sixth Commandment: **THOU SHALT NOT QUESTION ME.** Isn't it amazing how normally intelligent people become blind to the obvious effects of alcohol and drugs?

The Seventh Commandment: **THOU SHALT SUSPECT EVERYONE BUT ME.** Few people die more unsuspectingly than an alcoholic.

The Eighth Commandment: **THOU SHALT SEEK FORGIVENESS ONLY THROUGH ME.** Aware of all the losses of alcoholism, the alcoholic still seeks relief from pain with more alcohol.

The Ninth Commandment: **THOU SHALT NOT FORGIVE ME.** Even years after the last drink, cravings and vivid dreams of drinking live in the recesses of the brain.

The Tenth Commandment: **THOU SHALT MAKE OFFERINGS TO ME.** Call your church and ask how much was contributed in the past year and then call a successful bar and see how much more they earned from selling liquor – which god is more honored?

Answer a fool according to his folly, lest he be wise in his own eyes. (Psalm 26:5)

TODAY'S STEP: I ask God to help me understand and accept the full meaning of the disease of Alcoholism.

"In the life of the spirit, only he who does the work gets the bread." -- Soren Kierkegaard

As F. L. Rawson, the great English metaphysician, used to advise when engaging in spiritual treatment, don't think of material good. To do so is to drop the mind down into the welter of contrary suggestions. Think rather, of immaterial good. Rehearse in your mind all the highest truths you know. Recall scriptures which are meaningful to you, and such axiomatic statements as these:

"There is nothing good or bad, but thinking makes it so."

"It is not what happens to you, but what you think of what happens to you, that makes the difference between happiness and misery."

"Every thought tends toward its own embodiment."

"Every thought is nascent action."

"You have nothing to deal with but your thought."

"Let your opinion lie still and you do not suffer."

My Daily Prayer

God, I turn my will and my life over to You this day for Your keeping. Your will, Lord, not mine. I ask for Your guidance and direction. I will walk humbly with You and Your fellowman. You are giving me a grateful heart for my blessings. You are removing the defects of character that stand in my way. You are giving me freedom from self- will.

Let love, compassion, and understanding be in my every thought, word, and deed this day. I release those to You who have mistreated me. I truly desire Your abundance of truth, love, harmony, and peace. As I go out today to do Your bidding, let me help anyone I can who is less fortunate than I.

The fruit of the Spirit is love, joy, peace, patience, kindness, goodness, faithfulness, gentleness, and self-control... (Galatians 5:22-23)

TODAY'S STEP: Thankfulness today will help me see the miracles at work in my life and in the lives of others on the road to Recovery.

"I look back on my life like a good day's work, it was done and I am satisfied with it. I was happy and contented; I knew nothing better and made the best out of what life offered. And life is what we make it, always has been, always will be." -- Grandma Moses

Start With Yourself

The following words were written on the tomb of an Anglican Bishop (1100 A.D.) in the Crypts of Westminster Abby:

When I was young and free and my imagination had

no limits, I dreamed of changing the world. As

I grew older and wiser, I discovered the world

would not change, so I shortened my sights somewhat

and decided to change only my country.

But it, too, seemed immovable.

As I grew into my twilight years, in one last

desperate attempt, I settled for changing only my family,

those closest to me, but alas, they would have none of it.

And now as I lie on my deathbed, I suddenly realize:

If I had only changed my self first, then by example

I would have changed my family.

From their inspiration and encouragement, I would

Then have been able to better my country and, who

Knows, I may have even changed the world.

Anonymous

You will know them by their fruits. Do men gather grapes from thorn bushes or figs from thistles? Even so, every good tree bears good fruit, but a bad tree bears bad fruit. A good tree cannot bear bad fruit, nor can a bad tree bear good fruit. Every tree that does not bear good fruit is cut down and thrown into the fire. Therefore by their fruit you will know them. **(Matthew 7:16-20)**

TODAY'S STEP: There are so many ways in which I can improve the quality of my life. Instead of fretting about what I can't have or can't do, I'll take action to create something positive in my life today.

"The reason why worry kills more people than work is that more people worry than work." -- Robert Frost

"Live In the Now"

Problems are a fact of life and conflicts in relationships are too. But problem **solving** is also a fact of life. Learning to solve problems and negotiate differences propel us forward on our Recovery journey, whereas fear and worry keep us stuck.

Worry and fear can alter our perceptions until we lose all sense of reality. Because worry focuses on the future, if we can learn to stay in the present, living one day or one moment at a time, we can take positive steps toward warding off the effects of fear. Melody Beattie, **Beyond Codependency and Getting Better All the Time,** has a few suggestions for dealing with problems:

- Identify and accept the problem.
- Look for solutions in the best interest of the relationship.
- Be open to various solutions.
- Learn to combine emotion and reason.
- Don't take problems and differences personally.
- Don't deny an adversarial reaction if it's present, but don't assume one either.
- Learn to combine detachment with appropriate action steps.
- Practice deliberate, time-limited patience.
- Be clear about what you want and need.
- Consider the wants and needs of yourself and others as important.
- Separate issues from people.
- Communicate.
- Healthy boundaries are crucial to conflict negotiation.
- Consistently foregoing what you want and need isn't conflict negotiation.
- Avoid power plays. Don't waste time negotiating non-negotiables.

Do not worry about your everyday life . . . . Which of you by worrying can add a single moment to your life? . . . . Your heavenly Father knows all you need. (Matthew 6:25-32)

TODAY'S STEP: I ask my Higher Power to help me let go of fear, doubt and anxiety and to fill me with faith, trust and serenity.

"For souls in growth, great quarrels are great emancipations." -- Logan Pearsall Smith

Look at the *Recovery Check List* that follows. It can help you determine your strengths and weaknesses in Recovery, as well as help in setting your Recovery goals.

<u>*Recovery Check List**</u>

___ Maintaining appropriate daily routine

___ Personal care

___ Setting and sticking to limits with children and others

___ Choosing behaviors

___ Well-rested

___ Accepting (versus denying)

___ Open to appropriate criticism/feedback

___ Valuing wants and needs

___ Free of victim self-image

___ Free of worry and obsession

___ Faith in a Higher Power

___ Trusting and valuing self

___ Making appropriate decisions about trusting others

___ Mind clear and peaceful: logical thinking; free of confusion

___ Appropriately disclosing

___ Setting and achieving daily goals

___ Constructive planning

___ Appropriate decision-making and problem-solving efforts

___ Resentment-free

___ Not controlling others nor feeling controlled by them

___ Free of criticism of self/others

___ Not feeling excessively responsible for others

___ Maintaining Recovery routine (attending support groups, etc.)

___ Feeling and dealing appropriately with feelings, including anger

___ Needing people versus NEEDING them

___ Responsible expectations of self

*Based in part on "Relapse Warning Signs for Co-Alcoholism," developed by Terence T. Gorski and Merlene Miller, from *"Co –Alcoholic Relapse,"* in **Co-Dependency, An Emerging Issue.**

Teach me what I do not see. (Job 34:32)

TODAY'S STEP: Emotional health is from within, not without.

"We move from being at the mercy of any problem that comes along to an inner certainty that no matter what happens in our lives, we will be able to face it, deal with it, and learn from it with the help of our Higher Power." . . . . **In All Our Affairs**

<u>*Seven Powerful Prayers*</u>

The Bible is full of powerful prayers and treatments. Some of the best known chapters are really treatments for healing and inspiration.

Twenty-third Psalm. Use this chapter when you need something of importance. You know it by heart, but read it and get something new from it. This new inspiration brings the result.

Ninety-first Psalm. Read when you feel a sense of danger or apprehension. The note about the 23rd Psalm applies to this one also.

Daniel, Chapter 6. Read this chapter when your difficulties are actually with you, and seem to be almost immovable.

Hebrews, Chapter 2. This is the chapter for handling doubts and discouragement.

James, Chapter 1. Packed with psychology and metaphysics it is a course of instruction in itself. James is profound, very practical, and rather personal.

Exodus, Chapter 15. A song of triumph – of thanksgiving for prayer answered. Thanksgiving (before the demonstration arrives – or is in sight) is a most powerful form of prayer.

1 Corinthians, Chapter 13. This is the fulfilling of the law and the shortest cut to Health, Harmony, and Success.

You may know all of these prayers by heart, but the way to use them **effectively** is to read them over carefully, trying to get something new out of each verse. Getting something new in this way is really an expansion of consciousness, and it is the expansion of consciousness that brings results.

When you are praying, do not use meaningless repetition as the Gentiles do, for they suppose that they will be heard for their many words. (Matthew 6:7)

TODAY'S STEP: I connect with my Higher Power through prayer and meditation in the morning and at night, and anytime in-between.

"Why are you drinking?" demanded the little prince.

"So that I may forget," replied the tippler.

"Forget what?" inquired the little prince, who already was sorry for him.

"Forget that I am ashamed," the tippler confessed, hanging his head.

"Ashamed of what?" insisted the little prince, who wanted to help him.

"Ashamed of drinking!" The tippler brought his speech to an end, and shut himself up in an impregnable silence. Antoine de Saint-Exupery, *The Little Prince*

Do You Have A Problem With Alcohol?

1.   Do you drink because you have problems? To relax?

2.   Do you drink when you get mad at other people, your friends or parents?

3.   Do you prefer to drink alone, rather than with others?

4.   Are your grades starting to slip? Are you goofing off on your job?

5.   Did you ever try to stop drinking or drink less – and fail?

6.   Have you begun to drink in the morning, before school or work?

7.   Do you gulp your drinks?

8.   Do you ever have loss of memory due to your drinking?

9.   Do you lie about your drinking?

10. Do you ever get into trouble when your drinking?

11. Do you get drunk when you drink, even when you don't mean to?

12. Do you think it's cool to be able to hold your liquor?

Create in me a clean heart, O God. And renew a steadfast spirit within me. (Psalm 51:10)

TODAY'S STEP: I am finding the courage to face the Truth about myself.

"In my judgment such of us who have never fallen victims (to alcoholism) have been spared more by the absence of appetite than from any mental or moral superiority over those who have. Indeed, I believe if we take habitual drunkards as a class, their heads and their hearts will bear an advantageous comparison with those of any other class." Abraham Lincoln, Address to the Washington Temperance Society, 1842

A "Big-Book" Fourth Step

On pages 64 through 71 of **Alcoholics Anonymous, "The Big Book"** is the original approach suggested for a Fourth Step. This version calls for an honest taking stock of ourselves. It is simple and straightforward. We write down the names of people we resent, and why. We write down what part of our lives we feel those people have affected and harmed. On our list of resentments, we include "people, institutions or principles with whom we are, or were angry." For instance, "I'm resentful toward my friend because she doesn't call me often enough, and that affects my social life and my feelings of well-being."

We list our fears. Many of us learn fear is an underlying motive in our codependency. This Step is a way to ferret it out. "Sometimes we think fear ought to be classed with stealing -- it seems to cause more trouble," wrote the authors of **"The Big Book"** (p. 68).

We list our grudges and our injuries — real and imagined. "It is plain that a life, which includes deep resentment, leads only to futility and unhappiness. To the precise extent that we permit these, we squander the hours that might have been worthwhile -- for when harboring such feelings, we shut ourselves off from the sunlight of the Spirit" says **"The Big Book"** (p. 66).

We don't squelch or repress our anger and resentments. Our feelings may be long overdue. The purpose of this process is to get out into the light our deeply rooted feelings, so we can feel them and be done with them.

In this Fourth Step, we may want to cover all the troublesome areas of our lives — anger, fear, sex, and money — reviewing each area thoroughly and with an attitude of self-acceptance, not shame.

Look straight ahead with honest confidence . . . (Proverbs 4:25)

TODAY'S STEP: How do I feel today? How am I doing? If I can answer those questions truthfully, I am more likely to pursue the help I need and to share the happy times with others as well.

"Every human soul is worth saving; but . . . if a choice is to be made, drunkards are about the last class to be taken hold of . . . ."   J. E. Todd, "Drunkenness a Vice, Not a Disease"

Did You Grow Up With A Problem Drinker?

Al-Anon is for families, relatives and friends whose lives have been affected by someone else's drinking. Many adults question whether they have been affected by alcoholism. If someone close to you has, or has had a drinking problem, the following questions may help you in determining whether alcoholism has affected your life.

______ 1. Do you constantly seek approval and affirmation?

______ 2. Do you fail to recognize your accomplishments?

______ 3. Do you fear criticism?

______ 4. Do you overextend yourself?

______ 5. Have you had problems with compulsive behavior?

______ 6. Do you have a need for perfection?

______ 7. Are you uneasy when your life is going smoothly (anticipating problems)?

______ 8. Do you feel more alive in the midst of a crisis?

______ 9. Do you still feel responsible for others, as you did for the problem drinker?

______10. Do you care for others easily, yet find it difficult to care for yourself?

______11. Do you isolate yourself from other people?

______12. Do you respond with anxiety to authority figures and angry people?

______13. Do you feel that individuals /society in general are taking advantage of you?

______14. Do you have trouble with intimate relationships?

______15. Do you confuse pity with love, as you did with the problem drinker?

______16. Do you attract and seek people who are compulsive?

______17. Do you cling to relationships because you are afraid of being alone?

______18. Do you often mistrust your own feelings and the feelings of others?

______19. Do you find it difficult to express your emotions?

______20. Do you think parental drinking has affected you?

Do you not know that your body is a temple of the Holy Spirit . . . ? (1 Corinthians 6:19)

TODAY'S STEP: I am finding the courage to face the Truth about myself.

"As better knowledge and understanding of the actions of alcohol becomes available, more sensible attitudes regarding it are arising, [but] it is also interesting to observe how little the people wanted to learn about alcohol in a scientific way. They seem to prefer their violently differing emotional fantasies about it." Chauncey D. Leake, in a symposium called *"Alcoholism,"* 1957

<u>*Marriage on The Rocks*</u>

There are three statements in the alcoholism field with which there appears to be agreement:

1. Alcoholism runs in families. Rarely do we see a case in isolation. Someone, somewhere else in the family usually has been, or is currently, suffering from the disease.

2. Children of alcoholics run a higher risk of developing alcoholism than children in the mainstream of the population. There may have been some discussion of environment or genetics, or a combination of both, but the truth of the statement is without question.

3. Children of alcoholics tend to marry alcoholics. They rarely go into the marriage with that-awareness, but we see this phenomenon occur over and over again.

In **Marriage On The Rocks,** Dr. Janet Geringer Woititz talks about these and other qualities, which are prevalent among alcoholics, such as (a) excessive dependency; (b) inability to express emotions; (c) low frustration tolerance; (d) emotional immaturity; (e) high level of anxiety in interpersonal relationships; (f) low self-esteem; (g) grandiosity; (h) feelings of isolation; (i) perfectionism; (j) ambivalence toward authority; and, (k) guilt.

The family responds with: (a) denial; (b) protectiveness, pity – concern about the drinker; (c) embarrassment, avoiding drinking occasions; (d) shift in relationship – domination, takeover, self-absorptive activities; (e) guilt; (f) obsession, continual worry; (g) fear; (h) lying; (i) false hope, disappointment, euphoria; (j) confusion; (k) sex problems; (l) anger; and, (m) lethargy, hopelessness, self-pity, remorse, despair.

These additional statements further demonstrate the many undeniable links between the aspects of the family disease we call alcoholism.

If one falls down, his friend can help him up. But pity the man who falls and has no one to help him up. (Ecclesiastes 4:10)

TODAY'S STEP: God is helping me see more clearly.

"Calmly we look behind us, on joys and sorrows past,

We know that all is mercy now, and shall be well at last;

Calmly we look before us, -- we fear no future ill,

Enough for safety and for peace, if Thou are with us still." -- Jane Borthwick

<u>*Screening for Alcoholism*</u>

Researchers and clinicians have developed several screening tests to identify alcoholics. Screening tests have been used effectively with, for example, patients who have medical problems, such as pancreatitis, that indicate alcoholism. One of the more well-known is the **Michigan Alcoholism Screening Test (MAST).** The original instrument developed by Dr. Melvin Selzer contained 24 items, but a newer version of 13 questions (1975) has proven just as effective. The questions for the **Self-Administered Short Form of the MAST** are:

1. Do you feel you are a normal drinker? (By normal we mean you drink **less than** or **as much as** most other people.)
2. Does your wife, husband, a parent, or other near relative ever worry or complain about your drinking?
3. Do you ever feel guilty about your drinking?
4. Do friends or relatives think you are a normal drinker?
5. Are you able to stop drinking when you want to?
6. Have you ever attended a meeting of Alcoholics Anonymous?
7. Has drinking ever created problems between you and your wife, husband, a parent, or other near relative?
8. Have you ever gotten into trouble at work because you were drinking?
9. Have you ever neglected your obligations, your family, or your work for two or more days in a row because you were drinking?
10. Have you ever gone to anyone for help about your drinking?
11. Have you ever been in a hospital because of drinking?
12. Have you ever been arrested for drunken driving, driving while intoxicated, or driving under the influence of alcohol?
13. Have you ever been arrested, even for a few hours, because of other drunken behavior?

A response to any of the questions that corresponds to the following answers is given one point: 1. No, 2. Yes, 3. Yes, 4. No, 5. No, 6. Yes, 7. Yes, 8. Yes, 9. Yes, 10. Yes, 11. Yes, 12. Yes, 13. Yes. Alcoholism is suggested in people who score two points and assessed in people who score three or more points.

Now, if God so clothes the grass of the fields, which today is, and tomorrow is thrown into the oven, shall He not much more clothe you, O ye of little faith. (Matthew 6:30)

TODAY'S STEP: I am finding the courage to face the Truth about myself.

"We are here and it is now. Further than that, all human knowledge is moonshine."

    -- H. L. Mencken

<u>*A Time for Everything*</u>

"There is a time for everything, and a season for every activity under heaven:

A time to be born and a time to die, a time to plant and a time to uproot,

A time to kill and a time to heal, a time to tear down and a time to build,

A time to weep and a time to laugh, a time to mourn and a time to dance,

A time to scatter stones and time to gather them, a time to embrace and a time to refrain,

A time to search and a time to give up, a time to keep and a time to throw away,

A time to tear and a time to mend, a time to be silent and a time to speak,

A time to love and a time to hate, a time for war and a time for peace."

Ecclesiastes 3:1-9

How often do we waste our time and energy wishing we were someone else, were doing something else, or were someplace else. We wish our present circumstances were different. We needlessly confuse ourselves and divert our energy by thinking that our present moment is a mistake. But we are right where we need to be for now. Our feelings, thoughts, circumstances, challenges, tasks – all are on schedule.

To trust the process, to trust all of it, without hanging on to the past or peering too far into the future, requires a great deal of faith. Surrender to the moment. If you're feeling angry, get mad. If you're setting a boundary, dive into that. If you're grieving, grieve. Get into it. Step where instinct leads. If you're waiting, wait. If you have a task, throw yourself into the work. Get into the moment; the moment is right. We are where we are, and it's okay. It's right where we're meant to be to get where we're going tomorrow. And that place will be good, too – it has been planned in love for us – we need only wait in confidence.

TODAY'S STEP: I ask my Higher Power to help me let go of fear, doubt, and anxiety and to fill me with faith, trust, and serenity.

"God is a circle whose center is everywhere and whose circumference is nowhere." -- Timaeus of Locri

<u>*An Amazing Book*</u>

Which is by far the greatest of all books? – **The Bible.**

Which is the most widely circulated of all books; the world's all time best seller? – **The Bible.**

Which has been the most loved of all books? – **The Bible.**

Which is the most thrillingly interesting of all books? – **The Bible.**

Which is the best, clearest, and most useful book on practical psychology? – **The Bible.**

Which is the simplest and most effective textbook on metaphysics? – **The Bible.**

Which is the greatest of all story books? – **The Bible.**

What book contains the world's greatest and finest poetry? – **The Bible.**

Which is the world's best collection of well written, instructive, and inspiring biographies? – **The Bible.**

What book can one study to get a good command of forceful, convincing, and beautiful English? – **The Bible.**

Is there a short cut to the spiritual life? -- Yes, **The Bible.**

Which is the one book that no one anywhere can afford to neglect? – **The Bible.**

Remember that the greatest spiritual Power House is – **The Bible.**

Ye do err, now knowing the scriptures, nor the power of God. (Matthew 22:29)

TODAY'S STEP: I pray that my Higher Power gives me the courage and strength to recognize the Truth about myself and to help me accept that I am powerless.

"When the need is great, the help is near." -- German Proverb

What about AA?

AA offers social support based on a model of fellowship. Members help each other stay sober. At meetings members talk about their problems and gain guidance from each other. Each member also works through the "Twelve Steps". These steps give the recovering alcoholic a set of goals to be achieved. Some steps offer moral and ethical corrections to help you turn your life around. Other steps help you find peace in God or gain strength through God "as you understand Him."

AA has been helping alcoholics to stop drinking since 1935. Current membership is about one million in the United States, about two million worldwide. AA is probably the most recommended treatment for alcoholics today. Unfortunately, its success seems highly limited. In the United States, only about 5% of alcoholic drinkers choose to use AA.

Of course, if AA is right for you, it can work wonders. AA can help you in many ways. In addition to those already mentioned, here are some other ways AA can help:

- It offers total involvement in a nonalcoholic community. This makes it easier for you to break away from your total involvement with alcohol. When you join AA, you join a ready-made social scene to replace the alcoholic scene.
- As an AA member, you gain an important sense of belonging. When you belong to a valued organization, you feel more valued inside yourself.
- Group members lend mutual support for not drinking.
  This can be very helpful. As a popular song says, "We all need somebody to lean on."
- It's easy to make new friends in AA. You will have something in common with everyone you meet.
- AA destigmatizes alcoholism. You're not seen as a "disgusting drunk," but someone with a disease. More important, it's not your fault.
- You can count on it. You can find meetings all over the world at many different times during the day, seven days a week. Also, you're sponsor is available 24 hours a day.

Therefore encourage one another and build each another up, just as you also are doing. (1 Thessalonians 5:11)

TODAY'S STEP: I need to believe in myself and my dreams.

"Only those are deprived, who place in themselves an obstacle to grace." -- St. Thomas Aquinas

Response/Ability

the game we play
is let's pretend
and pretend
we're not
pretending

to avoid
punishment
or the loss of love
we chose to deny
our response/ability

we choose to
forget
who we are
and then forget
that we've
forgotten

pretending that
things just
happened
or that we were
being controlled
taken over

who are we really?

we put ourselves
down
and have become
used to this
masochistic
posture

the center
that watches
and runs the show
that can choose
which way
it will go

this weakness

the I AM
consciousness
the powerful
loving perfect
reflection
of the cosmos

this indecisiveness

but we are
in reality
free
a center
of cosmic energy

but in our attempt
to cope with
early situations
we choose or were
hypnotized into
a passive position

don't pretend
you don't have it
or you won't.

Bernard Gunther

For you, Lord, art good, and ready to forgive; and abundant in loving kindness to all who call upon You. (Psalm 86:5)

TODAY'S STEP: I do not run from myself, my circumstances, or my feelings.

"God often visits us, but most of the time we are not home." -- Joseph Roux

Faith is the practice of counting our blessings! No joy ever sprouts from the soil of cynicism. By contrast, the process of counting our blessings strengthens faith and produces contentment in the most adverse circumstances.

<u>*Lord, Forgive Me When I Whine*</u>

Today, upon a bus, I saw a lovely girl with golden hair, I envied her . . . she seemed so gay . . . and wished I were as fair.

When suddenly she rose to leave, I saw her hobble down the aisle;

She had one leg and wore a crutch; But as she passed . . . a smile!

Oh, God forgive me when I whine, I have two legs. The world is mine!

I stopped to buy some candy. The lad who sold it had such charm. I talked with him. He seemed so glad.

If I were late 'twould do no harm. And as I left he said to me, "I thank you. You have been so kind. It's nice to talk with folks like you. You see, "he said, "I'm blind."

Oh, God, forgive me when I whine, I have two eyes.

The world is mine.

Later, while walking down the street, I saw a child with eyes of blue. He stood and watched the others play. He did not know what to do. I stopped

a moment, then I said, "Why don't you join the others,

dear?" He looked ahead without a word, and then I

knew he could not hear. Oh, God forgive me when I

whine. I have two ears. The world is mine.

With feet to take where I'd like to go, with eyes

to see the sunset's glow. With ears to hear what I would

know . . . Oh, God forgive me when I whine. I'm blessed

indeed. The world is mine.

How precious also are Your thoughts to me, O God! How great is the sum of them! If I should count them, they would be more in number than the sand; When I wake, I am still with You. (Psalm 139:17-18)

TODAY'S STEP: My sense of humor helps me to carry – and to get – the message.

"Dreams are surely for the spirit what sleep is for the body." -- Friedrich Hebbel

"Act As If . . ."

Affirmations create space for reality to happen in. The concept of using affirmations in Recovery means replacing negative messages with positive ones: **we change what we <u>think</u>, so we can change what we <u>say</u> so we can change what we believe.** Recovery is a process, and it's a spiritual one. But aggressively working with affirmations is one of our parts in the process.

Using affirmations doesn't mean we ignore problems. That's denial. We need to identify problems, and we need to empower solutions. Affirmations won't eliminate problems from our lives, but they will help solve them. **If we want to change what happens, we change what we believe and expect.** Step by step we: (1) Surrender to what was and is; (2) Let go of our need to have these negative circumstances happen; (3) Change our behaviors; (4) Accept our present circumstances; and, (5) Create space for something different to happen. The following is a brief list of the many actions and activities which can be affirming:

- Regularly attending Twelve Step support groups and applying those Steps to our lives affirms us and our Recovery.
- The concept of "acting as if" is an affirmation. Another phrase for this concept is "faking it 'till we make it." It means treating ourselves as if we were already the person we want to become.
- Prayer is an affirmation.
- Listening to audiotapes, (pod casts, cd's) helps. Subliminal tapes are specifically designed so our subconscious hears the affirmations, bypassing any conscious resistance to the positive message.
- Using imagery or visualization is another method for inviting the positive. We create mental images of what we want to happen; we see ourselves as we want to be.
- Celebrating our successes and achievements is affirming.

But the word is very near you, in your mouth and in your heart, that you may observe it. (Deuteronomy 30:14)

TODAY'S STEP: There are so many ways in which I can improve the quality of my life. Instead of fretting about what I can't have or can't do, I'll take action to create something positive in my life today.

"There is only one way to put an end to evil, and that is to do good for evil." -- Tolstoy

The Benefits of Not Drinking

INSTRUCTIONS: Put a check next to the changes you've made and benefits you've been enjoying by not drinking. Consider how important these changes and these benefits are to you. Remind yourself over and over that the only way to get these benefits is to stay off the alcohol:

[ ]   I'm getting healthy again.

[ ]   I don't have as many headaches.

[ ]   I don't have as many physical pains.

[ ]   My liver is healing (no pains in my right side).

[ ]   My pancreas is healing (no pains in my left side).

[ ]   My stomach isn't always hurting. My ulcer is going away.

[ ]   My blood pressure is becoming normal.

[ ]   My heart feels stronger (my chest pains are going away).

[ ]   My eyes are healing. I can see more clearly.

[ ]   I feel more limber.

[ ]   My muscles don't ache as much.

[ ]   I'm beginning to eat normally again.

[ ]   I'm beginning to lose weight and look trimmer.

[ ]   I don't get as angry as I used to.

[ ]   I feel stronger inside.

[ ]   My concentration is better.

[ ]   My creativity is returning.

[ ]   I can go out and have a good time without making a fool of myself.

[ ]   I don't complain as much as I used to.

[ ]   I feel confident I can hold a job now.

I beseech you therefore, bretheren, by the mercies of God, that ye present your bodies a living sacrifice, holy, acceptable unto God, which is your reasonable service. (Romans 12:1)

TODAY'S STEP: Emotional health is from within not without.

"Far better it is to dare mighty things, to win glorious triumphs, even though checkered by failure, than to take rank with those poor spirits who neither enjoy much nor suffer much, because they live in the gray twilight that knows not victory nor defeat." Theodore Roosevelt, **Speech before the Hamilton Club**

<u>*"Progress, Not Perfection"*</u>

Recovery is a dynamic process. One of the values of any Fourth and Fifth Step is that we can and should gauge the progress we've made. We too often forget this is a program promoting "Progress, Not Perfection". Karen Casey, the author of **Each Day a New Beginning,** shares with us some principles, which she adopted through AA:

1. Along the way I've expanded my understanding of "The Program" only to discover that it will always invite yet a deeper level of commitment and understanding.
2. The past has no reality, no power over me except what I choose to give it. My thoughts, noisy and troubled or quiet and serene, are in my charge.
3. I believe my soul is on a journey, one made by choice. My stops along the way to my destination are not happenstance, but rather are assuring me of the growth that is mine to experience.
4. Each of us is unique and needed by those who are sharing our journey.
5. Following through on projects, disciplining myself to continue preserving, strengthens my evolving, healthy sense of self.
6. Listening intently to another's words promises me a connection to my God.
7. Any expression of gratitude gives me additional blessings in return.
8. Acknowledging God's presence in every situation, within every person I encounter, extinguishes my fear.
9. Slowing down to appreciate the moment's voice and dream enhances my serenity.
10. A quiet mind knows no fear, realizes all knowledge, and moves ahead with confidence and ease.

Forgetting what lies behind and reaching forward to what lies ahead, I press on toward the goal for the prize of the heavenly call of God. (Philippians 3:13)

TODAY'S STEP: I allow myself to recognize, name, and accept my feelings.

<u>**Step Five**</u>

<u>"Admitted to God, to ourselves, and to another human being the exact nature of our wrongs."</u>

In Step Five, we admit the exact nature of our wrongs to God, to ourselves, and to another human being. It is important to share as much as we possibly can, as the degree to which we cleanse ourselves determines the degree to which we will be ready to proceed with our lives. As our guilt and pain is relieved, we will feel as though a great weight has been lifted from us.

Step Five provides a pathway out of our isolation and loneliness. It is a step toward wholeness, happiness and a real sense of renewal. It tests our humility, in the sense that we see ourselves as we really are – one of many human beings, all children of God. As we develop humility, we will feel more secure and self-accepting when admitting to God the exact nature of our wrongs.

Step Five gives us the opportunity to say things out loud. It may be our first attempt at speaking the truth about ourselves as we now understand it. This can serve to assist us as a future positive communication skill.

In completing the Fifth Step, our final meeting with another person will first be "rehearsed" by admitting our wrongs to God and ourselves. This brings us closer to ultimately surrendering to a Higher Power – "Letting Go and Letting God". To attain this goal, we must give up our need to control things and offer ourselves, our desired outcomes and our lives to our compassionate Higher Power. Admitting our wrongs to God is not for God's benefit. It is an opportunity for us to know our Higher Power loves us and is patiently waiting for us to admit to and learn from our ineffective behavior. In doing this we experience an inner acceptance of our Higher Power and others.

Admitting to ourselves the exact nature of our wrongs is the least threatening part of Step Five and can be done with minimal risk. It does not test our honesty or expose our self-deception. Talking only to ourselves prevents us from having to place ourselves in a realistic perspective. Deceiving ourselves is a well-cultivated talent. In the past, we have manipulated our own thoughts and feelings so we saw only what we wanted to see. The most difficult part of Step Five is admitting our wrongs to another human being. Allowing another person to see parts of us that have been hidden even from ourselves can be a frightening experience. We may be concerned that we will be laughed at or rejected. This Step seriously challenges our ability to be completely honest and willing to accept the consequences.

FIFTH STEP PRAYERS

"Admitted to God, to ourselves, and to another human being the exact nature of our wrongs."

Higher Power, my inventory has shown me who I am, yet I ask for Your help in admitting my wrongs to another person and to You. Assure me, and be with me, in this Step, for without this Step I cannot progress in my Recovery. With Your help, I can do this, and I will do it.

In this moment, I will acknowledge myself for doing what was most difficult for me. I will rest in the accepting presence of my Higher Power. I know I have deepened my commitment to the journey for Recovery by opening my self and my heart to a fellow human being.

MEDITATIONS

Fill my day, dear Lord, with the strength to resist all that may offend Thee. Too often do I resort to my inner weaknesses. Teach me the beauty of inner strength, to know
the difference between selfishness and charitable actions. If it be Thy holy will, let me use my strength to help others. Allow me to be a fortress for those who seek comfort and solace. If today I am tempted to use my strength solely for my own purpose and pleasure, remind me and show me where my strength can best be used. Help me to use gentleness when I feel the need to force my opinions on others; grant me the patience to wait instead of pushing. I pray for true strength of character and long for the stillness of my material wants. Grant me the grace of knowing that true strength is faith in Thee

AFFIRMATIONS

Right now, even while I am telling my self these truths about me, I know I can succeed and I am succeeding. At this moment, if I think of any challenge in front of me, I know I will become even more a winner because of it.

I keep my chin up, my head held high. I look, act, sound, think, and feel like the winner I am! Anytime a problem starts to get me down, I get my self right back up! I tackle problems and I solve them. When frustration or defeat threatens me, I just become that much stronger, more positive, better organized, and more determined than ever!
No matter what it is that requires the very best of me, I can do it and I know I can.

"I used to spend so much time reacting and responding to everyone else that my life had no direction. Other people's lives, problems, and wants set the course for my life. Once I realized it was okay for me to think about and identify what I wanted, remarkable things began to take place in my life." -- Anonymous

Living and Loving Unconditionally

The first five steps in the program are about opening our lives to the acceptance of unconditional love. In Step One, we let go of false centers that keep us attached to a lifestyle of conditional love. In Step Two, we affirm our hope in God's loving care for us. In Step Three, we surrender our spiritual center to God's care. The moral inventory in Step Four allows us to be honest with ourselves about our values and how we have been living.

Then comes Step Five, here we are asked to tell God, ourselves, and another human being the exact nature of our wrongs. We do this by sharing our Step Four Inventory with God and with another person. For most of us, this is a frightening prospect. If we have done this in the past only to be put down, we question whether that might happen again.

The one who hears our Fifth Step is supposed to listen, accept, and validate in a nonjudgmental way the experiences we share. He or she may also offer moral or spiritual counseling, but this too should be done non-judgmentally.

Understanding the roots of our problems can help us recognize what we need in order to be healed. If conditional love is ultimately the problem, then it follows that unconditional love is ultimately the cure we need.

It helps to know that God accepts us as we are – even in our messiness, selfishness, imperfection, and brokenness. And if just one person can love us with no strings attached, we can more easily conclude that we are lovable. Step Five is our opportunity to find unconditional love and acceptance from God and at least one other person.

With the kind You show Yourself kind; With the blameless You show Yourself blameless; With the pure You show Yourself pure, and with the crooked You show Yourself astute. (Psalm 18: 25-26)

TODAY'S STEP: I do not run from myself, my circumstances, or my feelings. I am open to myself, others, my Higher Power, and to loving myself unconditionally.

"We should learn not to grow impatient with the slow healing process of time. We should discipline ourselves to recognize that there are many steps to be taken along the highway leading from sorrow to renewed serenity . . . . We should anticipate these stages in our emotional convalescence: unbearable pain, poignant grief, empty days, resistance to consolation, disinterestedness in life, gradually giving way . . . . to the new weaving of a pattern of action and the acceptance of the irresistible challenge of life." -- Joshua Loth Liebman

"Don't Quit – [Surrender]"

When things go wrong, as they sometimes will,

When the road you're trudging seems all uphill,

When the funds are low and the debts are high,

And you want to smile, but you have to sigh.

When care is pressing you down a bit –

Rest if you must, but don't you quit.

Life is queer with its twists and turns,

As every one of us sometimes learns,

And many a person turns about,

When they might have won had they stuck it out.

Don't give up though the pace seems slow –

You may succeed with another blow.

Often the struggler has given up,

When he might have captured the victor's cup;

And he learned too late when the night came down,

How close he was to the golden crown.

Success is failure turned inside out –

So stick to the fight when you're hardest hit –

It's when things seem worst that you mustn't quit..

Enter by the narrow gate; for wide is the gate and broad is the way that leads to destruction, and there are many who go in by it. Because narrow is the gate and difficult is the way which leads to life, and there are few who find it. (Matthew 7:13-14)

TODAY'S STEP: There are many things I can do to improve my life and further my Recovery, but I cannot heal myself. I need to continually ask God's help.

"O, World, thou choosest not the better part! It is not wisdom to be only wise, and on the inward vision close the eyes, but it is wisdom to believe the heart. Columbus found a world, and had no chart, save one that faith deciphered in the skies; to trust the soul's invincible surmise was all his science and his only art." George Santayana, **"O, World, Thou Choosest Not"**

It Might Be Possible . . .

Dr. Robert H. Schuller in his book, ***Tough Minded Faith for Tender Hearted People,*** tells us the word faith is a noun, but we must make it become a verb, an action in our lives on a daily basis. In fact, his book contains 366 faith-generating, human-motivating Bible verses to start off each day. Surely, steadily, slowly, but successfully his one-year spiritual fitness program will strengthen us and help us gain emotional freedom that will make it possible for us to go through tough times with surviving power!

According to Dr. Schuller, faith is applying positive thinking to solve problems, spot opportunities, and make decisions. Somehow we all "surmise" there is a Higher Power that can unlock the problems we're wrestling with.

It's strange, mysterious, marvelous, yes, miraculous how faith operates in our daily life. Once we turn our thinking in the direction of an "invincible surmise", we begin to imagine breakthroughs. We begin to think:

- "It might be possible **if . . .** "

- "It could be possible **when . . .**"

- "It might be possible **after . . .**"

- "It might be possible **in conjunction with . . .**"

- "It might be possible **for God . . .**"

- "It might be possible **but . . .**"

- "It might be possible so I'll keep on surmising – and I'll soon be surprising."

I am the Lord . . . there is no God beside Me. I will strengthen you, though you have not known Me . . . I am the Lord, and there is no other. (Isaiah 45:5-7)

TODAY'S STEP: God free me from emotional blockages and grant me the gift of a tough-minded faith.

"Each decision brings its own delays and days are lost lamenting over lost days . . . What you can do or think you can do, begin it. For boldness has Magic, Power and Genius in it." Johann Wolfgang Von Goeth

Walking the Walk

Faith is not folly. Dr. Robert H. Schuller, in his book, ***Tough Minded Faith for Tender Hearted People,*** says "It's a responsible confidence rooted in the assurance that a wiser providence maneuvers our lives. Confidence is not human arrogance. Rather, possibility thinking and self-assurance are the reflections of an abiding trust in the Lord who knows us perfectly. He has only our best interest in mind." Dr. Schuller believes our relationship with God allows us to be affirmative. He suggests two steps to exercise our growing faith (1) Meditate on the following declarations daily and (2) Pray the following prayer:

"I'm on the right road. I am walking the walk of faith. I have made the decision to follow the Lord."

"I have given my life to God and He is in control of it."

"The God who has command over my life is protecting me from hidden shoals that could sink the ship of my soul and spirit."

"God is opening doors that will surprise me with new opportunities."

"God is closing doors that I want to go through because He knows they will lead to my failure and destruction."

"Thank You, Father, for assuring me of success on my walk of faith. I know I'm on the right road. I thank You, Lord, for opening and closing doors, thereby guiding me on my daily walk. I sense my faith growing stronger and I declare my faith and affirm You as Lord of my life. Thank You, O God."

Examine yourselves as to whether you are in the faith. Test yourselves . . . (2 Corinthians 13:5)

TODAY'S STEP: Faith is recognizing that the longer I suffer under trying circumstances, the more certain I am to appreciate my deliverance.

"And acceptance is the answer to **all** my problems today. When I am disturbed, it is because I find some person, place, thing or situation – some fact of my life – unacceptable to me, and I can find no serenity until I accept that person, place, thing or situation as being exactly the way it is supposed to be at this moment. Nothing, absolutely nothing happens in God's world by mistake. Until I could accept my alcoholism, I could not stay sober; unless I accept life completely on life's terms, I cannot be happy. I need to concentrate not so much on what needs to be changed in the world as on what needs to be changed in me and my attitudes." -- **"The Big Book" – Page 449**

<u>"We Are Only As Sick As Our Secrets"</u>

After you have succeeded in identifying your core mistaken beliefs and your character defects in Step Four, then you are ready to discuss these things with other people – your refusal to do so will keep you sick. In order to change, you must share what you have learned about yourself. It's self-defeating to keep it a secret because keeping secrets forces us to live in isolation. If you don't know yourself, you can't really know anybody else. Your addictive self keeps you out of touch with yourself and isolated from other people. The Fifth Step is the path out of isolation if you:

1. Acknowledge you are living in isolation from other people and this isolation prevents you from achieving a comfortable sobriety.
2. Acknowledge that ego (the addictive self) is preventing you from sharing the results of your inventory (your deepest thoughts, feelings, and beliefs) with others.
3. Acknowledge that it is self-defeating to keep the results of your inventory and other distressing and humiliating memories secret by refusing to discuss them with another person.
4. Become willing to confide the results of your inventory to another person.
5. Select a person in whom you are willing to confide.
6. Discuss the results of your inventory openly and honestly with this person in private.
7. Listen to and accept advice and direction from the person in whom you confided.

Be of the same mind towards one another. Do not set your mind on high things, but associate with the humble. Do not be wise in your own opinion. *(Romans 12:16)*

TODAY'S STEP: I am not afraid because God is my courage and my strength; He helps me to face the Truth.

"Forgiveness is an answer, the divine answer, to the question implied in our existence. An answer is answer only for him who has asked, who is aware of the question." Paul Tillich, **To Whom Much Was Forgiven**

"What Goes Around, Comes Around"

The book **Alcoholics Anonymous** makes an astounding statement: "Resentment is the 'number one' offender. It destroys more alcoholics than anything else." "Surely," the casual reader thinks, "that must be a mistake: surely it is **alcohol** that destroys alcoholics." But "The Big Book" means what it says, and in the very next sentence explains why: "From [resentment] stem all forms of spiritual disease (p. 64)."

Resentment unites anger, fear, and sadness in a kind of closed-circle, scissors-paper-rock game. In the absence of resentment, anger, fear, and sadness tend to heal each other. Anger can act like a scissors, cutting through fear – the fear like an enveloping shroud wraps itself around and threatens to smother the rock that is sadness. But that very sadness, which rises from the realization of our own transience and the ultimate futility of our human efforts to control, is the only tool we have to blunt anger – to forestall the resentment that anger becomes if it is nourished even after our fears have been quelled.

Anger and sadness butt against each other, steel against stone. But just as scissors "take" paper and rock "takes" scissors, sadness will finally take anger – if we let sadness through. For sadness shared can heal. Anger storms in the hard passage between fear and sadness; cultivated, it turns into a jagged resentment that tears rather than trims and resists healing. Denying fear and scorning the sadness that is shared, resentment refuses the possibility of going through and beyond anger into forgiveness.

Forgiveness is not ours to give, but ours to receive. We cannot create it; we can be certain only that it is beyond our ability to will it into existence.

And be ye kind one to another, tenderhearted, forgiving one another, even as God for Christ's sake hath forgive you. (Ephesians 4:32)

TODAY'S STEP: I ask God to free me from feelings of bitterness, resentment, anger, envy and the desire for revenge in order that I receive the gift of forgiveness.

"Three things are necessary for the salvation of man: to know what he ought to believe; to know what he ought to desire; and to know what he ought to do." Saint Thomas Aquinas, **Two Precepts of Charity**

Sometimes we persevere with the help and compassion of friends and loved ones. Some-times we have to do it alone. This poem speaks a hard truth, but one we might as well accept nonetheless: pain is harder to share with joy. But if we have the wisdom to know we can and will endure, with God's help, we'll find more company along the way.

Solitude

Laugh, and the world laughs with you; weep, and you weep alone;

For the sad old earth must borrow its mirth,

But has trouble enough of its own.

Sing, and the hills will answer; sigh, it is lost on the air;

The echoes bound to a joyful sound, but shrink from voicing care.

Rejoice, and men will seek you; grieve, and they turn and go;

They want full measure of all your pleasure,

But they do not need your woe.

Be glad, and your friends are many; be sad, and you lose them all –

There are none to decline your nectared wine,

But alone you must drink life's gall.

Feast, and your halls are crowded; fast, and the world goes by.

Succeed and give, and it helps you live, but no man can help you die.

There is room in the halls of pleasure for a large and lordly train,

But one by one we must all file on through the narrow aisles of pain.

Ella Wheeler Wilcox

If any of you lacks wisdom, let him ask of God, who gives to all liberally and without reproach . . . . But let him ask in faith . . . for he who doubts is like a wave in the sea driven and tossed by the wind. (James 1:5-6)

TODAY'S STEP: My sense of humor helps me to carry – and to get – the message.

"Thinking is a kind of thanking. In thanking, we accept the gift of existence. In accepting ourselves, we become ourselves. As released, we gratefully enter into the play of which we are already a part. Release means 'homecoming.' Thinking as thanking means loving." Michael Zimmerman, **Eclipse of the Self**

<u>Thanks-Giving</u>

Gratitude's opposite – greed is the vision that everything is to be "gotten." Greed and misery go hand in hand; and misery arises inevitably from the belief that we are in control, that we can control everything and that anything we have, we deserve. Misery is the mind-set that we must get and get and get; it is the yearning for more, the push to acquire more, win more, have more. Misery is misery because it does not know the meaning of enough.

Those who lack gratitude's vision do not possess things; things possess them. And that is misery. Entitlement believes it "deserves".

Happiness – the joy of living – comes in the experience of gratitude flowing from a vision of one's life as a reality received, a gift given freely and spontaneously. Such a vision removes self from the center, thus healing self-centeredness by revealing the folly of the illusion of control.

"The Program" and the fellowship of Alcoholics Anonymous emphasize gratitude because AA members experience their sobriety as a gift. Each had tried, promised, struggled to "never drink again," or at least never get sickeningly, obnoxiously drunk again. And they meant it.

But all their will, all their effort and sincerity had gone for naught, had achieved nothing. And so they gave up, gave in, and in one way or another surrendered and came to Alcoholics Anonymous. And there, in AA, the first thing that they heard was that they could not stop drinking . . . on their own or by themselves. Some resisted that truth and kept up the struggle, now against AA as well as against booze. And so as long as they fought, they lost. So long as they tried to gain and to get – even to get sobriety – they lost. Finally, they gave up. Then and only then, was sobriety given to them.

Thanks be to God, who gives us the victory through our Lord Jesus Christ. (1 Corinthians 15:57)

TODAY'S STEP: I need to believe in myself and trust God.

"True happiness is to enjoy the present, without anxious dependence upon the future, not to amuse ourselves with either hopes or fears, but to rest satisfied with what we have, which is sufficient, for he that is so wants nothing. The great blessings of mankind are within us and within our reach. A wise man is content with his lot, whatever it be, without wishing for what he has not." Lucius Annaeus Seneca, **Epistles**

"First Things First"

Someone once said the things that are urgent are rarely important, and the things that are important are rarely urgent. Often we get so caught up in the trivial matters of day-to-day life that we forget to make time for more important pursuits. The Al-Anon slogan, which is most helpful in getting our priorities in order is "First Things First."

Today, maintaining our serenity is our first priority. Our connection with our Higher Power is the source of serenity, so maintaining that connection must come first.

If we imagine we are in a dark room and our a Higher Power is our only source of light, then our best hope for navigating around the furniture will be to bring that source of light with us as we move through the room. Otherwise, we may get through the room, but our passage is sure to be slow, confusing, and possibly painful.

Al-Anon helps us discover that our priorities are: To put God's will first, to be loyal to our values; to keep an open mind; to detach with love; to rid ourselves of anger and resentment; to express our ideas and feelings instead of stuffing them; to attend Al-Anon meetings and keep in touch with friends in the fellowship; to be realistic in our expectations; to make healthy choices; and to be grateful for our blessings.

We also have certain responsibilities to others: To extend a welcome to newcomers; to be of service; to recognize that others have a right to live their own lives; to listen, not just with our ears, but also with our hearts; and to share our joy as well as our sorrow.

Therefore give to Your servant an understanding heart to judge Your people, that I may discern between good and evil. *(The prayer of Solomon – 1 Kings 3:9)*

TODAY'S STEP: I focus on the power available to me by learning to wait with a good attitude.

"Anyone can carry his or her burden, however hard, until nightfall. Anyone can do his work, however hard, for one day. Anyone can live sweetly, patiently, lovingly, purely, till the sun goes down. And this is all that life really means." -- Robert Louis Stevenson

Tradition Five

Each Al-Anon Family Group has but one purpose: to help families of alcoholics. We do this by practicing the Twelve Steps of AA ourselves, by encouraging and understanding our alcoholic relatives, and by welcoming and giving comfort to families of alcoholics.

Tradition Five reminds us of our purpose. If we find our groups no longer carry out that purpose, we need to voice our concerns. Taking an inventory of our group practices is a good place to start. Are we following the principles of Al-Anon and thereby helping families and friends of alcoholics? If we are not, it's never too late to begin.

Tradition Five clearly states how we can help families of alcoholics. "We do this by practicing the Twelve Steps of AA ourselves, by encouraging and understanding our alcoholic relatives, and by welcoming and giving comfort to families of alcoholics." If we practice the Twelve Steps ourselves, which includes taking our inventories, admitting our wrongs and making amends, we will be in a better place to pass the message to others.

Groups are applying Tradition Five when their members treat the alcoholic with compassion and love, let newcomers know how important they are and pass the message to families and friends both inside and outside meetings. If members have done their best to apply Tradition Five without success, it may be necessary to move to another group, or perhaps, start a new one.

I lift up my eyes to the hills . . . where does my help come from? My help comes from the Lord, the Maker of heaven and earth. He [God] will not allow your foot to be moved, He who keeps you will not slumber. . . . The Lord will keep you from all harm . . . He will watch over your life; the Lord shall preserve your going out and your coming in . . . forevermore. *(Psalm 121:1-8)*

TODAY'S STEP: I focus on the power available to me by learning to wait with a good attitude for His will and timing.

"If a man has a talent and cannot use it he has failed. If he has a talent and uses only half of it, he has partly failed. If he has a talent and learns somehow to use the whole of it, he has gloriously succeeded, and won a satisfaction and a triumph few men ever know." Thomas Wolfe, ***The Web and the Rock***

Five Truths about Fear

"IF EVERYBODY FEELS FEAR WHEN APPROACHING

SOMETHING TOTALLY NEW IN LIFE,

YET SO MANY ARE OUT THERE 'DOING IT'

DESPITE THE FEAR,

THEN WE MUST CONCLUDE THAT

FEAR IS NOT THE PROBLEM"*

*Dr. Susan Jeffers, ***Feel the Fear and Do It Anyway***

Obviously, the real issue has nothing to do with the fear itself, but, rather, how we **hold** the fear. For some, the fear is totally irrelevant. For others, it creates a state of paralysis. The former hold their fear from a position of <u>power</u> (choice, energy and action), and the latter hold it from a position of <u>pain</u> (helplessness, depression and paralysis).

From this it can be seen that the secret in handling fear is to move ourselves from a position of pain to a position of power. The fact that we have the fear then becomes irrelevant. We can't escape fear, but we can deal with it. According to Dr. Jeffers, if we have not been successful in dealing with fear it's probably because we never learned the following **Fear Truths:**

1.   The fear will never go away as long as we continue to grow.
2.   The only way to get rid of the fear of doing something is to go out . . . and do it.
3.   The only way to feel better about ourselves is to go out . . . and do it.
4.   Not only are we going to experience fear whenever we're on unfamiliar territory, but so is everyone else.
5.   Pushing through fear is less frightening than living with the underlying fear that comes from a feeling of helplessness.

For God did not give us a spirit of timidity, but a spirit of power, of love and self-discipline. (2 Timothy 1:7)

TODAY'S STEP: I am not afraid because God is my courage and my strength; He helps me to face the Truth.

"One is happy as a result of one's own efforts, once one knows the necessary ingredients of happiness – simple tastes, a certain degree of courage, self-denial to a point, love of work, and, above all, a clear conscience. Happiness is no vague dream, of that I now feel certain. By the proper use of experience and thought one can even restore one's health . . . so let us live as it is, and not be ungrateful." -- George Sand

Success Is Within You

The most thoughtful among us <u>must</u> conclude at last that personal success <u>must</u> exist *inside* if it is to exist at all. It cannot be composed of outward signs or appearances, but only of intangible personal values stemming from a mature philosophy. One of the things which impressed the world about Mahatma Gandi was the published photograph of all his earthly possessions at the time he died: a pair of sandals, a pair of spectacles, a few simple garments, a spinning wheel, and a book. Yet the world knew, here had passed one of the richest men. Perhaps the world in the wells of its consciousness was somehow aware of what Henry David Thoreau had put into this simple sentence: "A man is rich in the proportions of things he can let alone."

Gandhi himself often spoke of the reduction of needs. Life to him seemed a process of gradual divestment of needs, so from a squalling infant in the cradle who needs everything, the human being, if he lives successfully, gradually matures into an adult who needs virtually nothing. Gandhi was himself an example of such growth, so rare an example that his life dramatized for the rest of us how short we fall of the human growth potential.

This is not to say poverty should be the goal, or an ascetic denial of material progress or possessions makes one a **mahatma**, a great soul. Many a great soul has been vastly surrounded by material possessions and formidably wealthy: Andrew Carnegie, Jacob Riis, Julius Rosenwald, Samuel Mather, the Guggenheims, and Russell Sage, to name a few. All these men achieved true personal success, in these cases, outward as well as inward.

Man shall not live by bread alone, but by every word that proceeds from the mouth of God. *(Matthew 4:4)*

TODAY'S STEP: I have faith that daily work on myself will result in my becoming the best person I can be.

"If we do not consciously and consistently focus on the spiritual part of ourselves, we will never experience the kind of joy, satisfaction and connectedness we are all seeking." Dr. Susan Jeffers, *Feel the Fear and Do It Anyway*

The Choice Is Mine

When I Am Tuned Into My Chatterbox:	When I Am Tuned Into My Higher Self:
I need	I love
I am insensitive	I care
I am in turmoil	I am at peace
I don't know I count	I count
I repel	I attract
I make a negative difference	I make a positive difference
I take	I give and receive
I am bored	I am involved
I am empty	I am filled up
I am filled with self-doubt	I am confident
I have tunnel vision	I see big
I am dissatisfied	I am content
I wait and wait	I live now
I am helpless	I am helpful
I never enjoy	I am joyful
I am always disappointed	I go with what is
I hold resentment	I forgive
I am tense	I am relaxed
I am a robot	I am alive
I am being passed by	love getting older
I am weak	I am powerful
I am a victim	I am protected

Search me, O God, and know my heart . . . And see if there is any wicked way in me, and lead me in the way everlasting. *(Psalm 139:23-24)*

TODAY'S STEP: With the help of a Higher Power, decision-making can be one of life's great adventures and I am capable of dealing with whatever comes my way.

"A man who fears suffering is already suffering from what he fears." -- Montaigne

<u>Children of Alcoholism</u>

Judith Seixas and Geraldine Youcha, authors of ***Children of Alcoholism: A Survivor's Manual*** believe that children brought up in an alcoholic household seem to have the following characteristics in common:

1. We become isolated and afraid of people and authority figures.

2. We become approval seekers and lose our identity in the process.

3. We are frightened by angry people and any personal criticism.

4. We become alcoholics, marry them, or both, or find another compulsive personality such as workaholic to fulfill our sick abandonment needs.

5. We live life from the viewpoint of victims and are attracted by that weakness in our love, friendship, and career relationships.

6. We have an overdeveloped sense of responsibility and find it easier to be concerned with others than with ourselves; this enables us not to look too closely at our faults or our responsibility to ourselves.

7. We feel guilty when we stand up for ourselves instead of giving in to others.

8. We became addicted to excitement.

9. We confuse love and pity and tend to "love" people we can "pity" and "rescue".

10. We have stifled our feelings from our traumatic childhoods and have lost the ability to feel or express our feelings because it hurts so much. This includes our good feelings such as joy and happiness. Being out of touch with our feelings is one of our basic denials.

11. We judge ourselves harshly and have low self-esteem.

12. We are dependent personalities who are terrified of abandonment and will do anything to hold on to a relationship in order not to experience the painful abandonment feelings we received from living with sick people who were never there for us emotionally.

We also rejoice in our sufferings, because we know that suffering produces perseverance; perseverance, character; and character, hope. *(Romans 5:3-4)*

TODAY'S STEP: I am finding the courage to face the truth about myself.

"Let love through all my conduct shine,
An image fair, though faint, of Thine;
Thus let me his disciple prove,
Who come to manifest Thy love."
Anonymous

<u>And Now, A Word About Your Sponsor . . .</u>

If you have never been to a Twelve Step Self-help Group — such as Alcoholics Anonymous (AA), Al-Anon, Overeaters Anonymous (OA), Narcotics Anonymous (NA), Adult Children of Alcoholics (ACoA), or Codependents Anonymous (CODA) – you might not be familiar with the concept of a sponsor.

A sponsor is a person you choose to be your advocate to guide you in your journey toward physical, emotional, psychological and spiritual Recovery. Since you are picking this person to be a surrogate mentor and teacher, he or she should already have gone where you have yet to go. This person must have a real handle on Recovery and must not be afraid to challenge you when you are getting off the track.

A sponsor needs to know how to stand toe-to-toe with the defiant members of our inner family: our inner child, who maybe confused, mistrustful, angry, hurt, lonely, guilty and ashamed; our inner parent, who likes to play God, act morally superior, and beat up on the little child in our spirit; and our inner adult, who is constantly trying to intellectualize, analyze, and pulverize every part of our moral and emotional being.

By asking someone to sponsor us, we express a willingness to experience more intimate relationships. When he or she is there for us, returning our calls, offering support, caring, we develop a basis for trust. Sponsors help us learn to receive love, but we also learn about giving. Someone who demonstrates unconditional love and still takes care of his or her own needs and who offers support without telling us what to do can be a wonderful role model. We can best put what we learn into practice by passing it on.

I am a real believer in self-help and the idea of sponsorship. If by chance you do not have a Twelve Step Group or a sponsor, I strongly suggest that you get at least one of each.

A new commandment I give unto you, That ye love one another; as I have loved you, that ye also love one another. *(John 13:34)*

TODAY'S STEP: I create a healthy atmosphere of love and nurturing around and within me. I accept the love and support of my sponsor and my group.

"Receive every inward and outward trouble, every disappointment, pain, uneasiness, temptation, darkness, and desolation, with both thy hands, as a true opportunity and blessed occasion of dying to self, and entering into a fuller fellowship with thy self-denying suffering Saviour. Look at no inward or outward trouble in any other view; reject every other thought about it; and then every kind of trial and distress will become the blessed day of thy prosperity. That state is best, which exerciseth the highest faith in, and fullest resignation to God." -- William Law

"I Can't Handle It God; You Take Over"

As children growing up in a troubled family we learn to use lots of indirect forms of behavioral expressions, such as running away from home, disobeying our parents, getting into fights, pouting, getting into trouble with the law, skipping classes, using drugs, being sexually promiscuous, getting pregnant, dropping out of school, lying or – at the other extreme – being a perfect child.

As adults who deny our thoughts and feelings, we also learn to communicate indirectly by having affairs, being sexually inappropriate, getting drunk, overeating, gambling, not paying bills, working too much, nagging, being violent or by neglecting, abandoning and abusing our children.

These dysfunctional adult patterns of behavior can point back to many things, but in most cases they boil down to the fact that we do not think we are okay and we do not love ourselves. This is the great revelation that most adult child/codependents run into on the road to Recovery. It is one thing to believe others do not think we are okay or do not love us, but it is quite another when we discover that we think and feel this way about ourselves. Like it or not, we are stuck with ourselves for the duration. As they say in the program, "Wherever you go, there you are."

Putting aside the dysfunctional patterns of avoidance, denial and repression is the only way to heal our emotional and/or spiritual wounds. Until we emancipate ourselves from the script of our troubled family we will continue to live out someone else's life. The individual who fails to confront the dysfunctional scripts of the past is destined to repeat them.

Beloved, think it not strange concerning the fiery trial which is to try you, as though some strange thing happened unto you; but rejoice, to the extent that ye are partakers of Christ's sufferings. (1 Peter 4:12-13)

TODAY'S STEP: I trust "The Program Works If I Work It" and I can be restored to wholeness with God's help.

"You don't have to suffer continual chaos in order to grow." -- John C. Lilly

A Wall of Shame

Inside the void I stood alone and questioned not the solemn tone. The voices spoke in anger clear, but never lent a loving ear.

It must be me, the thought occurred, the judgment made, the pictures blurred.

"That's right, it's me," a voice did say, "and mark my words, one day you'll pay."

Then hide I will behind this wall, its mortar strong and structure tall.

And in this place I know I'll find the time to heal and solve the crime.

Yet nothing changed from year to year because I chose to live in fear.

How wrong I was to build this frame that locked out love and nurtured stone.

For the child of my youth, you see, was innocent, but never free.

And through the lonely days that passed, I came to know the truth at last. No fault should I have placed on he, who worked so hard to rescue me.

Now on the road behind I see the emptiness that followed me.

Through wisdom gained across the years, I've finally learned to face my fears. United now, with child in hand, I've staked my claim and made my stand.

That wall of shame that once I knew has been replaced with love that's true. And now I'm whole, no longer bound, forgiven all and freedom found.   *Anonymous*

As thy days, so shall thy strength be. (Deuteronomy 33:25)

TODAY'S STEP: I face my problems squarely and without blame.

"Give what you have. To someone, it may be better than you think." -- Henry Wadsworth Longfellow

<u>Paradoxical Commandments</u> (Adapted)

1. People are illogical, unreasonable, and self-centered.
    Love them anyway.

2. If you do good, people will accuse you of selfish, ulterior motives.
    Do good anyway.

3. If you are honest, some people will laugh at you.
    Be honest anyway.

4. If you speak out for what you believe, people may make fun of you.
    Speak out anyway.

5. Think big and small-minded people will sneer at you.
    Think big anyway.

6. What you spend years building may be destroyed overnight.
    Build anyway.

7. People are crying out for help but may attack you if you help them.
    Help them anyway.

8. Some days there won't be a song in your heart.
    Sing anyway.

9. The world applauds top dogs.
    Fight for a few underdogs anyway.

10. Give the world the best you have, and most people will not even notice. Give this miraculous, fragile world the best you have -- **ANYWAY!**

Trust in the Lord, and do good; *Dwell in the land, and feed on His faithfulness.* **(Psalm 37:3)**

TODAY'S STEP: I trust God will bring out the best in me and others.

"Pure truth, like pure gold, has been found unfit for circulation, because men have discovered that it is far more convenient to adulterate the truth than to refine themselves." Charles Caleb Colton

"To Thine Own Self Be True"

This may be one of the most challenging steps we face in our Recovery process, but it can also be one of the most fulfilling in terms of removing us from our isolation. In order to accomplish Step Five, the three-part sharing it endorses must take place, i.e., all of what we discovered about ourselves in our Step Four Inventory is to be freely admitted to God, to ourselves, and to another human being. Step Five sharing is the beginning of the end of our isolation.

There are basically five types of wrongs we should share:

1. We need to acknowledge all of our addictions.

2. We need to acknowledge what went wrong in our families of origin to initiate our codependent love hungers.

3. We need to acknowledge the multi-generational wrongs that may have led to our family of origin situations. We need to understand and be compassionate toward the families our parents emerged from.

4. We need to acknowledge the wrongs that have occurred in all major relationships in our lives.

5. We need to acknowledge the specific ways in which we have wronged others by the practice of our addictions.

Perhaps the single greatest barrier to Recovery is the inability to be HONEST. In Step Five sharing, maybe for the first time in our lives, we open our deepest, darkest secrets and most private hurts to another human being.

Search me, O God, and know my heart; try me, and know my thoughts; and see if there be any wicked way in me, and lead me in the way everlasting. (Psalm 89:23-24)

TODAY'S STEP: How do I feel today? How am I doing? If I can answer those questions truthfully, I am more likely to pursue the help I need and to share the happy times with others as well.

"And, as the path of duty is made plain,

May grace be given that I may walk therein,

Not like the hireling, for his selfish gain,

With backward glances and reluctant tread,

Making a merit of his coward dread, --

But cheerful, in the light around me thrown,

Walking as one to pleasant service led;

Doing God's will as if it were my own,

Yet trusting not in mine, but in His strength alone!"

J. G. Whittier

"Thy Will, Not My Will"

Once we work the Fifth Step and share the results of our Fourth Step Inventory with others, we begin to realize that we're gaining more and more insight into the **why** of our addiction. With increasing clarity, we see that our own behavior has been the major cause of our unhappiness.

As we uncover the characteristics that led us down the path to our disease, we slowly realize it wasn't our life situation that was at fault. It wasn't our parents' fault. It wasn't "bad luck". It wasn't any person, place or thing that pushed us over the edge. The reality is we had begun to develop some dysfunctional habit patterns. At first they seemed innocuous enough. But in the end, it was these patterns that led to the chronic progression of our disorder.

The good news here is that the more we uncover and discover, and the more candid we become about sharing this with another person, the closer we are to our Recovery. Along the way we'll learn what looks like a catastrophe at first glance become a golden opportunity.

There are people today in the Twelve Step process who are able to accept things that we're still making ourselves miserable about. And they stand ready to help us work through every step of our Recovery. All we have to do is ask.

Pray for us unto the Lord thy God . . . that the Lord thy God may show us the way *in which we should walk and the thing we should do*. (Jeremiah 42:2-3)

TODAY'S STEP: I understand the true nature of humility. I recognize that the ability to develop and practice it is the basic foundation of the Twelve Steps.

> "Wherever He may guide me,
> No want shall turn me back;
> My Shepherd is beside me,
> And nothing can I lack.
> His wisdom ever waketh,
> His sight is never dim, --
> He knows the way He taketh,
> And I will walk with Him."
> A. L.. Waring

"Take What You Can Use and Leave the Rest"

There are certain Key Tasks in which we must attain at least some degree of mastery in this life, if we are not to waste our time. They are:

1. Making a personal contact with God.

2. Healing and regenerating our own bodies – demonstrating health.

3. Getting control of ourselves and finding our True Place.

4. Learning to handle other people both wisely and justly.

5. Perfecting a technique for getting direct personal inspiration for a general or a specific purpose.

6. Letting go of the past completely.

7. Planning the future definitely and intelligently.

To have made some real progress on each of these points, even though we may still be far short of mastery, is true success. Of course, we shall all advance farther in some of these directions than in others, but some progress must be made in each of them.

And that which fell among thorns are they, which, when they have heard, go forth, and are choked with cares, and riches and pleasures of this life, and bring no fruit to perfection. (Luke 8:14)

TODAY'S STEP: With the help of a Higher Power, decision-making can be one of life's great adventures. Each crossroad brings a new challenge, and I am capable of dealing with whatever comes my way.

"I would lie in bed at night and say the alphabet, counting all the things I had to be grateful for starting with the letter A . . . . This made a great change in my life." **As We Understood . . .**

"Gratitude Is the Attitude"

If we said, "Thank You, God" for each blessing we receive, we wouldn't have time to do anything else. Yet giving thanks for just a few blessings is a great way to realize our constant connection with God.

"Thank You, God, for Your healing life that flows throughout my body. I am continually strengthened and renewed by Your energy and power."

"Thank You, God, for wisdom and understanding. Your light shines brightly on my path, guiding me and showing me the way."

"Thank You, God, for this lovely world, for peace, security, and the inner knowing that You are always with me. I love You, God, and I appreciate the wonder You have created."

"If the only prayer you said in your whole life was, 'Thank You,' that would suffice."

> Meister Eckhart

Today I will practice gratitude. I will think of some of the things, big or small, for which I am truly grateful. Maybe I'll even put this list in writing or share it with a 12-Step friend. Sometimes a tiny action can be a great step toward seeing my life with increasing joy. When we take time for gratitude, we can perceive a better world. Today I will appreciate the miracles around me.

Give thanks to the Lord, call on his name; make known His deeds among the people. Sing unto Him, sing psalms unto Him; talk ye of all his wondrous works. Glory ye in His Holy name; let the heart of them rejoice that seek the Lord. (Psalm 105:1-3)

TODAY'S STEP: Thankfulness today will help me seed the miracle at work in my life and in the lives of others on the road to Recovery.

"An earnest and concentrated study of the Al-Anon program, in depth, will help us to become more tolerant, confident, and loving, teaching us to accept the faults of others as we seek to correct shortcomings in ourselves." *The Dilema of the Alcoholic Marriage*

"Principles before Personalities"

Daily practice of the Al-Anon program can help us become more tolerant of other people. For example, when we take our own inventory and examine our motives, we recognize the same shortcomings we once eagerly pointed out in others. It is easier to accept the limitations of others when we acknowledge our own.

When we finally recognize our own thinking has been distorted and our behavior inconsistent, then we can also appreciate the fact that because the perceptions of ourselves have been so inaccurate, then how reliable can our perceptions of others be? We really don't know what anyone else is thinking or feeling or going through; therefore, we can not justify intolerance.

Regular, dedicated practice of the principles of "The Program", keeps us feeling good about ourselves. This permits us to be increasingly open-minded and considerate toward everyone in our lives.

Each of us puts the Al-Anon program into practice in our lives as best we can, moving at the pace that is right for us. That is why we avoid speaking harshly, using phrases such as "get off the pity-pot" or "quit feeling sorry for yourself." Perhaps someone needs more time to work through a painful situation than we do. Their story may sound repetitious to us, but who are we to judge?

When we're struggling with our difficulties, we can be grateful that no one in Al-Anon is standing over us with a stopwatch, telling us we are taking too long to learn our lesson. A non-judgmental, listening ear can be a great blessing, and we can learn to offer it more freely by trying to extend to our fellow members the respect, patience, and courtesy that we want for ourselves.

You can see the speck in your friend's eye, but can't see the log in your own eye. (Luke 6:41)

TODAY'S STEP: I let go of old ideas about myself and discover a new self through Recovery. . I stop taking other people's inventory and focus on my own.

"We must learn to lean on others, and sometimes accept others' leaning on us . . . .
We can't do it alone." *Alateen – Hope for Children of Alcoholics*

Self-Help Groups

A self-help group is any gathering of people who meet to give each other mutual
support. There is no professional leadership, but trust and safety develop so people
can speak out and can find that they are understood; their dignity is recognized, for
they all have a problem in common. Self-help groups offer a natural support system
for rape victims, the bereaved, dialysis patients, Lesbians, child abusers, addicts, and
epileptics to name a few. Twelve Step programs share the following common
properties with self-help groups:

1. Members all share the same problem; therefore no one feels unique.

2. There is an unlimited amount of mutual support and help.

3. There is a sense of altruism among members that enables the giver to enjoy
   the sense of giving and serves to reduce a person's undue self-absorption and
   to enhance sensitivity to others.

4. The group enables members to feel a reinforced sense of normality – they are
   not different or deviant.

5. There is a collective will power. Each member, simply because of the fact that
   he or she is there, encourages others in their determination to do whatever
   needs doing.

6. There is an exchange of information, some of which may not be available from
   books or experts.

7. There is constructive action toward shared goals.

Alcoholics Anonymous is the prototype of self-help groups and serves all of the
functions named above, but it is not considered traditional group therapy. Rather, it is
a "fellowship of men and women whose only purpose is to stay sober and to help
other alcoholics get sober."

Be kindly affectionate to one another with brotherly love. (Romans 12:10)

TODAY'S STEP: Community, rather than loneliness, will define our lives. We will know
that we belong, we are welcome, we have something to contribute—and that is
enough.

"We don't need more strength or more ability or greater opportunity. What we need is to use what we have." -- Basil S. Walsh

"Identify Don't Compare"

There are a few more stumbling blocks to our continued progress we need to add to our inventory. These are: (1) Rebellion, (2) Self-Deception, (3) Sentimentality, (4) Defiance, (5) Blaming, and (6) Phony Remorse.

How do we turn these negatives into positives? Steps Six, Seven, Eight and Nine will give us guidelines in clearing them away. For now these blocks simply act as clues to help us do a thorough job of Step Five. Let's define them clearly:

1. **Rebellion**: Are we resisting making a totally clean breast of our failings?

2. **Self-Deception**: Are we still seeing ourselves as victims?

3. **Sentimentality:** Do we persist in dwelling on the memory of how good it once was?

4. **Defiance:** Are we belligerently defensive about past actions?

5. **Blaming:** Do we believe it's what other people have done to us that caused our problems?

6. **Phony Remorse:** Are we working this step in a self-deprecating way, saying we were totally to blame when we really believe we were not?

The deeper we dig, the more we'll find things we want to acknowledge and discard. We need to examine all the hidden blocks that get in the way of completing Step Five. In uncovering our defects, we discover how they can become assets. As we admit our faults, the barriers to wholeness come down. As we listen to others tell the truth we find the courage to stop defending and pretending.

Let us not therefore judge one another any more: but judge this rather, that no man put a stumbling block, or an occasion to fall, in his brother's way. (Romans 14:13)

TODAY'S STEP: I avoid making excuses for my own or someone else's behavior.

> "Discouraged in the work of life,
> Disheartened by its load,
> Shamed by its failures or its fears,
> I sink beside the road; --
> But let me only think of Thee,
> And then new heart springs up in me."
> Samuel Longfellow

"Try Not to Place Conditions on Your Recovery"

There is a definite catharsis that occurs when we rid ourselves of our secrets. And yet, some of us may experience a sensation of our secrets. And yet, some of us may experience a sensation of emptiness or loss. In time, this will change as we pursue our resolve. We'll discover our identity needs to be re-formed to fit into a positive Recovery mode.

When we question how we can turn negatives into positives, we need to remind ourselves **Failure Is Not Final.** It simply means we've missed the mark. As we move on in Recovery, we begin to understand that what caused us to feel guilt and shame was due more to chronic progression of our disease than our character. And once we're free of our compulsive addiction, we'll have no need to repeat those negative patterns of the past.

It's a paradox that the very qualities that were defeating us can now become our greatest assets. Both our elaborate denial system and our persistent self-deception can be made to serve us by alerting us to the necessity of letting go of past attitudes, reactions, and behavior. As we unearth and admit to these defects, we begin to understand how to monitor the trigger mechanisms that caused us to act in an unproductive manner.

When we see our failures as only temporary setbacks, we realize we are finally learning how to be kind to ourselves. By taking each negative in turn, and examining its effects and admitting its exact nature to ourselves and another human being, we develop personal responsibility.

And he said unto me, My grace is sufficient for thee: for my strength is made perfect in weakness. Most gladly therefore will I rather glory in my weaknesses, that the power of Christ may rest upon me. Therefore I take pleasure in weaknesses in insults, in necessities, in persecutions, in distresses for Christ's sake: For when I am weak, then I am strong. (2 Corinthians 12:9-11)

TODAY'S STEP: By calling on my Higher Power for help daily I can turn failure into success.

"Once to every man and nation comes the moment to decide, in the strife of Truth with Falsehood, for the good or evil side." James Russell Lowell, ***The Present Crisis***

"Important Guidelines for Preparing Your Fifth Step"

The book ***The 12 Steps A Way Out: A Working Guide For Adult Children From Addictive And Other Dysfunctional Families*** has the following helpful suggestions for persons preparing for the Fifth Step (either as a communicator or listener):

- Begin with prayer, asking your Higher Power to be present as you prepare to go through your Fourth Step revelations and insights. Ask God to guide and support you in what you are about to experience.
- Allow ample time to complete each thought and stay focused on the subject. Discourage unnecessary explanations.
- Eliminate distractions. Telephone calls, children, visitors and extraneous noises should be eliminated.
- Remember Step Five asks only that we admit the exact nature of our wrongs. It is not necessary to discuss how the wrongs came about or how changes will be made. You are not seeking counsel or advice.
- As the listener, be patient and accepting. You are your Higher Power's spokesperson and are communicating unconditional acceptance.
- When Step Five is completed, both parties can share their feelings about the experience. It is now possible to extend to each other the love our Higher Power extends to us individually.
- Observe confidentiality. What you have shared is personal. Nothing defeats honesty and changes relationships faster than a betrayed confidence.

After completing your Fifth Step, take time for prayer and meditation to reflect on what you have done. Thank your Higher Power for the tools you have been given to improve your life. Spend time rereading the first five Steps and note anything you have omitted. Acknowledge that you are laying a new foundation for your life. The cornerstone is your relationship with your Higher Power and your commitment to honesty and humility.

I have wiped out your transgressions like a thick cloud and your sins like a heavy mist. Return to Me, for I have redeemed you. (Isaiah 44:22)

TODAY'S STEP: I have courage to go forward; to meet the new day, to handle whatever confronts me. Peace is coupled with courage, now and forever.

" All happy families resemble one another; every unhappy family is unhappy in its own way." -- Count Leo Tolstoy, *Anna Karenina,* Part 1, Chap. 1.

"Are You Codependent?

Once a person begins the downward cycle to addiction, those closest to him/her (family, friends, and even co-workers) begin compensating to try to reestablish balance. Without knowing it, they develop behavior patterns, which allow the dependency to continue. The following is a list of typical questions posed by addictions therapists and organizations established to help the dependent's family and friends. (**NOTE:** Yes to five or more of the above questions may indicate a dependency problem --seek out a professional for an accurate assessment.)

YES   NO

[ ]   [ ]   1. Has the person's drinking or using ever caused you embarrassment?

[ ]   [ ]   2. Does this person's drinking or using make the atmosphere uncomfortable and tense?

[ ]   [ ]   3. Has this person ever had a loss of memory as a result of drinking or using?

[ ]   [ ]   4. Are you concerned about this person's association with other heavy drinkers or drug users?

[ ]   [ ]   5. Has this person made and broken numerous promises to stop drinking or using?

[ ]   [ ]   6. Does this person expect you to lie and make excuses to cover up his/her drinking or using?

[ ]   [ ]   7. Has this person's use of alcohol or drugs caused difficulty on the job, at home, or socially?

[ ]   [ ]   8. Has this persons drinking or using ever caused a medical, legal, or financial problem?

[ ]   [ ]   9. Is this person's drinking or using affecting his or her reputation?

[ ]   [ ]   10. Has anyone outside the family ever expressed concern about this person's use of alcohol or drugs?

[ ]   [ ]   11. Does this person consider holidays, weekends, and special events as drinking or drugging celebrations?

[ ]   [ ]   12. Does this person use drinks or drugs in response to good news and bad news?

Do not be afraid...For I am with you to deliver you. (Jeremiah 1:8)

TODAY'S STEP: God help me believe in myself and help me let go of old beliefs and feelings that are hurting me.

"Our spiritual growth is unlimited and our reward endless if we try to bring this program into every phase of our daily lives." **The Twelve Steps And Traditions**

<u>"Unity, Recovery, and Service"</u>

The Twelve Steps and Traditions are guides for personal growth and group unity. The Twelve Concepts are guides for service. They show how Twelve Step work can be done on a broad scale and how members of a World Service Office can relate to each other and to the groups, through a World Service Conference, to spread Al-Anon's message worldwide.

1. The ultimate responsibility and authority for Al-Anon World Services belongs to the Al-Anon groups.
2. The Al-Anon Family Groups have delegated complete administrative and operational authority to their Conference and its service arms.
3. The Right of Decision makes effective leadership possible.
4. Participation is the key to harmony.
5. The Rights of Appeal and Petition protect minorities and assure that they be heard.
6. The Conference acknowledges the primary administrative responsibility of the Trustees.
7. The Trustees have legal rights while the rights of the Conference are traditional.
8. The Board of Trustees delegates full authority for routine management of the Al-Anon Headquarters to its Executive Committees.
9. Good personal leadership at all service levels is a necessity. In the field of world service, the Board of Trustees assumes the primary leadership role.
10. Service responsibility is balanced by carefully defined service authority and double-headed management is avoided.
11. The World Service Office is composed of standing committees, executives, and staff members.
12. The spiritual foundation of Al-Anon's World Services is contained in the General Warranties of the Conference, Article 12 of the Charter.

I will bless the Lord, who has given me counsel. (Psalm 16:7)

TODAY'S STEP: If I want to become skillful at applying "The Program" to my life, I need to do more than go to an occasional meeting. I must make a commitment and practice, practice, practice.

"The real fault is to have faults and not to amend them." -- Confucius

<u>"Courage to Change . . ."</u>

In Step Five it says we "admitted to God . . . the exact nature of our wrongs." The authors of the book ***The 12 Steps for Adult Children: From Addictive and Other Dysfunctional Families*** offer the following helpful information for completing our Fifth Step with God:

- Step Five is for our own benefit – our Higher Power already knows us. We are beginning a process of living a life of humility, honesty and courage. The result is freedom, happiness and serenity.

- Imagine your Higher Power sitting across from you in a chair.

- Start with a prayer: e.g., "Higher Power, I understand you already know me completely. I am now ready to openly and humbly reveal myself to you – my hurtful behaviors, self-centeredness and traits. I am grateful to you for the gifts and abilities that have brought me to this point in my life. Take away my fear of being known and rejected. I place myself and my life in your care and keeping."

- Speak out loud, sincerely and honestly sharing your understanding of the insights you gained from your Fourth Step Inventory. Be aware that emotions may surface as part of the powerful cleansing experience taking place.

- The objective is balance. Remember each of your character traits has strength and a limitation. Begin with resentments and fears, then proceed to those traits you have included in your Fourth Step Inventory.

Acknowledge your courage for proceeding to this point. This and every part of this process releases excess emotional baggage you have carried around because of low self-worth. Congratulate yourself for having the courage to risk self-disclosure, and thank your Higher Power for the peace of mind you have achieved.

And what does the Lord require of you, but to do justly, and to love mercy, and to walk humbly with your God. (Micah 6:8)

TODAY'S STEP: I have courage to go forward; to meet the new day, to handle whatever confronts me. Peace is coupled with courage, now and forever.

"The welfare of each is bound up in the welfare of all." -- Helen Keller

The Wife of Noble Character

This tribute to wifehood and womanhood from the book of Proverbs (31:10-31) is an ideal portrait, not a checklist of performance expectations. No one woman should feel she is required to live up to all of these standards. Nevertheless, the passage is a powerful affirmation of women's diverse gifts and abilities. Contrary to what we may have learned in our dysfunctional homes, there are few if any areas of life in which women cannot participate.

A wife of noble character
who can find?
She is worth far more than rubies.
Her husband has full confidence
in her and lacks nothing of value.
She brings him good, not harm
all the days of her life.
She selects wool and flax and
works with eager hands.
She gets up while it is still
dark; she provides food for her family.
And portions for her servant girls.
She considers a field and buys
It; out of her earnings she plants a vineyard.
She sets about her work vigorously;
her arms are strong for her tasks.
She sees that her trading is profitable,
and her lamp does not go out at night.
In her hand she holds the distaff
and grasps the spindle with her fingers.
She opens her arms to the poor
and extends her hands to the needy.

When it snows, she has no fear
for her household; for all
of them are clothed in scarlet.
She makes coverings for her bed;
She is clothed in fine linen and purple.
Her husband is respected at the
city gate, where he takes
his seat among the elders of the land.
She makes linen garments and sells
them, and supplies the merchants
with sashes.
She is clothed with strength and dignity;
she can laugh at the days to come.
She speaks with wisdom, and faithful
instruction on her tongue.
She watches over the affairs of her
household and does not eat the
bread of idleness.
Her children arise and call her blessed;
her husband also, and he praises her:
"Many women do noble things, but you
surpass them all."

And this also we wish, that you be made complete. (2 Corinthians 13:9)

TODAY'S STEP: I understand the true nature of humility. I recognize that the ability to develop and practice it is the basic foundation of the Twelve Steps.

Step Six

<u>"Were entirely ready to work in partnership with God to remove our ineffective behavior."</u>

"A radiant, confident personality exists in each of us, hidden under a welter of confusion, uncertainty and discontent. If someone were to ask if we wanted to be freed from these hindrances, there could be only one answer, that we were entirely ready to have God remove them." -- ***Al-Anon's Twelve Steps & Twelve Traditions***

Our willingness to work Steps One through Five indicates our readiness to complete Step Six. Steps One and Two prepared us for Step Three, at which time we made a decision to turn our will and our lives over to the care of God as we understood God. Steps Four and Five helped us uncover our behavior flaws, facing them courageously and sharing them with God, ourselves and another human being.

Our current ineffective behavior stems from many of the traits we have identified. We probably acquired many of these behaviors in childhood, and as adults we continue to use them as a means to survive the chaos and imbalance in our lives. As we become more aware of these behaviors and accept them without fault-finding, we can better deal with them from a position of choice. With the help of our Higher Power, we can use our decision-making ability to perform and express ourselves in a more positive way. By being honest with ourselves and our Higher Power, and trusting we will experience healing, we develop a foundation of strength and hope as we meet life's challenges.

The task of removing our ineffective behavior is more than we can handle alone. Step Six does not indicate we are the ones to do the removing; all we have to do is be "entirely ready" for it to happen. It is a state of being, not something that we actually do. We reach this state of being by faithfully working "The Program," whether or not we feel we are making progress. When we are "entirely ready," our reservations about letting God assist us in removing our shortcomings will have lessened.

__"Were entirely ready to have God remove all these defects of character."__

Dear God,

I am ready for Your help in removing from me the defects of character which I now realize are an obstacle to my Recovery. Help me continue being honest with myself and guide me toward spiritual and mental health.

In this moment, I am entirely ready to be freed of all my shortcomings. In this moment, I am ready to surrender these defects of character to God, knowing the power of willingness to heal is great. Each new step I take in my Recovery, no matter how small it may appear, is an affirmation of my wholeness.

__MEDITATIONS__

My love for Thee, dear Father, is so inconstant, it seems easy to appreciate my blessings when all is well with me. Grant me the courage to reach out into the dark of my own misdemeanors. Life is ever changing, and I need the wisdom to understand the seasons of my life. Help me understand how to accept these changes, for I am weak and sometimes feel I don't know how to cope. I feel insecure and long for love and yet it seems I continually struggle and try to do it on my own. I turn to Thee, dear Father, as I approach this new day. Fill me with faith and trust in the almighty mercy of Thy love. Teach me to accept graciously, knowing Thou wilt take it from me if the burden is too heavy. Teach me to pray and retain the courage Thou placeth within me.

__AFFIRMATIONS__

My mind is constantly in tune with the positive – it is bright, cheerful, enthusiastic – and full of good, positive thoughts and ideas.

My mind focuses its attention only on those things I can do something about. If I cannot affect it or direct it – I accept it.

I choose to look at the world around me in the bright, healthy light of optimism and self- assurance.

"I've started to realize that waiting is an art, that waiting achieves things. Waiting can be very, very powerful. Time is a valuable thing. If you can wait two years, you can sometimes achieve something that you could not achieve today, however hard you worked, however much money you threw up in the air, however many times you banged your head against the wall . . . " -- Dennis Woley, *The Courage to Change*

"Turn It Over"

To know that justice, harmony, and love are supreme in the universe is likewise to know that all adverse and painful conditions are the result of our own disobedience to Eternal Law. Such knowledge leads to strength and power, and it is upon such knowledge alone that a true life and an enduring success and happiness can be built.

To be patient under all circumstances, and to accept all conditions as necessary factors in your training, is to rise superior to all painful conditions, and to overcome them with an overcoming which is sure, and which leaves no fear of their return, for by the power of obedience to law they are utterly slain. Such an obedient one is working in harmony with the law, had, in fact, identified himself with the law, and whatsoever he conquers he conquers for ever; whatsoever he builds can never be destroyed.

The cause of all power, as of all weakness, is within: the secret of all happiness as of all misery is likewise within. There is no progress apart from unfoldment within, and no sure foothold of prosperity or peace except by orderly advancement in knowledge.

If you would become truly and permanently prosperous, you must first become virtuous. It is therefore unwise to aim directly at prosperity, to make it the one object of life, to reach out greedily for it. To do this is to ultimately defeat yourself. But rather aim at self-perfection, make useful and unselfish service the object of your life, and ever reach out hands of faith toward the supreme and unalterable God.

Wait on the Lord: Be of good courage, and He shall strengthen thine heart: Wait, I say, on the Lord. (Psalm 27:14)

TODAY'S STEP: I will focus on the power available to me by learning to wait.

"In order to arrive at what you do not know
You must go by a way which is the way of ignorance.
In order to possess what you do not possess
You must go by the way of dispossession.
In order to arrive at what you are not
You must go through the way in which you are not.
And what you do not know is the only thing you know
And what you own is what you do not own
And where you are is where you are not."

-- T. S. Eliot, "East Coker" [**Four Quarters** (New York, Harcourt Brace & Co., 1943) p.15]

"Do You Need Therapy?"

Because children of alcoholics have so much trouble trusting their own judgment and a lot of difficulty knowing what is normal, they may have doubts about their needs for therapy.

Perhaps you think the way you feel is normal enough and you just want to do a patch job on yourself, but skip any major excavation. One way to tell if you really need outside help is to listen to those close to you. If a friend, spouse, or loved one has hinted that you do, you should seriously consider it. Some people feel that seeking out help or therapy is a sign of weakness, shame or guilt. Recognizing the need for help, however, is really a strength. It shows a self-awareness and a willingness to grow.

Some of the clues to knowing you need help are feelings of depression, uncontrollable anger, and incapacitating fears or disorientation. Or you may repeatedly find yourself involved in interpersonal difficulties. If so, a professional counselor may be able to determine with you whether the stress under which you live can be diminished by therapy.

Sometimes just one or two sessions are enough to help you make a decision. One young man described his dilemma: "My life was like a puzzle. I couldn't get all the pieces together. What's more, many pieces were blank and some weren't even there – they were missing! In therapy, as time went on, all the parts appeared and at some point they began to fit together." Another said, "I was ready to commit suicide. A friend suggested I make an appointment with a therapist. So I went. And I'm still here."

Great in counsel and mighty work: For thine eyes are open upon all the ways of the sons of men. (Jeremiah 32:19)

TODAY'S STEP: I pray my Higher Power gives me the courage and strength to recognize the Truth about myself and help me accept that I am powerless.

"I was angry with my friend:

I told my wrath, wrath did end.

I was angry with my foe:

I told it not, my wrath did grow."

-- from *"A Poison Tree"* by William Blake

The Poison Tree

Anger and resentment work like poison in our lives. When we give way to anger and resentment, their poison seems to spread through our whole being, just as water taken in through the roots spreads upward through a tree. Our body is numbed by the poison of resentment, our mind is numbed, our whole being is concentrated on the terrible wrong we believe we have suffered and our resulting "righteous" anger. If we were a real tree we would turn from green to black and just start rotting.

Unless, that is, we act immediately to dispel the poison of resentment. This we do by talking over our resentment with the person who aroused it. Just as Blake says, we treat the person who angered us as a friend, not a foe. We indicate the relationship is important and we don't want it to suffer because of something said or done.

We have to give ourselves the opportunity to heal. Otherwise we face the terrible possibility of turning black with our resentment, and getting numb, and rotting away. As we reflect on people who have inflicted emotional pain on us, we realize some of these people may never change. We're tempted to hold on to our resentment toward these people, perhaps even to take revenge. But doing so may actually increase the damage to ourselves. That's why God wants us to leave the judgment and retribution up to Him. He will carry it out, in His way – in His time.

When troubled by feelings of resentment we need to pray:

God, bring any resentments that are hidden within

Me to the surface, and help me become ready to

Let go of them.

For if you forgive men when they sin against you, your heavenly Father will also forgive you. But if you do not forgive men their sins, your Father will not forgive your sins. (Matthew 6:14, 15)

TODAY'S STEP: I am seeking a saner approach to everything I encounter. The slogans are a valuable source of sanity in chaotic situations. If I am tempted to act out of anger or frustration, I will remember "Easy Does It."

"God can exercise His mercy when we avow our defects. Our defects acknowledged, instead of repelling God, draw Him to us, satisfying His longing to be merciful. As this is understood through meditation, the person realizes that those things by which he feels unlovable are exactly what he has to offer God to attract Him." Raphael Simon, *Studies in Formative Spirituality*

<u>Identifying Character Defects</u>

There are several common ways in which we try to make ourselves okay:

- "I'll be okay when . . . I'm in control" (meaning when I don't experience or demonstrate painful feelings).

- "I'll be okay when . . . other people approve of me – or are impressed with me."

- "I'll be okay when . . . I'm perfect" (meaning I no longer make mistakes).

- "I'll be okay when . . . I don't need others" (so they can't hurt me).

Control, approval, perfectionism, and autonomy are the four character defects most commonly observed. We believe attaining these values will make us okay – but, of course, they won't.

It is impossible to be in control, approved, perfect, and autonomous. In trying to make ourselves okay by being in control, approved, perfect, and autonomous, we continue to generate fear, shame, and resentment. These, in turn, compel us toward the use of fixes such as drugs, alcohol, sex, food, etc.

It is a shock to us when we finally discover it is not life that is giving us shame, fear, and resentment, but we are doing it to ourselves. It is the way we react to life that keeps us stuck in pain. Without judging ourselves as bad, dumb, or stupid for getting caught up in defects of character, we can accept responsibility for changing our self-defeating attitudes by affirming to ourselves the good news – God loves us **just as we are!**

How often shall my brother sin against me, and I forgive him . . . . Jesus said to him, . . . "up to seventy times seven." (Matthew 18:21-22)

TODAY'S STEP: I ask God to free me from feelings of bitterness, resentment, anger, envy, and the desire for revenge in order that I receive the gift of forgiveness.

"Addiction keeps a person in touch with the god . . . At the very point of the vulnerability is where the surrender takes place – that is where the god enters. The god comes through the wound." Marion Woodman, ***Parabola***

Eliminating Character Defects

The people who put together the Twelve Step Program of Alcoholics Anonymous learned it was emotional pain that fueled the compulsion to drink. By working the first Five Steps, they began to move out of emotional pain. Later, we shall see how Steps Eight and Nine enable the healing process to deepen.

After some degree of relief from pain has been experienced, however, the issue becomes how to **stay out of pain.** This is where Steps Six and Seven come in. These two Steps address the issue of defects of character, which are at the root of our emotional pain. It is because of defects of character that we actually produce emotional pain in our minds. This is true for everyone, not only alcoholics. If we want to be free from emotional pain and the self-centeredness that accompanies it, we must eliminate our defects of character.

Emotional pain leaves us feeling we are "not okay" inside. The feeling part of our nature tells us something is wrong, and that something is **us!** This is an intolerable situation for the mind to endure. Something must be done to right the wrong. The intellectual part of our nature takes up the challenge and attempts to right the wrong by reversing its cause. Since the wrong is thought to be us, however, the project we undertake must be one of "making us okay." Thus the feeling attitude "I'm not okay" becomes balanced by the intellectual attitude "But I'll be okay when . . . ."

The attitude "I'll be okay when . . ." places our happiness in a future that doesn't even exist. Only "now" exists. If we're not okay now, we'll never be okay, for the future will be just another now that "I'll be okay when . . ." forbids us to experience.

Commit your way to the Lord. Trust also in Him, and He shall bring it to pass. (Psalm 37:5)

TODAY'S STEP: I am beginning to understand that surrender is not defeat and I welcome my powerlessness.

"We must always remember why we are here, and never use the group to promote our pet projects, or our personal interests in outside causes." -- ***Twelve Steps & Twelve Traditions of Alateen***

Tradition Six

Our Al-Anon Family Groups ought never endorse, finance, or lend our name to any outside enterprise, lest problems of money, property and prestige divert us from our primary spiritual aim. Although a separate entity, we should always cooperate with Alcoholics Anonymous.

Tradition Six tells us that "Our Al-Anon Family Group ought never endorse, finance, or lend our name to any outside enterprise, lest problems of money, property, and prestige divert us from our primary spiritual aim."

I've had occasion to refer to this Tradition many times while doing service work at our local Al-Anon Information Office. I often receive requests for Al-Anon's endorsement from various research projects, charities, and treatment programs. These requests always pique my interest, and many appear to have merit.

As an individual, I am free to participate in any cause I support. As an Al-Anon member, I am free to send information about our fellowship to outside organizations. But I cannot consider affiliating my group with these outside enterprises, no matter how worthy they may be. Doing so could divert us from our primary spiritual aim of our program, which is to help families and friends of alcoholics recover from the effects of alcoholism.

We come to Al-Anon to receive the spiritual benefit of the meetings, principles, and fellowship. We must be vigilant to ensure we are not diverted from our primary aim.

But take care and watch yourselves closely, so as neither to forget the things that your eyes have seen, nor to let them slip from your mind all the days of your life. (Deuteronomy 4:9)

TODAY'S STEP: If I want to become skillful at applying "The Program" to my life, I need to do more than go to an occasional meeting. I must make a commitment and practice, practice, practice.

"That saints will aid if men will call: For the blue sky bends over all!"
Samuel Taylor Coleridge, *The Rime of the Ancient Mariner*

Desiring to Change

To be successful with Step Six, we must sincerely desire to change our disabling behaviors. Our past has been dominated by our self-will, through which we sought to control our environment. We victimized ourselves, rarely calling on God for help. By recognizing our life condition and being honestly determined to eliminate our behavior flaws, we see that self-will has never been enough to help us. We must be ready to accept help and relinquish our self-destructive natures.

At this point in our Program, we see that change is necessary to live life to the fullest. Recognizing the need for change and being willing to change are two different matters. The space between recognition and willingness can be filled with fear. As we move toward willingness, we must let go of our fears and remain secure in the knowledge that with God's guidance everything will be restored to us.

As we reflect on people who have inflicted emotional or physical pain on us, we realize some of these people may never change. We're tempted to hold on to our resentment toward these people, perhaps even to take revenge. But doing so may actually increase the damage to ourselves. That's why God wants us to leave the judgment and retribution up to Him. He will carry it out, in His way – in His time!

When we are ready, we begin to see the possibilities available to us once we change our behavior. The excitement of this revelation will help us do whatever may be necessary to achieve the results we want. From now no, there will be no turning back!

But if men are bound in chains, held fast by cords of affliction, he tells them what they have done – that they have sinned arrogantly. He makes them listen to correction and commands them to repent of their evil. If they obey and serve Him, they will spend the rest of their days in prosperity and their years in contentment. But if they do not listen, they will perish by the sword and die without knowledge. (Job 36:8-13)

TODAY'S STEP: I visualize myself achieving my goal of changing for the better.

"... man occupies a middle position in the universe, between the infinitesimal and the infinite; he is an All in relation to Nothingness, a Nothingness in relation to the All. This middle position of man is the final and dominant fact of the human condition . . . . It is also a perfect image of the finitude of human existence . . . . Man is his finitude."

William Barrett, *Irrational Man: A Study in Existential Philosophy*

The Willingness to Change

One way to do a Sixth Step is to make a list of our character defects, including the problems and benefits experienced from each of them.

It should come as no surprise that character defects cause us problems. But many people deny the problems. They prefer to look the other way or to blame the problems on someone or something else. To get ready to give up a character defect, we must carefully examine the problems it causes.

Working Step Six involves the completion of six tasks:

1.　We acknowledge that in sobriety our character defects often drive us into self-defeating behaviors with problematic consequences.

2.　We acknowledge our character defects give us temporary pleasure we enjoy.

3.　We identify the character defects we are ready to give up.

4.　We ask for the willingness to do what is necessary to remove the character defects that we are ready to give up.

5.　We identify the character defects we are still unwilling to give up.

6.　We ask for the willingness, at some time in the future, to give up the character defects we still choose to hold on to.

The Lord knows the days of the upright, And their inheritance shall be forever. (Psalm 37:18)

TODAY'S STEP: I have faith that daily work on myself will result in my becoming the best person I was created to be.

"Every man has to seek in his own way to make his own self more noble and to realize his own true worth. You must give some time to your fellow man. Even if it's a little thing, do something for those who have need of help, something for which you get no pay, but the privilege of doing it. For remember, you don't live in a world all your own. Your brothers are here too." Albert Schweitzer, ***On Receiving The Nobel Prize***

The Lord's Prayer

In the Sermon on the Mount, Jesus gave what came to be called the Lord's Prayer as a daily practice of forgiveness. Unfortunately, the poor translations of Jesus' original Aramaic words into Greek and then into English obscured some of the richness of his teachings. Compare the King James Version of the Lord's Prayer to the far more sensitive and factual excerpts from the translation by Neil Douglas-Klotz from ***Prayers of the Cosmos: Meditations on the Aramaic Words of Jesus:***

> Pray then like this:
>
> Our Father which art in heaven. [O Birther!
>
>> Father-Mother of the Cosmos.]
>
> Hallowed be thy name.
>
> Thy Kingdom come.
>
> Thy will be done, on earth as it is in heaven.
>
> Give us this day our daily bread. [Grant what we
>
>> need each day in bread and insight.]
>
> And forgive us our debts, as we forgive our debtors.
>
>> [Loose the cords of mistakes binding us, as we
>>
>> Release the strands we hold of other's guilt.]
>
> And lead us not in temptation, but deliver us from evil.
>
>> [Do not let surface things delude us, but free us
>>
>> From what holds us back.]
>
> For thine is the kingdom, and the power, and the glory, forever. (Matthew 6:9-13)

Out of the depths have I cried unto Thee, O Lord. Lord, hear my voice: Let Thine ears be attentive to the voice of supplications. If Thou, Lord, shouldest mark iniquities, O Lord, who shall stand? But there is forgiveness with Thee, that Thou mayest be feared. I wait for the Lord, my soul doth wait, and in His word do hope. (Psalm 130:1-6)

TODAY'S STEP: When faced with difficult or painful situations, I remember that a loving God is always here for me, always available as a source of comfort, guidance and peace.

"Dear God – help me to get up. I can fall down by myself." -- Anonymous

"We Are Not Alone"

Among all the beautiful and heart searching prayers of the Bible there is none that surpasses the wonderful poem that we call the **Forty-Sixth Psalm**. This is an inspired tool that will enable us to overcome any kind of difficulty; if we can tune ourselves in to the level of consciousness to which it attains. It is the supreme Bible tool against fear. **We are not alone, God is always with us!**

1. God is our refuge and strength, a very present help in trouble.

2. Therefore we will not fear, though the earth be removed, and though the mountains be carried into the midst of the sea;

3. Though the waters roar and be troubled, though the mountains shake with its swelling. Selah.

4. There is a river, the streams whereof shall make glad the city of God, the holy place of the tabernacles of the most High.

5. God is in the midst of her; she shall not be moved; God shall help her, just at the break of dawn.

6. The nations raged, the kingdom were moved; he uttered His voice, the earth melted.

7. The Lord of hosts is with us; the God of Jacob is our refuge. Selah.

8. Come, behold the works of the Lord, who has made desolations in the earth.

9. He makes wars to cease to the end of the earth; he breaks the bow, and cuts the spear in two he burns the chariot in the fire.

10. Be still, and know that I am God: I will be exalted among the nations, I will be exalted in the earth.

11. The Lord of hosts is with us; the God of Jacob is our refuge. Selah.

TODAY'S STEP: I am not afraid because God is my courage and my strength; He helps me to face the Truth.

"Sleeping at last, the trouble and turmoil over,
Sleeping at last, the struggle and horror past,
Cold and white, out of sight of friend and of lover,
Sleeping at last." Christina Georgina Rossetti, *Sleeping at Last*

There is absolutely no reason to fear death. The same God is on the other side of the grave as on this side – as Dick William so beautifully expresses it in his famous prayer – "We remember. O Lord the slenderness of the thread which separates life from death and the suddenness with which it can be broken. Help us also to remember that on both sides of that division we are surrounded by your love."

RESURGAM

There is no death! Our stars go down
To rise upon some fairer shore;
And bright in heaven's jeweled crown
They shine for evermore.

There is no death! The dust we tread
Shall change beneath the summer showers
To golden grain or mellow fruit,
Or rainbow-tinted flowers.

The granite rocks in powder fall,
And feed the hungry moss they bear
The fairest leaves drink daily life
From out the viewless air.

There is no death! The leaves may fall,
The flowers may fade and pass away;
They only wait through wintry house
The coming of the May.

And, ever near us, though unseen,
The fair immortal spirits tread;
For all the boundless universe
Is life; there are no dead!   -- Attributed to Bulwer Lytton

Death is swallowed up in victory. O death, where is thy sting O grave, where is thy victory? (1 Corinthians 15:54-55)

TODAY'S STEP: I am not afraid because God is my courage and my strength; He helps me to face the Truth.

"Truth is within ourselves; it takes no rise from
Outward things, what e'er you may believe.
There is an inmost center in us all,
Where truth abides in fullness; and around,
Wall upon wall, the gross flesh hems it in,
This perfect clear perception – which is truth.
A baffling and perverting carnal mesh
Binds it, and makes all error; and to know
Rather consist in opening out a way
Whence *the imprisoned splendour* may escape,
Than in effecting entry for a light
Supposed to be without."   Robert Browning, ***Paracelsus***

The Imprisoned Splendour

Step Six offers us a chance to accept ourselves as we really are – a chance to own and acknowledge our defects and assets. And this puts us in a splendid position to divest ourselves of our negative characteristics.

Life is a package deal. It is not enough to look only at the parts we like. It is necessary to face the whole picture so we can make realistic choices for ourselves and stop setting ourselves up for disappointment. Living with alcoholics, many of us coped with an ever-

shifting situation in which our sense of reality changed from one minute to the next. We adapted by taking whatever part of reality suited us and ignored the rest.

Our lives will remain unmanageable as long as we pretend that only half of the truth is real -- that's why sharing is such an important Twelve Step tool! When we share what is really going on with our group members, we cut through our denial and anchor ourselves in reality. While it may be difficult to face certain facts, when we allow ourselves to confront them, we cease to give our own denial the power to devastate us at every turn.

"There is a radiant, confident personality in each of us, hidden under a welter of confusion, uncertainty and discontent. If someone were to ask if we wanted to be freed from these hindrances, there could be only one answer; that we were entirely ready to have God remove them (***Al-Anon's Twelve Steps & Twelve Traditions***, p. 41).

Keep therefore the words of this covenant, and do them, that ye may prosper in all that ye do. (Deuteronomy 29:9)

TODAY'S STEP: I search for my own Truth, and I allow others to do the same.

"Life holds so much — so much to be so happy about always. Most people ask for happiness on condition. Happiness can be felt only if you don't set conditions."
Arthur Rubinstein

"You Get What You Need"

Consider this story: A woman was going through a very difficult time in her life. Her husband had just died suddenly. Though she was earning a modest salary at her job, she feared that she would not be able to afford needed house repairs. Her own health was troublesome and she suffered from severe headaches. She was very discouraged. Exhausted, she asked the Lord to carry her burdens — not forever, but for a while, so she could rest. Immediately, she felt as if a leaden weight had been lifted from her shoulders.

The wonderful part of asking the Lord to help you is that God is strong enough to bear your load — for a few hours, for a night, for as long as you need. If you try to do this, you may not feel a flood of relief, but be assured of the Lord's help. When you ask God to carry the burden of your hopelessness, you are actually taking the first step toward reviving your hope, because trusting in the Lord is the basis for hope.

It is important you form a partnership with God. One person running a business has to shoulder all the responsibilities. Having a partner means the burdens are shared. One person dealing with despondency can be overwhelmed. Why struggle alone without a partner? The divine Power is there for the asking!

The expression, "Let Go And Let God," has become very popular as a means of handling problems. It is a simple task — letting go of your problems and letting God step in. It doesn't mean you give up your working and struggling. You simply try to see your challenge as not totally your own. Allow the Lord to be there for you.

Come to me, all you who labor and are burdened, and I will give you rest. Take my yoke upon you and learn from me, for I am meek and humble of heart; and you will find rest for yourselves. For my yoke is easy, and my burden light. (Matthew 11:28-30)

TODAY'S STEP: There are so many ways in which I can improve the quality of my life. Instead of fretting about what I can't do, I'll take action to create something positive in my life today.

"I fled Him, down the nights and down the days;
        I fled Him, down the arches of the years;
I fled Him, down the labyrinthine ways
        Of my own mind; and in the midst of tears
I hid from Him, and under running laughter.
        Up vistaed hopes I sped;
        And shot, precipitated,
Adown Titanic glooms of chasmed fears,
        From these strong Feet that followed, followed after."

God's Pursuit

These are the opening words of **The Hound of Heaven** by Francis Thompson. In this poem almighty God is identified as The Hound of Heaven who relentlessly pursues his prey who is running away from the grace of God. Thompson was a down-and-outer, at the end of his rope when he achieved sanity and projected his thinking into the lens of his poem.

"In the midst of tears I hid from Him." No one knows the remorse of the alcoholic, but the alcoholic himself or those in his fellowship. The tears shed; the remorse felt; yet the tears flow so copiously they fog the eyes which cannot perceive God's nearness.

"I hid from Him under running laughter." Alcohol produces laughter, sometimes hollow, sometimes boisterous, but as many a clown has been sad, very sad, beneath his laughter, so also is the alcoholic who appears to be bright and to the world. His laughter is only a cover-up to blanket out the grace of God which seeks to reclaim him to sobriety and to peace and happiness.

"Yet was I sore adread, lest, having Him, I must have naught besides." Francis Thompson could hear the insistent beat of the feet of The Hound of Heaven seeking him out, yet he was afraid to give up what he had, the comfort and euphoria of his drugs. The Higher Power sought him out, but he kept running away and The Hound of Heaven kept up his unhurried pursuit. Finally, Thompson allows his Higher Power to catch up with him. He then realizes his gloom and sadness and misery were but the shadow of the hand of God outstretched to bless him. **"Rise, clasp my hand, and come!"**

O Lord God of our fathers . . . Power and might are in Your hand, and no one can stand against You. (2 Chronicles 20:6)

TODAY'S STEP: When faced with difficult or painful situations, I remember a loving God is always here for me, always available as a source of comfort, guidance and peace.

"Alcoholics Anonymous is a terribly imperfect society because it is made up of very imperfect people. We are all dedicated to an . . . ideal of which, because we are very human and very sick, we often fall short. I know because I constantly fall short myself."
-- Bill Wilson, **Not-God** [p. 121]

"Another Friend of Bill W's"

"Honesty gets us sober," Bill Wilson once observed, "but tolerance keeps us sober." Such tolerance, AA members know, is not a grudging putting-up-with, but a loving identification with imperfection. When we accept ourselves in all our weakness, flaws, and failings, we can begin to fulfill an even more challenging responsibility: accepting the weaknesses, limitations, and mixed-up-ness of those we love. Then and only then, it seems, do we become able to accept the weaknesses, defects, and short-comings of those we find it difficult to love.

Learning how to live with other human beings is one of the grand, classic problems. Most of us "tolerate" each other by identifying with and seeking out those with whom we share strengths. But Alcoholics Anonymous and other Twelve Step groups are founded on a different truth: Human beings connect with each other most healingly, most healthily, not on the basis of common strengths, but in the very reality of their shared weaknesses.

Shared weakness: the shared honesty of mutual vulnerability openly acknowledged. That's where we connect. It is our weakness that makes us alike; it is our strengths that make us different. Acknowledging shared weakness ~~thus~~ creates a rooted connectedness, a sense of common beginnings, a sense of community. Participants in such a setting learn to appreciate rather than resent the strength in others because they know, at bottom, they are the same – flawed and imperfect. Those who do not share a weakness find in other's strengths a threat. But those who recognize shared weakness see in other's strengths a hope: the hope your strengths might also support me. With a shared weakness as a common bond, we can rejoice in another person's strengths rather than be threatened by them.

I do not have a Higher Power who cannot sympathize with my weaknesses, but was in all ways tempted as I am... (Hebrews 4:15)

TODAY'S STEP: I let go of old ideas about myself and discover a new self through Recovery.

"Just for today I will find a little time to relax and to realize what life is and can be." -- **Alcoholism, The Family Disease**

"Just For Today"

Just for today I will try to live through this day only, and not tackle my whole life's problems all at once. I can do something for twelve hours that would appall me if I felt that I had to keep it up for a lifetime.

Just for today I will be happy. This assumes to be true what Abraham Lincoln said, that "Most folks are as happy as they make up their minds to be."

Just for today I will adjust myself to what is, and not try to adjust everything else to my own desires. I will take my "luck" as it comes, and fit myself to it.

Just for today I will try to strengthen my mind. I will study; I will learn something useful; I will not be a mental loafer; I will read something that requires effort, thought, and concentration.

Just for today I will exercise my soul in three ways: I will do somebody a good turn, and not get found out; if anybody knows of it, it will not count; I will do at least two things I don't want to do – just for exercise. I will not show anyone that my feelings are hurt; they may be hurt, but today I will not show it.

Just for today I will be agreeable. I will look as good as I can, dress becomingly, talk low, act courteously, criticize not one bit, not find fault with anything, and not try to improve or regulate anybody except myself.

Just for today I will have a program. I may not follow it exactly, but I will have it.

Just for today I will have a quiet half hour all by myself, and relax. During this half hour, sometime, I will try to get a better perspective on my life.

Just for today I will be unafraid. I will enjoy that which is beautiful, and will believe that as I give to the world, so the world will give to me.

Whenever I am afraid, I will trust in Thee. (Psalm 56:3)

TODAY'S STEP: I trust that God will bring out the best in me and others.

"To be truly rich, a person must acknowledge that money is a sacred trust from God to be employed wisely and not wasted." Glenn Bland, *Legend of the Golden Scrolls*

The True Person's Creed

1. I will be fruitful and earn money, to labor six days and rest the seventh, to make money multiply as a grain of corn multiplies when planted in fertile soil, as to gain dominion over the power of money's essence, so that my riches may be used for worthy purposes.
2. I will refrain from love of money, for such passion causes every sort of iniquity to manifest from the heart, attracting weighty troubles.
3. I will respect and follow the higher laws of Divine order, which bring about the fulfillment of my worthy aspirations by making my efforts fruitful and by giving me increase and dominion regarding monetary matters.
4. I will walk in the counsel of wise men who possess a special gift for managing money and have the experience of many bountiful harvests.
5. I will not pursue ill-gotten monetary gains, for such profits bear an inescapable consequence that is a thousand fold greater than the misery of living in poverty.
6. I will enact every monetary transaction with honesty and integrity, so my heart may remain pure and my mind content that I might lie down in peace and sleep in safety.
7. I will refrain from passion for wine, pleasure, and luxury, for they are not conducive to making my fortune grow.
8. I will always measure the value of my fellow man with far greater importance than the temporal value of my riches.
9. I will respect the authority of the laws of the land, under God, regarding the corporeal matters of life.
10. I will let a humble spirit be my hallmark, rejecting the temptation to become puffed up with pride and brimming with haughtiness because of my affluence.
11. I will be generous in all ways, choosing not to hoard riches that would be detrimental to me and a grievous evil toward mankind.
12. I acknowledge the Almighty owns everything that exists, including all of the wealth of the world and, therefore, assumes the responsibility ownership invokes; consequently, my primary aim is to be God's spiritual possession, for all of the other details of life shall then be orderly and blessed.

Seek first God's kingdom and His righteousness, and all these things shall be yours as well. (Matthew 6:33)

TODAY'S STEP: I trust truth, my instincts, and my ability to ground myself in reality.

"I have often thought that the best way to define a man's character would be to seek out the particular mental or moral attitude in which, when it came upon him, he felt himself most deeply and intensely active and alive. At such moments there is a voice inside which speaks and says: 'This is the real me!'" William James, *The Letters of William James*

"Wherever You Go, There You Are"

The key words in this step are "entirely ready". We find for most of us, being "entirely ready" is an awesome and difficult step to take. We know blaming others for our shortcomings is a character defect, but never blaming others means we have to take total responsibility for what happens to us. It means we have to accept the fact that we cannot change or control anyone/thing other than OURSELVES!

To have God remove a character defect we need to study it and ask, when do we use it? What can we do instead that will be more helpful? We need to become aware of why we think such behavior is necessary. Many defects are considered defects only because we carry the behavior too far. For example, honesty is an admirable trait, but carried to the degree of brutal frankness it is cruel and hurtful.

Trying to do our best is great, but perfectionism is a defect and causes us to become very judgmental of others. Being a perfectionist is also saying, "I am God!" We can lose a lot of friends that way!

Sometimes we are in love with a character defect; we have had it for so long it is a part of us. In this case, "Pray for help to become entirely ready." Remember it took many years to get where we are, change will not come overnight. Be patient, work at this day after day. A helpful way to do this Step is to work on the most harmful defect first, continuing down with the worst defects one by one. When you run into difficulty, PRAY – God will help, if you ask.

For thus says the High and Lofty One who inhabits eternity, whose name is Holy; I dwell in the high and holy place, with him also who has a contrite and humble spirit, to revive the spirit of the humble, and to revive the heart of the contrite ones. (Isaiah 57:15)

TODAY'S STEP: I am willing to turn my will and my life over to my Higher Power, to let go of willfulness and to surrender myself to Recovery.

"Every man's condition is a solution in hieroglyphic to those inquiries he would put. He acts it as life, before he apprehends it as truth." – Ralph Waldo Emerson

<u>Healthy Relationships</u>

The prerequisites for intimacy are:

- Loving someone (being loving)
- while staying with yourself and
- fully participating in your own life.

Intimacy is not static. It is always moving to a new level. It is an energy flow with no barriers. Intimacy cannot be controlled. Like a feeling, it cannot be held on to or reproduced at will. We notice intimacy. We do not produce it. Intimacy is:

- knowing and being known by another
- sharing information openly
- a mutual hug or touch
- not necessarily romantic or sexual
- being alive and sharing that sense of aliveness
- being intimate with self first
- experience life together – developing a common history
- involving all the senses
- not brought about by techniques
- not confined to time and space – one can remain intimate without contact, allowing the other to go away when she or he needs to

- magical, beyond language, a hologram
- varied – one kind does not diminish another kind
- talking vs analyzing
- a lot of paradoxes – requires working at, yet cannot be worked at
- a gift.

Adapted from *The Good Sex Book: Recovering and Discovering Your Sexual Self,* by Sherry Sedgwick (CompCare Publishers, 1992)

And when ye stand praying, if ye have anything against anyone, forgive, that your Father in heaven may forgive you your trespasses. But if ye do not forgive, neither will your Father which is in heaven forgive your trespasses. (Mark 11:25-26)

TODAY'S STEP: Emotional health is from within not without.

"Our main business is not to see what lies dimly at a distance, but to do what lies closely at hand." -- Thomas Carlyle

"Believe in God or Be God"

Back in the days of sailing ships, a young and inexperienced seaman was sent aloft in a storm to disentangle the snarled ropes of the mainmast. He accomplished the ascent with the quickness of the young. Nevertheless, the descent frightened him as he gazed down at the tossing ship far below. The lurching deck rocking in the wind and storm froze him to the mast. All he could see was the fury of the storm in tossing of the boat and the force of the wind. The captain below, sensing his danger, shouted: "Don't look down, son look up!" The boy looked above him. The heavens were stable and quite immovable. By looking up to God in His heaven, the boy forgot the fury of the storm and the tossing of the boat and easily made his descent to safety.

The alcoholic who has attained sobriety has weathered the greatest storm of his life. Yet, the winds of compulsion do not cease to blow because he has weathered a major storm. There will be other big storms in his life. It is this failure to realize other storms will arise which often accounts for the slips of the alcoholic. He must realize he will be an alcoholic until he dies. The progress of alcoholism continues despite months and years of sobriety. Lack of belief in this truth will result in slipping back.

Wouldn't it be grand if there were no more storms in your life? However, this is not so. It is better to admit you are powerless over alcohol, for the very storms that blew during the days of wine and roses will continue to buffet you in the years ahead. When the winds blow, look up to God and be neither terrified nor hurt by the storms of compulsion and temptation. This is an area where it's helpful to have expectations. Expect the storms!

You must have faith that God can help you. You must have faith that God will help you. It is this faith in a Higher Power that is the cornerstone of 12 Step Programs. God loves you and will help you, but you must turn to Him through prayer and meditation.

Now faith is the substance of things hoped for, the evidence of things not seen. (Hebrews 11:1)

TODAY'S STEP: Faith is recognizing that the longer I suffer under trying circumstances, the more certain I am to appreciate my deliverance.

"In the march towards Truth, anger, selfishness, hatred, etc., naturally give way, for otherwise Truth would be impossible to attain. A man who is swayed by passions may have good enough intentions, may be truthful in word, but he will never find the Truth." Mohandas Karamchand [Mahatma] Gandi

<u>Do's and Don'ts When You're Angry</u>

1.   **Do** speak up when an issue is important to you.

2.   **Don't** strike while the iron is hot.

3.   **Do** take time out to think about the problem and to clarify your position.

4.   **Don't** use "below-the-belt" tactics.

5.   **Do** speak in "I" language. Learn to say, "I think …" "I feel …" "I want . …"

6.   **Don't** make vague requests. Let the other person know specifically what you want.

7.   **Do** try to appreciate the fact that people are different.

8.   **Don't** participate in intellectual arguments that go nowhere.

9.   **Do** recognize that each person is responsible for his or her own behavior.

10. **Don't** tell another person what she or he thinks or feels or "should" think or feel.

11. **Do** try to avoid speaking through a third-party.

12. **Don't** expect change from hit-and-run confrontations.

Adapted from ***The Dance of Anger: A Woman's Guide to Changing the Patterns of Intimate Relationships***, by Harriet Goldhor Lerner (Harper & Row, 1985).

He who is slow to anger is better than the mighty; and he that rules his spirit than he that takes a city. (Proverbs 16:32)

TODAY'S STEP: I am seeking a saner approach to everything I encounter. The slogans are a valuable source of sanity in chaotic situations. If I am tempted to act out of anger or frustration, I will remember that "Easy Does It."

"Prefer a loss to a dishonest gain; the one brings pain at the moment, the other for all time." -- Chilton

"P.L.O.M. = Poor Little Old Me"

As we come to terms with loss and change, we may blame ourselves, our Higher Power, or others. The person may be connected to the loss, or he or she may be an innocent bystander. We may hear ourselves say: "If only he would have . . . ." If I wouldn't have done that . . . . Why didn't God do it differently?"

For some people guilt and responsibility are nonexistent. When bad things happen in life, something or someone else is always blamed. Most of us used to be like that. We had an alibi or excuse for everything. Evading responsibility and avoiding blame became our way of life. In Recovery, the watchwords are self-responsibility and personal accountability. Eventually we finally recognize blame doesn't help and that surrender and self-responsibility are the only concepts that can move us forward – but to get there we may need to allow ourselves to feel angry and to occasionally indulge in some blaming.

It is helpful, in dealing with others, to remember they, too, may need to go through their angry stage to achieve acceptance. To not allow others, or ourselves, to go through anger and blame may slow down the grief process.

Trust yourself and the grief process. You won't stay angry forever. But you may need to get angry for awhile as you search over what could have been, to finally accept what is. When we face ourselves and see our own part in our misery, our burden of guilt can be removed – but we can't lay down a burden we refuse to carry or see.

"God, help me accept my own and other's anger as part of achieving acceptance and peace. Within that framework, help me strive for personal accountability."

This if the fate of those who trust in themselves, and of their followers, who approve their sayings. Like sheep they are destined for the grave, and death will feed on them. The upright will rule over them in the morning; their forms will decay in the grave, far from their princely mansions. But God will redeem my life from the grave; he will surely take me to himself. (Psalm 49:13-16)

TODAY'S STEP: I face my problems squarely and without blame.

"If you take good things for granted, you must earn them again. For every right you cherish, you have a duty to fulfill. For every hope you entertain, you have a task to perform. For every privilege you would preserve, you must sacrifice a comfort. Freedom will always carry the price of individual responsibility and the just rewards of your own choices." Dennis Waitley, ***Empires of the Mind***

"Let Go of Old Ideas"

Here are some "new ideas" and "re-engineering" action steps from Dennis Waitley's book, ***Empires of the Mind: Lessons to Lead and Succeed in a Knowledge-Based World*** to help you gain more personal responsibility in your business/personal life:

1. Carry this affirmative motto with you: **My rewards in life will reflect my service and contribution.**
2. Invest in developing your own knowledge and skills.
3. Take fifteen minutes each day for yourself alone. Think about how you can best spend your time for achieving what's important to you.
4. Set your **own** standards rather than comparing yourself to others. Successful people know they must compete with themselves, not with others – run your own race!
5. Learn to depend on yourself. Don't rely on other people, material rewards, or a prestigious job title to give you your self-worth. No one can take away your self-respect when it comes from within.
6. "No excuses, Sir" is a West Point motto. When you make a mistake or fail an assignment, avoid making excuses.
7. Use another motto for your self-analysis: **Life is a do-it–yourself project.** When your subordinates or team-mates bring you a problem, first ask them what **they** think should be done to resolve it.
8. Let your team-mates, subordinates, and children make mistakes without fear of punishment or rejection. Show them that mistakes are stepping stones to success.
9. Take the blame for your position in life honestly and openly – and share the credit for your success with those who deserve it.
10. Be more curious about your world. Observe nature's wonder and abundance. Get out of your comfortable rut.

I delight to do Thy will, O my God. Thy law is within my heart. (Psalm 40:8)

TODAY'S STEP: I do not run myself, my circumstances, or my feelings. I am open to myself, others, my Higher Power, and to loving myself unconditionally.

"The difficulties of life are intended to make us better, not bitter." -- Anonymous

"Pain Is Optional"

One of the most desirable attitudes of an employee, leader, manager, or individual is an ability to see challenges as opportunities, setbacks as temporary inconveniences. This positive attitude also welcomes change as friendly, and is not upset by surprises, even negative surprises. How we approach challenges and problems is a crucial aspect of our decision-making process, whether in business or in our personal lives. Here are some action ideas to help you avoid negative attitudes by framing your expectations in a positive way:

1. Visualize, think of, and speak well of your health. Don't dwell on your ailments or they'll reward you by visiting more often and staying longer.
2. Read and listen to the news and reports of professional growth, but resist the temptation to pollute your mind with the sordid details of other's tragedies.
3. Select more friends and associates who are optimists and highly motivated leaders.
4. Find a positive lesson and a positive reason for all your personal relationships. Accentuate the blessings and knowledge gained from each.
5. Learn to unhook your prejudices, especially in the new multicultural working environment. Make it a point to be more open and friendly with each and every person.
6. Learn to stay relaxed and friendly no matter how much pressure you're under. Be constructively helpful instead of unhelpfully critical.
7. Make a list of your current wants and desires and jot down the benefits you will get when you achieve them.
8. When dealing with your associates and subordinates, don't criticize failures in front of others. Correct mistakes in private, as conceivable innovations.
9. Instead of comparing yourself to others, set your own standards for achievement.
10. Above all, put your wishes and goals in positive terms. Live to greet success, not to avoid failure.

...It has not yet been revealed what we shall be --- (I John 3:2)

TODAY'S STEP: There are so many ways in which I can improve the quality of my life. Instead of fretting about what I can't have or can't do, I'll take action to create something positive in my life today.

"This is something really mysterious, something for which reason can provide no explanation, and for which no basis can be found in practical experience. It is nevertheless of common occurrence, and everyone has had the experience. It is not unknown even to the most hard-hearted and self-interested. Examples appear every day before our eyes of instant responses of this kind, without reflection, one person helping another, coming to his aid, even setting his own life in clear danger for someone whom he has seen for the first time, having nothing more in mind than that the other is in need and peril of his life." -- Arthur Schopenhauer

"Do You Just Belong?"

Are you an active member,
The kind that would be missed?
Or are you just contented
That your name is on the list?

Do you attend the meetings
And mingle with the flock?
Or do you meet in private
And criticize and knock?

Do you take an active part
To help the work along?
Or are you satisfied to be
The kind that just belongs?

Do you work on committees?
To this there is no trick;
Or leave the work to just a few,
And talk about the clique?

Please come to the meeting often,
And help with hand and heart.
Don't just be a member
But take an active part.

Think this over, members,
You know what's right from wrong.
Are you an active member?
Or do you just belong? -- Anonymous

For God so loved the world, that He gave His only begotten Son, that whosoever believes in Him should not perish, but have everlasting life. (John 3:16)

TODAY'S STEP: God will strengthen me when life gets hard.

"Are you willing to be sponged out, erased, cancelled, made nothing? Are you willing to be made nothing? Dipped into oblivion? If not you will never really change." -- D. H. Lawrence

Checklist to Help Co-Sex Addicts

1. Do you have money problems because of someone else's sexual behavior?
2. Do you tell lies to cover up for someone else's sexual behavior?
3. Do you think your loved one's behavior is caused by his/her companions?
4. Do you make threats, such as "If you don't stop, I'll leave you?"
5. Are you afraid to upset your partner for fear he or she will leave you?
6. Have you been hurt or embarrassed by the addict's behavior?
7. Do you find yourself searching for hidden clues that might be related to the sexual behavior of a loved one?
8. Do you feel alone in your problems?
9. Have you ever gotten someone out of jail who was there as a result of the person's sexual behavior?
10. Does sex play and all-consuming role in your relationship?
11. Do you feel responsible for the addict's behavior?
12. Do you fantasize and obsess about the addict's problems?
13. Do you find yourself being sexual with the addict to prevent him/her from being sexual with others?
14. Do you find yourself engaging in self-defeating or degrading behavior?
15. Have you ever thought about or attempted suicide because of someone's sexual behavior?

Hear me when I call, O God of my righteousness: Thou hast relieved me in my distress; have mercy upon me, and hear my prayer. O ye sons of men, how long will ye turn my glory into shame? (Psalm 4:1-2)

TODAY'S STEP: God help me to believe in myself and help me let go of old beliefs and feelings that are hurting me.

"Being human is difficult. Becoming human is a life-long process. To be truly human is a gift." Abraham Heschel

<u>Guidelines for Daily Maintenance and Progress In Recovery</u>

Emotional Self-Care

- Talk to someone on a personal level every day. Develop close relationships. Maintain them with frequent contact, and mend them when there is a problem.
- Stop every day to tune in to your feelings. Let your self feel them, talk to someone about them, and listen to how others feel. All feelings are acceptable.
- Be honest with yourself and others. Honesty is the foundation of mental health and Recovery.
- Avoid self-pity. Life is difficult, and self-pity distracts you from the real work of life and Recovery.

Physical Self-Care

- Do aerobic activity at least three or four times a week for a minimum of twenty minutes. Exercise vigorously enough to increase your breathing and heart rate. Try walking, running, biking, or swimming.
- A daily stretching routine will help you relax and stay fit and flexible. You may combine it with moderate sit-ups, push-ups and weight-lifting.
- Eat well. A healthy diet contains foods low in fat, salt, and sugar and high in fiber and complex carbohydrates.

Spiritual Self-Care

- Take the risk to believe you can recover. Remind yourself once a day your life can be better, you can have self-esteem. If you don't believe it, then act as if you do so you can proceed with your Recovery.
- Find your refuge. Identify a place or an activity you know will help you relax and feel safe. It might be special music, sports, nature, talking to friends, etc.
- Take twenty minutes each day to meditate, pray, or do creative visualization. It relaxes you, helps develop a connection with your Higher Power, and trains you in concentration and letting go.

In returning and rest shall ye be saved; in quietness and in confidence shall be your strength. (Isaiah 30:15)

TODAY'S STEP: Emotional health is from within not without.

"Try not to become a man of success,
Rather become a man of value." -- Albert Einstein

Don't Be Afraid to Fail

You've failed many times although you may not remember.

You fell down the first time you tried to walk.

You almost drowned the first time

You tried to swim, didn't you?

Did you hit the ball the first time you swung a bat?

Heavy hitters, the ones who hit the most home runs, also strike out a lot.

Babe Ruth struck out 1,330 times, but he also hit 714 home runs.

R.H. Macy failed seven times before his store in New York   caught on.

English novelist John Creasy got 753 rejection slips before he published 564 books.

Don't worry about failure.

Worry about the chances you miss when you don't even try.

A message as published in the **Wall Street Journal** by United Technologies Corporation, Hartford, Connecticut, 1982.

But now, thus says the LORD, your Creator, O Jacob, and He who formed you, O Israel, "Do not fear, for I have redeemed you; I have called you by name; you are Mine! (Isaiah 43:1)

TODAY'S STEP: By calling on my Higher Power for help daily I can turn failure into success.

"The other great antidote to greed is gratitude. If you contemplate all that you have, and all the blessings you have been given, gratitude will arise and drive out greed."
Laurence and Barbara Tarlo

Following a suggestion I frequently heard at meetings, I made a list of the things for which I was grateful – my health, my job, my family, etc. When I finished, I didn't **feel** very grateful, but the seed of gratitude was planted and I started to experience the rewards of "The Program".

<u>The Twelve Rewards</u>

1. Hope instead of Desperation.

2. Faith instead of Despair.

3. Courage instead of Fear.

4. Peace of Mind instead of Confusion.

5. Self-Respect instead of Self-Contempt.

6. Self-Confidence instead of Helplessness.

7. The Respect of Others instead of Pity and Contempt.

8. A Clean Conscience instead of Guilt.

9. Real Friendship instead of Loneliness.

10. A Clean Pattern of Living instead of a Purposeless Existence.

11. The Love and Understanding of our Families instead of Doubts and Fears.

12. The Freedom of a Happy Life instead of the Bondage of Alcoholic Obsession.

And I heard a great voice out of the heaven saying, Behold, the tabernacle of God is with men, and he will dwell with them, and they shall be his people, and God himself shall be with them, and be their God. And God shall wipe away all tears from their eyes; and there shall be no more death, neither sorrow, nor crying, neither shall there be any more pain: for the former things are passed away. (Revelation 21:3-4)

TODAY'S STEP: Thankfulness today will help me see the miracles at work in my life and in the lives of others on the road to Recovery.

"Freud was once asked what he thought a normal person should be able to do well. The questioner probably expected a complicated, 'deep' answer. But Freud simply said, 'Lieben und arbeite' (to love and to work). It pays to ponder on this simple formula; it grows deeper as you think about it." Erik Erikson, *Identity, Youth and Crisis*

Love and Work: A Transition Checklist

Love relationships and work are the two most important factors through which a person's inner changes become visible – each represents a new cluster of roles the person is ready to explore. Use this checklist to discover what these changes may mean to you.

1. **Take your time.** The outer forms of our lives can change in an instant, but the inner orientation that brings us back into a vital relation to people and activity takes time. Everything doesn't come to a standstill while we wait for self-renewal, inner change is slow, we can't rush it.

2. **Arrange temporary structures.** We need to work out ways of going on while the inner work is being done. We may need to get a temporary job while we look for a real job.

3. **Don't act for the sake of action.** Temporary situations are frustrating and there is the temptation to "do something – anything." We need to stay in transition long enough to complete the process and not to abort it prematurely.

4. **Recognize why you are uncomfortable.** Distress is not a sign something has gone wrong, but that something is changing. Expect times of fear and anxiety – they'll pass.

5. **Take care of yourself in little ways.** Be sensitive to your smallest needs and don't force change on yourself.

6. **Explore the other side.** Change has costs or benefits depending on whether it is chosen or not, we need to look at both sides of the situation and weigh the consequences.

7. **Talk to someone.** Whether you choose a professional counselor, sponsor, or just a good friend, when you are going through a transition in your work-life or relationships it's important to talk to someone about your feelings.

8. **Find out what is waiting in the wings.** Transitions clear the ground for growth of potentialities within us – use it to develop new interests and talents.

Adapted from William Bridges, *Transitions: Making Sense of Life's Changes.* Reading, MA: Addison-Wesley Pub. Co., 1980.

I waited for the Lord; and He inclined unto me, and heard my cry. (Psalm 40:1)

TODAY'S STEP: I visualize myself achieving my goal of changing for the better.

Step Seven

<u>"Humbly asked God to help us remove our shortcomings."</u>

The emphasis in Step Seven is on our ability to develop humility. This occurs as we develop consciousness with our Higher Power and regularly seek guidance in the affairs of our lives. Shifting our focus enables us to have our needs met in a healthy non-codependent way. This shift produces harmony with our Higher Power and other people. As we grow in "The Program," we begin to understand humility is a necessary ingredient for our healing. Only by a deepening understanding of this requirement can we adequately prepare to ask God's help in removing our shortcomings.

Positive preparation for removing our shortcomings demonstrates our willingness to let go of our destructive behaviors and cooperative with our Higher Power in the healing process. We cannot expect our circumstances to change if we continue to behave in ways that are hurtful to ourselves and others, while simply waiting for God to do all the work.
Even though we have turned it over to God and have asked for help, we should be aware of our tendency to repeat old behaviors. If we do become aware of "old behaviors" at work, we can simply observe them and not be overly judgmental with ourselves. God loves us the way we are, and the realization that we are repeating destructive behavior patterns is an opportunity for us to forgive ourselves as God forgives us.

Letting go of old negative behavior patterns, however destructive they may be, can create a sense of loss and require time to grieve. It is normal to grieve the loss of something we no longer have. If, in our childhood, people or "things" were taken from us before we were ready to release them, we may be overly sensitive and thereby resist experiencing feelings accompany the loss of familiar behaviors. Rather than using our own ineffective strategies to avoid or deny our fears, we can turn to our Higher Power for help and support. Even though our childhood learning did not adequately prepare us to handle the grieving for adult losses, our love and trust in God can heal our memories, repair the damage and restore us to wholeness.

Practicing the Steps on a daily basis until they become routine will help us reach our goals of peace, serenity, happiness and manageability. We will begin to trust our thoughts and feelings as a result of our conscious contact with God. We will learn that the guidance we receive from our Higher Power is always available; all we need to do is listen and act in spite of our fear.

"Humbly asked God to remove our shortcomings."

"My Creator, I am now willing that You should have all of me, good and bad. I pray that You now remove from me every single defect of character which stands in the way of my usefulness to You and my fellows. Grant me strength, as I go out from here to do Your bidding." (*Alcoholics Anonymous,* p. 76)

In this moment, I ask my Higher Power to remove all of my shortcomings, relieving me of the burden of my past. In this moment, I place my hand in God's, trusting the void I experience is being filled with my Higher Power's unconditional love for me and those in my life.

MEDITATIONS

The labors of yesterday will be justified in this new day. I am weak, dear Father, and afraid of the consequences of my own actions. It is terrible to know fear and allow it to blind me to Thy mercy. I need Thee by my side to face any justice bestowed upon me. When others judge me, open my eyes and let me understand the reasons why. Help me not to be quick to judge the acts of others. May I represent kindness and mercy when others condemn. When this night falls, may the love and understanding I show today give another soul comfort and happiness. As I start this new day, may this prayer rest in my heart and find its way to thee.

AFFIRMATIONS

I willingly, and without fail, take care of the duties and obligations which I have accepted for my self. I commit only to those responsibilities I know I can fulfill and which contribute to my well-being and to the well-being of others.

I automatically, and always, think in a decisive and determined way. I am full of conviction and resolution, and the absolute assurance of the best possible outcome in everything that I do.

All of my thoughts create healthiness within me. My mind dwells only on those thoughts which create more harmony, balance, and well-being within me, and in the world around me.

I am calm, confident, and self-assured.

"Failure is the condiment that gives success its flavor." -- Truman Capote

"No Pain . . . No Gain"

Why do we so often see ourselves as being the very personification of failure? What are the ingredients of failure? How do we analyze it?

F: Fear. Frustration. Futility. Falling short. False pride. Fallacies. Fallibility. Foul-ups. Frailty. Forgetfulness.

A: Anger. Animosity. Adversity. Arrogance. Anxiety. Arbitrariness. Antipathy. Alienation.

I: Indifference. Impulsiveness. Isolation. Ill will. Incapacity. Impatience. Impropriety.

L: Lethargy. Lying. Lechery. Laziness. Lugubriousness. Lust.

U: Unworthiness. Unctuousness. Undutifulness. Unfaithfulness. Unsociability. Uselessness.

R: Resentment. Regret. Remorse. Rationalization. Rage. Revenge. Rebellion. Recklessness. Regression.

E: Envy. Extremism. Egotism. Elitism.

Some of these characteristics are probably very familiar to us. The goal of Step Seven is that having already identified them, we now petition our Higher Power for help in removing them.

He leads me beside the still waters. He restores my soul; He leads me in the paths of righteousness for His name's sake. (Psalm 23:2-3) Righteousness means right thinking, and I know that to think rightly about my condition means healing and safety. Christ in me, my Good Shepard, is now guiding me in the path of Right Thought; so all will be well. The nature of God is all-powerful, omnipresent good, boundless love. I know this Boundless Love is now taking care of me, and arranging all my affairs.

Even though I walk through the valley of the shadow of death, I will fear no evil: for You are with me. (Psalm 23:4)

TODAY'S STEP: By calling on my Higher Power for help daily I can turn my failures into steps on a successful journey.

"Humility has its origin in an awareness of unworthiness, and sometimes too in a dazzled awareness of saintliness." -- Sidonie Gabrielle Colette

<u>"I Can't . . . God Can . . . I Think I'll Let Him"</u>

Humility, what is it? It's the opposite of arrogance or Pride. What is arrogance?

- Arrogance assumes that because you can't imagine how something can be done, you can declare without reservation that it's impossible!

- Arrogance does all the talking and none of the listening.

- Arrogance rejects advice, simply because someone else said it or because your mind is already made up or you don't want anybody else to get the credit.

- Arrogance is refusal to accept help unless you've earned it, and inability to accept a compliment when you have earned it.

- Arrogance stubbornly refuses to change a mind when it knows it is wrong.

- Arrogance is "one-up", better than, grandiose, labeling others.

- Arrogance spouts off without reservation: "There is no heaven. There is no hell."

- Arrogance is an unwillingness to consider the possibility of making the 360-degree turn in your life that will allow a Higher Power to come into your life.

Humility is giving up your rights, not expecting another to do it "right" or "correctly". The root cause of pride is selfishness. Pride says: "I want it my way".

We turn away from arrogance and seek humility because we realize it is the only way to achieve peace, serenity, happiness and manageability in our lives. Our desire to be maturing, growing, useful and joyous persons requires an inner calm, even in a turbulent, unbalanced world. Learning to accept things we cannot change, and asking God for the courage to change the things we can, helps us to achieve these desires.

Whoever humbles himself as this little child is the greatest in the kingdom of heaven. (Matthew 18:4)

TODAY'S STEP: I understand the true nature of humility. I recognize the ability to develop and practice it is the basic foundation of the Twelve Steps.

"We know that God can and will do anything that is for our ultimate good, if we are ready to receive His help." Anonymous

The Twelve Steps and Traditions

The Seventh Step of the Twelve Steps of Alcoholics Anonymous originally read: "Humbly on our knees asked Him to remove our shortcomings." Just before the publication of the AA ***Big Book*** (out of the same concern that led to the addition of the phrase 'as we understood Him' after the mention of **God** in Steps Three and Eleven) the phrase 'on our knees' was dropped.

Although the phrase was dropped, the advising of the posture remains as a bit of frequently bestowed sponsorly wisdom, -- "Get down on your knees in the morning and ask for help, and get down on your knees at night and say 'Thanks'."

"Getting down on your knees" might signify the experience of submission, of openness, or of vulnerability. But whatever the experience – however represented, however phrased, however conceived, however "felt" – this positioning of one's whole being connects the core spiritual act of the cry for help that admits one's flawed imperfection with some sort of experience of fitting-in, of connectedness to others and to a greater whole, a Higher Power, God.

Step Seven Commitment

"Dear Higher Power,
I am "entirely ready," to let go of
that which is in me and interferes with
my cooperating in doing your work.
I humbly seek to be restored to wholeness;
to love and be sensitive to my inner-child
and relate to others in a wholesome way.

My life is yours,
As I continue to do your bidding.
Thank you for helping me heal.

It is a good thing to give thanks unto the Lord . . . to declare thy loving kindness in the morning, and thy faithfulness every night. (Psalm 92:1-2)

TODAY'S STEP: When faced with difficult or painful situations, I remember a loving God is always here for me, always available as a source of comfort, guidance and peace.

"We do not do what we want and yet we are responsible for what we are – that is the fact." Jean Paul Sartre, **Situations**

The Addict's Declaration of Freedom and Responsibility*

My name is ___________. I am an addict, and I am responsible for my addiction. Nobody laid it on me. I brought it on myself.

No matter how sick or crazy I get, I am a free spirit, a child of God, and a responsible human being. My addiction was caused by taking alcohol or drugs, of my own free will, in such a way that I got hooked and lost the use of my free will. I lost it, and with the help of God I can regain it.

My addiction is the result of my own ignorance and my own perverseness. I am responsible for acting perversely, that is, doing wrong when I knew it was wrong. I am also responsible for acting ignorantly, that is, doing wrong when I did not know it was wrong. Ignorance is no excuse, and I do not claim it as an excuse. I blame nothing and nobody for my trouble. Granted, the society is often wrong, and other people are often wrong, but that is not what made me an addict. I made me an addict.

I am responsible for my Recovery. Nobody is going to do it for me. I need help and will seek and accept help, but I will not turn my helpers into leaning posts or crying towels. With the help of God and my already-recovered brother and sister addicts, I can and will live one day at a time in total abstinence and freedom from alcohol or addictive drugs. It is beneath my dignity as a human being to become a leech upon the society, a guinea pig for the scientists, or a ward of the government.

Walking daily in the strength of the truth of God, and in the love of my brothers and sisters, I will live honestly, honorably, and responsibly, and I will go forward to the discovery and fulfillment of the real meaning of life.

*Burns, John 1990 **The Answer to Addiction: The Path to Recovery from Alcohol, Drug, Food, and Sexual Dependencies.** New York, NY: The Crossroad Publishing Company, p.135.

I will go before you and make the crooked places straight. (Isaiah 45:2)

TODAY'S STEP: I do not run myself, my circumstances, or my feelings. I am open to myself, others, my Higher Power, and to loving myself unconditionally.

"It is clear that persons who live close to their capacity, who continue to activate their potential, have a pronounced sense of well-being and considerable energy. They see themselves as leading purposeful and creative lives." -- Hebert Otto

The Change Process

The road to success in any undertaking is usually marked by highs and lows. Sometimes there are twists and turns and we may feel we have lost our way. Sometimes we are filled with zeal and enthusiasm and other times we simply quietly ponder our next step. Sometimes we seem to be on an accelerated path, at other times it seems as if we are traveling in slow-motion. Wise is the person who maintains his self-confidence and finds some good in even the unexpected along the way.

There is no magical formula for change. But there are some helpful principles:

First of all, change happens little by little. Our capacity for trust grows more and more, and our ability to love and to receive love increases. These changes, like all of the most important changes in life, do not happen as a one-time event. An important change may require us to make a decision at a certain moment, but it also requires a process that takes place over months and years.

Second, change is not a race. The change process cannot be rushed. We often want to hurry it up, but we can't. Change that is real and long-lasting requires patience and perseverance. When we have been practicing our dysfunctions for decades, we can expect that unlearning them will also take time.

Third, change requires we practice the disciplines of honesty and fellowship. There is no Recovery unless we find ways to move out of denial and isolation. What a wonderful gift it is to be able to share our struggles and victories with people who will "always thank God for us" and who will encourage us, affirm us and hold us accountable.

. . . old things are passed away, behold, all things are becoming new. (2 Corinthians 5:17)

TODAY'S STEP: I am willing to change. I visualize myself achieving my goal of changing for the better.

"Do your work. Not just your work and no more, but a little more for the lavishings' sake — that little more which is worth all the rest. And if you suffer, as you must, and if you doubt, as you must, do your work. Put your heart into it, and the sky will clear. Then, out of your very doubt and suffering will be born the supreme joy of life." -- Dean Briggs

"Live and Let Live"

Sometimes we live our lives as if we were on a ladder. We think everyone is either above us – to be feared, envied – or below us – to be pitied. And God is way, way at the top, beyond our view. This is a hard, lonely way to live, because no two people can stand comfortably on the same rung for very long.

When we finally get into a Twelve Step program, we find a lot of people who have decided to climb down from their ladders into the "circle of fellowship." In the circle we are all on equal terms, and God is right in the center, easily accessible. When Newcomers arrive we don't have to worry about rearranging everyone's position, we just widen the circle.

Today we can decide not to look up to some people or down on others. We can look each person in the eye, squarely and honestly. Today, we can decide to be humble and climb down from the "ladder of judgment" of ourselves and others, and take our rightful place in a worldwide circle of love and support.

Our thoughts are our teachers. We need to ask ourselves if they are teaching us to love and appreciate ourselves and others, or are they teaching us to practice isolation? Today we can choose our teachers with greater care.

"Live and Let Live" sets us free from the compulsion to criticize, judge, condemn, and retaliate . . . which can damage us far more than those against whom we use such weapons. The Steps teach us patience and tolerance rooted in love.

Let the morning bring me word of your unfailing love, for I have put my trust in you. Show me the way I should go, for to you I lift my soul. (Psalm 143:8)

TODAY'S STEP: I focus on the power available to me by learning to wait with a good attitude.

"I can support my group in a number of ways. When the basket is passed, I can give what I can. Just as important, I can give any time and moral support to help make ours the kind of group I **want** to belong to." ***Alateen – A Day At A Time***

<u>Tradition Seven</u>

Every group ought to be fully self-supporting, declining outside contributions.

"Alcoholics are certainly all-or-nothing people. Our reactions to money prove this. As AA emerged from it infancy into adolescence, we swung from the idea that we needed vast sums of money to the notion that AA shouldn't have any. On every lip were the words 'You can't mix AA and money. We shall have to separate the spiritual from the material.'"

"We took this violent new tack because here and there members had tried to make money out of their AA connections, and we feared we'd be exploited. Now and then, grateful benefactors had endowed clubhouses, and as a result there was sometimes outside interference in our affairs. We had been presented with a hospital, and almost immediately the donor's son became its principal patient and would-be manager. One AA group was given five thousand dollars to do with what it would. The hassle over that chunk of money played havoc for years. Frightened by these complications, some groups refused to have a cent in their treasuries."

"Despite these misgivings, we had to recognize the fact that AA had to function. Meeting places cost something. To save whole areas from turmoil, small offices had to be setup, telephones installed, and a few full-time secretaries hired. Over many protests, these things were accomplished. We saw that if they weren't, the man coming in the door couldn't get a break. These simple services would require small sums of money which we could and would pay ourselves. At last the pendulum stopped swinging and pointed straight at Tradition Seven as it reads today."

Taken from ***Twelve Steps and Twelve Traditions,*** p. 161-162.

Now, O Lord God, You are God, and Your words are truth, and You have promised this good thing to Your servant. (2 Samuel 7:28)

TODAY'S STEP: I allow myself to recognize and accept whatever feelings pass through me.

"The ability to simplify means to eliminate the unnecessary so that the necessary may speak." -- Hans Hofman

True Needs

Philip St. Roman, in ***Twelve Steps to Spiritual Wholeness: A Christian Pathway,*** tells us if we are able to renounce false needs, what is left will be true. False needs are the "fixes" discussed in Step One and the defects of character in Step Six. "Fixes are not true needs; they are addictive needs. Defects of character are not true needs; they are ego needs."

In Step Seven, after making a decision to stop indulging in behaviors that support our defects of character, we can do the following with regard to each one:

1. **Approval.** We realize we do not need the approval of others. We are loved by God just as we are. There is no need for others to let us know we are okay. **Our true need is awareness of God's unconditional love for us.**

2. **Perfection.** We realize it is human to make mistakes; it is not a sin. We give ourselves permission to make mistakes. **Our true need is to do the best we can at whatever we do, knowing we will make mistakes – and it's okay.**

3. **Control.** We recognize we control nothing but our attitude about what is happening. **Our true need is not to be in control, but to be here-now-in love.** This means a willingness to give and to receive, to be strong and vulnerable, to be real, not phony.

4. **Self-sufficiency.** We realize it's okay to depend on others. **Our true need is to provide prudently for our needs, knowing it's okay to ask for help.**

After letting go of false needs associated with approval, control, perfection and self-sufficiency, we can discover our true needs – letting go brings us peace and serenity.

May the God of hope fill you with joy and peace in believing, so that you will abound in hope by the power of the Holy Spirit. (Romans 15:13)

TODAY'S STEP: I acknowledge my wants and needs, then turn them over to my Higher Power.

"We choose to behave with personal integrity, not because it will make someone else feel better, but because it reflects a way of living that enriches and heals us." *. . . In All Our Affairs*

"This Too Shall Pass"

Destructive behavior patterns that remain with us after we complete Step Seven may never be eliminated, but may need to be transformed. We have an opportunity to convert these aspects of our character into positive traits and learn to use them in a healthy way.

Leaders may be left with a quest for power but with no desire to misuse it. Lovers will be left with exquisite sexuality to refrain from causing pain to those they love. People who are materially wealthy may continue to be, but will set aside their greed and possessiveness. With the help of the Lord, all aspects of our personal life can be rewarding. By continuing to practice humility and accepting the tools God is giving us, we will eventually begin to aspire to sharing with others the love we have received.

For "The Program" to be successful, we must practice the Steps on a daily basis. When we have moments of inner struggle, we can simply say "This too shall pass"; "I will let go and let God"; "I fear no evil"; or "I choose to see the good in this experience". Depression, guilt and anger can be acknowledged and understood to be temporary.

We also need to stop from time to time and affirm ourselves for our commitment to Recovery. Note how our determination enables us to break the bonds of our unhealthy habits and behaviors. Accept the positive, spontaneous thoughts and feelings that occur and see that they stem from our personal relationship with God. The guidance we receive from Him is always available; all we need to do is listen, receive and act without fear. God does not put any challenges before us that we are unable to face. The comfort we find in that knowledge is sufficient to overcome our fears.

But we have this treasure in jars of clay to show that this all-surpassing power is from God and not from us. We are hard pressed on every side, but not crushed; perplexed, but not in despair; persecuted, but not abandoned; struck down, but not destroyed.   (2 Corinthians 4:7-10)

TODAY'S STEP: I let consequences and responsibility fall where they belong.

"This measure of a man is not determined by his show of outward strength, or the volume of his voice, or the thunder of his action. It is to be seen, rather, in terms of the nature and depth of his commitments, the genuineness of his friendship, the sincerity of his purpose, the quiet courage of his convictions, his capacity to suffer, and his willingness to continue "growing up." -- Grady Poulard

"Sponsors: Have One – Use One – Be One"

Sober

Person

Offering

Newcomers

Suggestions

On

Recovery

One day I received a call from a newcomer to Al-Anon. We had exchanged telephone numbers at a meeting, but I never thought he would call. We chatted for a while about a problem he was having and then he asked if I would be his sponsor. I was shocked! I never expected he would ask me!

I felt humble, fearful and grateful all at the same time. But had I grown enough to help someone else? What did I have to give? Could I be there for someone else without losing myself? I was paralyzed. I didn't know what to say. Then I remembered that he was not asking me to be his savior, only his sponsor. He was asking me to share my "experience, strength, and hope" to help him with his Recovery.

I know my Higher Power brings people into my life who can help me to grow. So I said a quick prayer, asking to be worthy, and answered that I would be honored to sponsor him.

Being a sponsor is as much a commitment to myself as it is to someone else. It is not a favor. Sponsorship gives me a chance to share intimately, to care, to practice detaching with love, and to apply the Al-Anon principles more consciously than ever. And, if I listen to my own words, I find I usually tell those whom I sponsor exactly what I myself need to hear.

Let brotherly love continue. (Hebrews 13:1)

TODAY'S STEP: I move forward in confidence, knowing my steps are guided.

"A person with a half-volition goes backward and forward, and makes no way on the smoothest road; but the person with a whole volition advances on the roughest , and will reach his purpose, if there be even a little wisdom in it." -- Robert Carlyle

False Ego Needs

In the book *Twelve Steps to Spiritual Wholeness: A Christian Pathway,* Philip St. Romain identifies our attachments to control, perfection, approval, and self-sufficiency as ways of trying to make ourselves okay. He notes that ultimately each of these attachments is unattainable, leaving us with a deep sense of not being okay. He believes attachments set us up for conditional happiness. It is only as a result of working Step Six and realizing these truths about attachments, that we become ready to lead a different life.

To work Step Seven, we have to give up these behaviors. When we find ourselves thinking about them, we check our thoughts, check our will, and decide to act differently. To begin meeting our true needs, we must stop indulging in behavior oriented toward approval, control, perfectionism, and self-sufficiency. St. Romain gives us the following examples of such behavior:

1. **Approval.** Doing things to impress people; trying not to upset people (even when they need to be upset); doing things to please people, even if it goes against our values.

2. **Perfectionism.** Judging ourselves and others harshly because we or they make mistakes; procrastinating about something because we're afraid it might not come out right.

3. **Control.** Checking up on people; nagging; not letting others know our vulnerability; not letting others be themselves.

4. **Self-Sufficiency.** Refusing to ask for help from others; striving for total security.

Come to me all you who are weary and burdened, and I will give you rest. (Matthew 11:28)

TODAY'S STEP: There are many things I can do to improve my life and to further my Recovery, but I cannot heal myself. I need to continually ask God's help in becoming free of all that blocks me from my true self.

"All the wonders you seek are within yourself." -- Sir Thomas Browne

<u>NACOA</u>

The National Association for the Children of Alcoholics (NACOA) has established the following facts about children of alcoholics:

- An estimated 28 million Americans have at least one alcoholic parent.
- More than half of all alcoholics have an alcoholic parent.
- One in three families currently reports alcohol abuse by a family member.
- Children of alcoholics are at the highest risk of developing alcoholism themselves or marrying someone who becomes alcoholic.
- Medical research has shown that children born to alcoholics are at the highest risk of developing attention-deficit disorders, stress-related medical problems, fetal alcohol syndrome, and other alcohol-related birth defects.
- In up to 90 percent of child-abuse cases, alcohol is a significant factor.
- Children of alcoholics are also frequently victims of incest, child neglect, and other forms of violence and exploitation.
- Children of alcoholics often adapt to the chaos and inconsistency of an alcoholic home by developing an inability to trust, an extreme sense of responsibility and denial of feelings, all of which result in low self-esteem, depression, isolation, guilt, and difficulty in maintaining satisfying relationships. These and other problems often persist throughout adulthood.
- The majority of people served by Employee Assistance Programs are adult children of alcoholics.
- The problems of most children of alcoholics remain invisible because their coping behavior tends to be approval-seeking and social acceptance. However, a disproportionate number of those entering the juvenile justice system, courts, prisons, and mental-health facilities, and referred to school authorities are children of alcoholics.

I pray that Thou should take them out of the world, but that Thou should keep them from the evil one. (John 17:15)

TODAY'S STEP: I accept who I am, where I am, and I continue to reach forward one day at a time.

"I was created in love. For that reason nothing can express my beauty nor liberate me except love alone." -- Mechtild of Magdeburg

<u>"Love One Another, As I Have Loved You!"*</u>

By Helen Steiner Rice

"Love one another as I have loved you"
May seem impossible to do –
But if you will try to trust and believe
Great are the joys that you will receive . . .
For love makes us patient, understanding and kind,
And we judge with our hearts and not with our mind . . .
For as soon as love enters the heart's open door,
The faults we once saw are not there anymore,
And the things that seemed wrong begin to look right
When viewed in the softness of love's gentle light . . .
For love works in ways that are wondrous and strange,
And there is nothing in life that love cannot change,
And all that God promised will some day come true
When you love one another the way He loves you.

(*Used with permission of the Helen Steiner Rice Foundation, Cincinnati, Ohio)

"Just for today . . . I will do somebody a good turn and not get found out; if anybody knows of it, it will not count." What a terrific exercise! It helps me break free of the habit of doing kind or generous things in order to get something back. Only when I perform a loving act with no expectations will I reap the true reward of giving.

I am learning that giving doesn't have to take away from me or anyone else – if there are not strings attached, everyone stands to benefit. Every good and loving gesture soothes my soul and contributes to a healthier world. These anonymous, positive actions are the building blocks of a flourishing spiritual well-being.

Today I will put unconditional love into action. When I give freely, without expecting anything in return, I always receive more than I give.

If a man say, I love God, and hates his brother, he is a liar: for he that loves not his brother whom he has seen, how can he love God whom he has not seen? (1 John 4:20)

TODAY'S STEP: I create a healthy atmosphere of love and nurturing around and within me. I accept the love and support of my sponsor and my group.

".. . Al-Anon helped me to accept the fact that, although I have no control over other people's reactions or thoughts, I can change the way I react." **. . . In All Our Affairs**

Loose It and Let It Go

By Helene Peterson

I carried a secret sorrow
And cherished it in my breast
Though it robbed me of peace of
Mind by day,
Made of night one long unrest.
Yet I could not solve the problem
That harried and plagued me so,
Till I harked to the voice of wisdom
To loose it and let it go.
It had ridden me like a nightmare
And driven me to despair,
Till I uttered the word of freedom
And loosed it upon the air.
For no one but God could solve it,
None other could understand,
But 'twas lifted fully and freely
At the spoken word of command.
We may speak the word into the ether,
In confidence, loud and clear,
Or whisper it quietly, softly –
The Father will surely hear.
Of ourselves, we may see but dimly
And darkly, as through a glass,
But say: "It is done. So be it."
And God "will bring it to pass."

Today I will take time to clear my mind and focus on what is essential. I will release any unimportant thoughts. I will then allow myself to be guided toward the best action I can take for today. Regardless of how simple the answers may seem, I will listen without judgment. I will not take my thoughts for granted, for they may be my only guide.

You will guide me with Your counsel, and afterward receive me to glory. (Psalm 73:24)

TODAY'S STEP: I acknowledge my wants and needs, then turn them over to my Higher Power.

"You get to the point where your demons, which are terrifying, get smaller and smaller and you get bigger and bigger." -- August Wilson

"Look for Similarities Rather Than Differences"

According to the Children of Alcoholics Foundation, Inc., 1 out of every 8 Americans is the child of an alcoholic. Of the 28 million children in the U.S., 7 million are under 18.

How Do Children of Alcoholics Feel?

- Guilty and responsible for parental drinking and unaware that alcoholism is a disease which they didn't cause, can't control, or cure.
- Invisible and unloved, since family life revolves totally around the alcoholic parent.
- Insecure, due to consistent inconsistencies in parental behavior, attitudes, and rules.
- Fearful the alcoholic parent will become ill, have an accident, or die.
- Embarrassed by the public behavior of alcoholic parents.
- Ashamed because of the stigma society attaches to alcoholism and the need to keep it a family secret.
- Frightened by family conflict, violence, and abuse.

How Do Children of Alcoholics React?

As youngsters, children of alcoholic parents may be more likely to:
- Have learning difficulties, do poorly in school, be truant or delinquent.
- Have fewer friends.
- Suffer psychosomatic illness.
- Be victims of neglect, child abuse, or incest.

As teenagers, children of alcoholic parents may be likely to:
- Be expelled from school or drop out due to early marriage, pregnancy, or institutionalization.
- Abuse alcohol or other drugs.
- Have serious behavior problems, anxiety or depression.
- Attempt suicide.

As adults, children of alcoholics may be more likely to:
- Have problems with interpersonal relationships.
- Experience difficulties in the workplace.
- Overuse medical facilities.
- Become alcoholic, suicidal, or mentally ill.

Open my eyes, that I may behold wonderful things from Your law. (Psalm 119:18)

TODAY'S STEP: God help me believe in myself and help me to let go of old beliefs and feelings that are hurting me.

"This is the beginning of a new day. I have been given this day to use as I will. I will use it for good, because I am exchanging a day of my life for it. When tomorrow comes, this day will be gone forever, leaving in its place something that I have traded for it. I want it to be gain, and not loss; good and not evil; success, and not failure; in order that I shall rejoice in the price that I paid for it." -- Anonymous

The 23rd – ½ Psalm

The Lord is my sponsor! I shall not want.

He maketh me to go to many meetings.
He leadeth me to sit back, relax, and listen with an open mind.
He restoreth my soul, my sanity, and my health.
He leadeth me in the paths of sobriety, serenity, and fellowship for mine own sake.
He teacheth me to think, to take it easy, to live and let live, and to do first things first.
He maketh me honest, humble, and grateful.
He teacheth me to accept the things I cannot change, to change the things that I can, and giveth me the wisdom to know the difference.

Yea, though I walk through the valley of despair, frustration, guilt, and remorse, I will fear no evil, for Thou art with me; the Program, thy way of life, the Twelve Steps, they comfort me.

Thou preparest a table before me in the presence of mine enemies: rationalization, fear, anxiety, self-pity, and resentment.

Thou anointest my confused mind and jangled nerves with knowledge, understanding, and hope.

No longer am I alone; neither am I afraid, nor sick, nor helpless, nor hopeless.

My cup runneth over.

Surely sobriety and serenity shall follow me every day of my life, twenty-four hours at a time, as I surrender my will to Thine and carry the message to others; and I will dwell in the house of my Higher Power, as I understand Him, daily.

Forever and Ever.
    -- Anonymous

Hath the Lord as great delight in burnt-offerings and sacrifices, as in obeying the voice of the Lord? Behold, to obey is better than sacrifice. (1 Samuel 15:22)

TODAY'S STEP: I move forward in confidence, knowing my steps are guided.

"I cannot imagine a God who rewards and punishes the objects of his creation [and] is but a reflection of human frailty. – Albert Einstein

"H.A.L.T. = Don't Get Too Hungry, Angry, Lonely or Tired"

Anger that sours turns to bitterness. Revengeful people suffer from intense bitterness. They have not been able to find an appropriate way to express their anger, and it has turned against them. George Washington Carver said, "I will not allow another person to ruin my life by hating them."

Are you that way? Are you driven by unforgiveness so much that it robs you of the joy of life? That kind of rage and anger destroys you. It affects you physically and emotionally. God doesn't tell you to forgive for the other person's sake; it is simply the best thing you can do for yourself. Pursuing revenge will destroy you in the end.

Give your desire for revenge to God. Fully acknowledge your anger to yourself, express it to people as appropriate, and leave the rest to God. Spending your life hating others robs you of the vitality of life.

Anger can be properly balanced by compassion. Many times the people we are most angry with need the most compassion. Balance is the key. There is a need for compassion toward others in the healthy life. Learn to balance your anger towards others with compassion for them. See them as valuable, significant people when you express your anger.

God has valid reasons for anger with us, but he also has compassion and forgiveness for us. Learning to control your wrath and forgive others feels good. You can express compassion instead of anger. When you feel angry today, think of a way to be compassionate to that person. The world tells you to be aggressive when you are wronged to keep it from happening again. Compassion is the opposite of aggression. It has amazing power in your life as well as in the lives of those to whom you are compassionate.

Yet he was merciful and forgave their sins and did not destroy them all. Many times he held back his anger and did not unleash his fury! For he remembered that they were merely mortal, gone like a breath of wind that never returns. (Psalm 78:38-39)

TODAY'S STEP: I am seeking a saner approach to everything I encounter. The slogans are a valuable source of sanity in chaotic situations. If I am tempted to act out of anger or frustration, I will remember "Easy Does It."

"To get everything, you must let go of everything." -- Taoist Proverb

The Principles of The Program

Step One - **Honesty.** We admitted our powerlessness – an act that found us beginning to understand the strength of humility and the curative power of surrender.

Step Two - **Hope.** We recognized our behavior lacked sanity and balance and conceded there might be some power – somewhere – that could restore us to sanity.

Step Three - **Faith.**   We again, admitted our powerlessness and accepted that fact by becoming willing to turn our will and lives over to a power greater than ourselves.

Step Four – **Courage.** We tackled this step accepting the shame and pain of self-assessment and were scrupulously honest about detailing all the wrongs we had committed.

Step Five – **Integrity.** We strengthened the commitment we made in Step Three by admitting to the God of our understanding, to ourselves, and to another person everything we discovered about ourselves in Step Four.

Step Six and Step Seven – **Willingness and Humility.**   We are more aware of the havoc our addictive/compulsive behavior has created in our lives and in other people's lives. We turn to our Higher Power to help rid us of these defects.

Step Eight and Step Nine – **Brotherly Love and Justice.** We listed all those who had suffered as a result of our behavior and with courage and determination we try to make restitution.

Step Ten – **Perseverance.** We took stock of our behavior each day. We checked to see where we were in error and promptly admitted it so we could keep our own house in order.

Step Eleven – **Spiritual Awareness.** We took the essence of each preceding step and brought it into play in this step of re-affirmation and re-dedication.

Step Twelve – **Service.** We accepted these steps as a blueprint for our life and tried to practice these principles in all our affairs.

I go from strength to strength. (Psalm 84:7)

TODAY'S STEP: When I rely on my Higher Power's help I can achieve.

"Be useful where thou livest, that they may
Both want and wish thy pleasing presence still.
. . . Find out men's wants and will,
And meet them there. All worldly joys go less
To the one joy of doing kindness. G. Herbert

Pettiness Prayer

Keep us, Oh God, from pettiness.
Let us be large in thought, in word, in deed.
Let us be through with fault-finding
and leave off self-seeking.
May we put away all pretense and meet each
other face to face,
without self-pity or without prejudice.
May we always be patient, never hasty
`in judgment and always tolerant.
Teach us to put into action our better
impulses straightforward and unafraid.
Let us take time for all things, make us
calm, serene and gentle.
Grant that we may realize that it is the
little things in life that create the
differences, than in the big things,
we are as one.
And may we strive to touch and to know
the greatest common heart of us all.
And, Oh God, let us not forget to be kind.

"Small kindnesses, small courtesies, small considerations, habitually practiced in our social intercourse, give a greater charm to the character than the display of great talents and accomplishments." -- M.A. Kelty

No eye pitied you . . . to have compassion on you; but you were thrown out into the open field . . . on the day you were born. And when I passed by you and saw you struggling in your own blood, I said to you . . . "Live!" . . . I made you thrive like a plant in the field; and you grew, matured, and became very beautiful. . . . you were naked and bare. When I passed by you again and looked upon you, indeed your time was the time of love; so I spread My wing over you and covered your nakedness. Yes, I swore an oath to you and entered into a covenant with you, and you became Mine. (Ezekiel 16:5-8)

TODAY'S STEP: I focus on the power available to me by learning to wait.

"As long as we feel victimized, we have lost the power to change." -- Anonymous

<u>"Stay In Recovery for Yourself"</u>

Growing-up in a dysfunctional home often causes us to take on certain roles. Through these roles, which are really ways of reacting to and masking pain, we pass on our dysfunction. Usually each member of the family confines him/herself to one major role, although some vacillate between roles. These include:

- The **Hero,** who excels outside the family to prove the family's worth by achieving

- The **Placater,** who shuttles diplomatically between family members, refereeing and smoothing feathers;

- The **Scapegoat,** who either gets blamed for the problems in the family or creates new ones that rival those of the problem person in magnitude;

- The **Mascot,** who cheers the hurting family by joking and otherwise diverting attention from the problem;

- The **Martyr,** who is usually but not always the spouse of the problem person, suffering on his or her behalf;

- The **Rescuer,** who leads the family in saving the problem person from the consequences of his abuse;

- The **Lost Child,** who fades into the background masking his/her pain silently by living in a neglected, unconnected, withdrawn and isolated world;

- The **Victim,** who sometimes receives the brunt of the problem person's anger; and,

- The **Abuser,** who is usually (though not always) a parent or parent-figure.

If I am to bring about healing, I must make a conscious effort to break these roles. Higher Power, show me how to quit being a role and start being a person – freely choosing to follow you and to live a healthy life.

Call upon Me in the day of trouble; I will deliver you, and you shall glorify Me. (Psalm 50-15)

TODAY'S STEP: I trust that "The Program" works if I work it and I can be restored to wholeness with God's help.

"The foundation I have developed in Al-Anon not only makes me grateful when things are going well, but also makes me realize that the program works especially when things go badly." -- **. . . In All Our Affairs**

<u>"Addiction Is an Equal Opportunity Destroyer"</u>

Pain and loss are part of life. No matter what we do, we will not be able to change this fact. But with the fellowship to support us and the Steps to guide us, we are able to face, and grow through, anything that comes our way.

In "The Program" – as in life – we've found nothing in our past was a wasted effort. Over time, we realize the seemingly bad frequently turn out to be a force for good. Our many negative memories have transformed themselves into guidelines pointing us toward a more positive approach to living.

Many among us have been faced with bankruptcy; with loss of a spouse, children, or home; with loss of a job; loss of a car; loss of prestige and social standing in our community – even with imprisonment and confinement. These are symptoms and consequences of losing ourselves.

But despite these losses, all of us who have hung on to "The Program," and whenever possible to our group, have found ourselves in a better position than we've ever occupied before. We've been able to clean the slate, write a new script and settle into a comfortable position in which we're able to love ourselves and accept ourselves for all that we are.

We certainly do not discount the material possessions or positions of prominence that many of us enjoy. But we've learned that these things are not the top priorities on our list of happiness-producing factors.

Don't store up treasures here on earth, where moths eat them and rust destroys them, and where thieves break in and steal. Store your treasures in heaven. Wherever your treasure is, there the desires of your heart will also be. (Matthew 6:19-22)

TODAY'S STEP: There are many things I can do to improve my life and to further my Recovery, but I cannot heal myself. I need to continually ask God's help in becoming free of all that blocks me from my true self.

"The first time I ever heard the Twelve Steps read at a meeting, I became very still. I felt I was not breathing . . . I was just listening with my whole being . . . I knew deep within me that I was home." -- *As We Understood . . .*

"Learn to Listen & Listen to Learn"

The goal of listening is understanding. It is the best gift you can give to anyone, and perhaps the best way to communicate love and respect. The next time you have an opportunity to give this gift, remember the following points:

The Listening Ladder

L: Look at the person speaking

A: Ask questions for clarification

D: Don't change the subject

D: Don't interrupt

E: Express emotions with control

R: Responsibility to listen

You, as a good listener, look into the eyes of whomever is speaking and see that person for whom he or she is. You devote your energy to taking in what the speaker has to say, withholding evaluation of the message and not judging it or overreacting to it. The good listener in you does not interrupt or change the subject, but when feedback is requested, you will give it, clearly and sincerely. You are tolerant and don't let a person's manner of speaking turn you off. You concentrate on facts but listen for the feelings behind what is being said, and you don't let emotion-arousing words disrupt the listening process. If someone is having difficulty expressing emotion, lean back. If someone is really desperate to be heard, lean forward. Responsibility for listening also means letting people know if you don't have time to listen rather than faking attentiveness.

... I no longer walk in the futility of my mind. The Gentiles are darkened in their understanding, alienated from the life of God because of the ignorance that is in them, due to their hardness of heart. They have become callous and have given themselves up to sensuality, greedy to practice every kind of impurity. But that is not the way you learned Christ! — assuming that you have heard Him and were taught by Him . . . (Ephesians 4:17-21)

TODAY'S STEP: I pray my Higher Power gives me the courage and strength to recognize the Truth about myself and help me accept I am powerless.

"Today is only a small manageable segment of time in which our difficulties need not overwhelm us. This lifts from our hearts and minds the heavy weight of both past and future." ***One Day at a Time in Al-Anon***

Affirmation for a Troubled Mind

Step back from your hectic life, your troubling thoughts and take a few minutes just to relax and be good to yourself by closing your eyes and repeating the following affirmation:

> I know the quality of what I have
> > and it cannot be devalued.
> I know the source of all my strength
> > and have tapped into its power.
> I know the beauty of my soul
> > and that it can't be altered
> I know I am God's child
> I know I am God's child.
>
> I know I am a treasure and preciousness is
> > real
> I know these feelings in me now are only
> > passing through
> I know that it's my right to be joyous and
> > be free
> And I know I am God's child.
> I know I am God's child.
>
> I feel the power of a love that is constant
> > and all-giving.
> I feel the pull to goodness within me even now
> I feel your strength embrace me as I tremble in
> > This time
> I can comfort my own child
> I can comfort my own child.
> > -- Anonymous

Jesus answered them, Is it not written in your law, I said, Ye are gods? If he called them gods, unto whom the word of God came, and the scripture cannot be broken. (John 10:34-35)

TODAY'S STEP: I pray my Higher Power gives me the courage and strength to recognize the Truth about myself and help me accept my powerlessness.

"No mistake is fatal unless you make it so." -- Anonymous

"Remember: Addiction Is Incurable, Progressive, and Fatal"

The best way to look at our patterns of addiction is to look at a typical list of symptoms and indicators of addiction used by professionals to determine **whether** we are addicted and **how strongly** we are addicted. The following are some of the major indicators on the **continuum** of addiction:

1. **Preoccupation With The Addictive Agent:** Thinking about it, talking about it, looking forward to it, being distracted because of it, not being to "be" with others because of the preoccupation.
2. **Increased Tolerance For The Addictive Agent:** We need more and more of the chemical or experience to achieve the desired effect. The more we use, the less the effect.
3. **Loss Of Control:** We can't have "just one".
4. **Withdrawal:** When we stop using whatever it is we're addicted to, we have symptoms of withdrawal, such as irritability, depression, moodiness, hostility, etc.
5. **Sneaking:** Hiding bottles, having a few drinks or pills before going out to be sure there's enough in the bloodstream in case we can't get more later.
6. **Denial:** It includes defensiveness about use and one's symptoms, as well as the consequences of one's actions.
7. **Personality Changes And Mood Swings:** Up, down, moody, temperamental, elated, irritable, sad, etc.
8. **Blaming:** It's everyone else's fault. There is a powerful inability to accept responsibility for our own life.
9. **Blackouts:** With chemical addictions, these occur when we can't remember what we did while we were under the influence – we don't remember driving home, etc.
10. **Physical Symptoms:** These depend upon the addiction – with non-chemical addictions, they are most often the stress disorders, such as headaches, ulcers, etc.
11. **Rigid Attitudes:** Black-and-white thinking; intolerance of other's compulsiveness, and all-or-nothing thinking.
12. **Loss Of Personal Values:** We stop caring as our addiction progresses. We don't take care of ourselves and we don't care about others. Apathy sets in.
13. **Disability And/Or Death:** Death comes either through physical damage due to a drug or chemical, or stress-related illness, such as cancer or heart attack.

What shall we do, that we might work the works of God? (John 6:28)

TODAY'S STEP: Emotional health is from within not without.

"There is a principle which is a bar against all information, which is proof against all arguments and which cannot fail to keep a man in everlasting ignorance – that principle is contempt prior to investigation." -- Herbert Spencer

"E.G.O. = Edging God Out"

What we give to God's work comes back multiplied, and with a blessing. What we withhold from God's work can hardly bring us any good. The way of God is always open if we are open too.

A problem is not a barrier. It is a challenge. The appearance of a problem of any kind in our life means the time has come to take a step forward; and the taking of that step will, of course, be prompted by the solving of the problem.

The real step forward is always a mental step. The only progress we ever make is mental progress. All things are ready if our minds are, and this means all progress is a change of mind. The universe is always ready when we are.

Man discovered fire as an answer to the challenge of cold. If the whole world had been tropical he would probably not have discovered it. Man designed tools to overcome the many practical problems of daily living. The telephone and the automobile and the airplane are answers to the problems of space and time.

In our personal lives, a problem is not a barrier saying, "You shall not pass" – there is a solution – there is nothing in life that need confound us. With our Higher Power's help, we can find the answer to any problem we face. This knowledge gives us courage to follow through with action. We need only be willing to accept the answer we receive.

How blessed is the man who does not walk in the counsel of the wicked, Nor stand in the path of sinners, Nor sit in the seat of scoffers! But his delight is in the law of the LORD, and in His law he meditates day and night. He will be like a tree firmly planted by streams of water, which yields its fruit in its season and its leaf does not wither; and in whatever he does, he prospers. (Psalm 1:1-4)

TODAY'S STEP: I avoid making excuses for my own or someone else's behavior. I practice keeping an open mind, to God, others and situations.

"Many of us find that as we practice treating others fairly, with love and respect, we ourselves become magnets for love and respect." -- . . . **In All Our Affairs**

<u>"To Keep It, You Have to Give It Away"</u>

Forgiveness is a release of feelings: we must feel them, deal with them, and give them up, so the space they took up can be filled with love. We don't have to forgive everyone at once, only as we can. When we want love more than hate, we will be willing to make the exchange.

Forgiveness is the key to loving ourselves. If we can choose not to forgive and hold on to our pain, we can also choose to let go, for there are two sides to everything. Mary A. Dombroski, Ph.D., has developed a helpful acronym for the forgiveness process called **ADDS:**

> **Awareness** means crossing the threshold of denial and acknowledging that the wrongs inflicted happened and that they hurt.

> **Discovering** means sharing those feelings with others, for communicating them make them real. We have been carrying the burden of our secret, and sharing that secret does away with it just as a sunrise does away with the night. Once a secret is shared, it loses its power and becomes real.

> **Decision** means a willingness to let go. Holding on to the discovery will give it power again. Detaching from it is a choice to make for health.

> **Serenity** is the healing gift of forgiveness.

Humility is about forgiving. It's learning to come to everyone with love, even people who have wronged us. It doesn't matter what people do. It's more important what we do!!!

Be kind to one another, tender-hearted, forgiving each other, just as God in Christ also has forgiven you. And walk in love, just as Christ also loved you and gave Himself up for us. (Ephesians 4:32; 5:2)

TODAY'S STEP: I search for Truth, and I allow others to do the same.

"If you have built castles in the air, your work need not be lost; that is where they should be. Now put foundations under them." -- Henry David Thoreau

"If Only . . . "

At a recent CODA meeting we were asked to fill in the blank in this statement: "If only ___________ would happen, I would be happy." Many of us were tempted to answer that we would be happy if our loved ones got sober or handled themselves differently. But the truth is other *"If only's"* also kept us feeling deprived: If only my boss, family, job, health, government, finances, would change in the way that I want, I would be happy. It became clear that many of us have put our happiness on hold for things beyond our control.

So we applied the First Step, and admitted that we were powerless over these people, places, and things. These *"If only's"* made our lives unmanageable, but a Power greater than ourselves could restore us to sanity. Many of us decided to surrender our 'if only's" to a Higher Power. When we did, we stopped acting like victims, waiting for things to change. We chose to take a more active role in seeking happiness in the here and now.

In Step Seven we concentrate on ridding ourselves of old tapes, old ideas and old patterns. Our objective is to open our minds and emotions to new possibilities; to think of ourselves as competent human beings whose capabilities and talents are continually developing and emerging.

In order to make room for positive action and reaction, we first need to rid ourselves of the old behaviors and characteristics that stand between us and our growth and well-being. These stumbling blocks have been in place for some time and removing them can be a tough task. We fall into old habits and old ideas so automatically, that it takes constant reappraisal to see where we are.

There are many areas of our lives we cannot change. What we can change is our attitude. Today we can accept our life as it is. We can be grateful and happy, here and now, with what we have.

...Rebellious people walk in a way that is not good, according to their own thoughts. (Isaiah 65:2)

TODAY'S STEP: Day by day, I entrust my problems to a power greater than myself.

"Today I'll use the slogan, "How important is it?" It will help me think things through before I act and it will give me a better picture of just what is important in my life." – **Alateen – A Day at a Time**

"How Important Is It?"

Are my priorities in order? Am I so busy with smaller, less meaningful concerns that I run out of time for the really important considerations? Am I taking time to enjoy the present moment? Am I becoming the person I want to be? Am I in touch with my Higher Power?

There are certain key tasks in which we must attain at least some degree of mastery in this life, if we are not to waste our time. They are:

1. Making a personal contact with God.

2. Healing and regenerating our own bodies.

3. Getting control of ourselves and finding our <u>True Purpose</u>.

4. Learning to handle other people both wisely and justly.

5. Perfecting a technique for getting direct personal inspiration for a general or specific purpose.

6. Letting go of the past completely.

7. Planning the future quantitatively and qualitatively, as led by my Higher Power.

To have made some real progress on each of these points, even though we may still be far short of mastery, is true success. Of course, we shall all advance farther in some of these directions than in others, but some progress must be made in each of them. Happiness, peace of mind, prosperity, and real health are within the reach of all who sincerely want them, and who are willing to pay the price, i.e., "to go to any lengths to achieve victory over ourselves."

For what is a man profited, if he shall gain the whole world, and lose his soul? Or what shall a man give in exchange for his soul? (Matthew 16:26)

TODAY'S STEP: I practice the discipline of H.O.W. – Honesty, Open-mindedness and Willingness everyday.

"The world cannot be discovered by a journey of miles ... only a spiritual journey ... by which we arrive at the ground at our feet, and learn to be at home." -- Wendell Berry

"Stick With the Winners"

A Scientist is one who asks, "How?"
A Philosopher is one who asks, "Why?"
A Mystic is one who sees life from the inside.
A Materialist is one who sees life from the outside.
A Poet is one who is a master of language.
A Politician is one who puts his party or his own career first.
A Statesman is one who puts his country first.
A Patriot is anyone who puts his country's interest above his own.
An Artist is one who makes beauty a religion.
A Hero is one who does the kind of thing that others are content to admire.
A Gentleman is one who never takes an advantage.
A Coward is one who sees the higher and chooses the lower.
A Fool is one who thinks that the Great Law can be evaded.
A Thief is one who tries to take something, which he has not earned.
A Gambler is one who thinks he can gain something which does not belong to him by
          right of consciousness.
An Adult is a person who has learned to control his emotions.
A Youthful person is one who is never bored.
An Elderly person is one who has lost the capacity for wonder.
A Saint is one who loves God more than he loves anything else.
A Pharisee is one who loves God to glorify himself.
A true Optimist is one who knows that there is only One Cause.
A Pessimist is really one who believes in many causes.

So watch yourselves. If your brother or sister sins against you, rebuke them; and if they repent, forgive them. Even if they sin against you seven times in a day and seven times come back to you saying 'I repent,' you must forgive them. (Luke 17: 3-4)

TODAY'S STEP: I practice the discipline of H.O.W. — Honesty, Open-mindedness and Willingness everyday.

"The only wisdom we can hope to acquire is the wisdom of humility; humility is endless."
-- T.S. Eliot, **Four Quarters, East Coker**

<u>Humbly Asked . . .</u>

In order for us to experience life-changing humility we must be aware that:

1. What we accomplish, amass, or achieve materially will never bring us true contentment nor the satisfaction of our innermost spiritual hunger; and

2. Surrender to God's leadership cannot occur until we acknowledge our own limitations and need for His guidance. We must surrender the leadership role to God.

What is entailed in this conversion? We admit and yield every character distortion to God's transforming touch. We open our every relationship to His guidance. We surrender to His care and discipline all addictive and compulsive behavior patterns. We ask without restraint that He be the God of our lives.

We need humility for three reasons:

1. So we can recognize the severity of our defects. One aspect of our addictions is we tend to deny and minimize the pain they inflict. Therefore, as we try to assess our character defects, we may, unless we take a very humble approach, underestimate their severity.

2. So we can acknowledge the limits of human power in addressing these character defects. We cannot do it on our own. We cannot do it by sheer willpower. We cannot do it by our own intellect and reasoning.

3. So we can appreciate the enormity of God's power to transform lives.

You younger men, likewise, be subject to your elders; and all of you, clothe yourselves with humility toward one another, for God is opposed to the proud, but gives grace to the humble. Therefore humble yourselves under the mighty hand of God, that He may exalt you at the proper time, casting all your anxiety on Him, because He cares for you. (1 Peter 5: 5-7)

TODAY'S STEP: I understand the true nature of humility. I recognize the ability to develop and practice it is the basic foundation of the Twelve Steps.

"You are asking yourself, as all of us must: 'Who am I?' . . . 'Where am I?' . . . 'Whence do I go?' The process of enlightenment is usually slow. But, in the end, our seeking always brings a finding. These great mysteries are, after all, enshrined in complete simplicity." -- Bill W., *Letter,* 1955

"We Demand Less and Give More"

In *The Big Book,* Bill W. talks about the five major factors involved in our spiritual fulfillment – (1) Strength, (2) Humility, (3) Understanding, (4) Emotional Stability, and (5) Peace of Mind.

1. Spiritual strength develops from our recognition of a Higher Power and our faith in its healing. It also develops from thinking through a personal spiritual philosophy.

2. We find humility when we follow the Twelve Step program, give up our obsession with control and management, and truly accept our equality as human beings.

3. Understanding comes when we break through denial and self-absorption and realize others struggle as we do.

4. Giving up our focus on our addiction, and allowing ourselves to accept love, care, and support of our Higher Power and the community of Twelve Step followers can bring us emotional stability.

5. And surrendering to powerlessness over our addiction and emotional pain, together with faith in the healing potential of our Higher Power, can give us peace of mind.

All discipline for the moment seems not to be joyful, but sorrowful; yet to those who have been trained by it, afterwards it yields the peaceful fruit of righteousness. (Hebrews 12:11)

TODAY'S STEP: The Steps offer me a road map for living that leads to a spiritual awakening and beyond. I can't skip ahead to the end of the journey – which can at times be a tough one – but I can put one foot in front of the other and follow the directions I've been given, knowing others who have gone before me have received more along the way than they had ever dreamed.

<u>**Step Eight**</u>

<u>"Made a list of all persons we had harmed, and became willing to make amends to them all."</u>

The first seven Steps are personal, in that they focus on examining our past behavior patterns and making us aware of our personal strengths and limitations. Step Eight begins the process of making adjustments to our lives as a result of what we have discovered in the previous Steps. By the time we reach this point in Recovery, we realize how important it is for us to let go of the painful memories of our past and the circumstances surrounding them. Releasing the past opens the door to healing and to a new life for us, a life based on living one day at a time in harmony with ourselves and others.

Step Eight brings us to the end of isolation from ourselves, our community and our Higher Power, and sets the course for restoring our relationships. We release the need to blame others for our misfortune and accept responsibility for our own lives. Our Step Four inventory revealed how our behavior caused injury to us as well as to others. In Step Eight, we document our personal conflicts with others, citing the dates and listing the names of all the people involved. We cannot effectively change our behaviors until we look at our past and eventually make restitution where needed. This is accomplished through careful examination and thoughtful analysis of what happened, when and to whom.

If we have conscientiously worked the first five Steps, we are usually aware of the harm we have caused to others by the time we reach Step Eight. We may even see we have become our own worst enemies, by allowing our attitudes toward ourselves to create excessive self-blame, guilt and shame. Guilt is remorse over having done or not done something we believe to be important. It is often an appropriate response to the regret we feel for actions or inactions that conflict with our personal values. Shame is a feeling of being deeply flawed or defective as a person, and causes us to view ourselves as bad or worthless. These are all unhealthy views of ourselves that can lead us into severe depression.

Step Eight helps us identify the damage we have done and prepares us for Step Nine. Our continued growth requires that we make amends, in order to reduce the likelihood of repeating our unhealthy patterns of behavior. A forgiving attitude will assist us with this work. If we do not accept and forgive ourselves, we cannot accept and forgive others. If we do not accept and forgive others as they are, we cannot make amends with dignity, self-respect and humility.

"Made a list of all persons we had harmed, and became willing to make amends to them all."

Higher Power, I ask Your help in making my list of all those I have harmed. I will take responsibility for my mistakes, and be forgiving to others as You are forgiving to me. Grant me the willingness to begin my restitution. This I pray.

In this moment, I see the impossible become not only possible but real. As I forgive myself for my shortcomings, I am able to forgive others, opening the way for a true and lasting change in my behavior. Thank you God.

MEDITATIONS

Faith has been the strength of saints and can withstand all cruel reasoning. The simplicity of faith is my need for today. Grant me this gift, dear Lord: When things go wrong, let me have faith; when I am challenged let me show faith; when I seek for answers, let me ask in faith. I put my day into Thy divine order, I ask Thee to be a part of all I do today. Let faith shine through my eyes so others in need of faith may share it. I will not demand answers today, I will not be concerned, for my faith is in Thee. I offer my day to all who are in need of Thy word. Let this day be an example to all and a worthwhile offering to my heavenly Father.

AFFIRMATIONS

My personal relationships are warm, meaningful, and richly rewarding. I am genuine and sincere at all times and with all people I meet – regardless of the situation or their relationship to me.

My friendliness is genuine and my sincerity is real. Because I like, enjoy, and accept others, friendliness and sincerity are habits with me.

Every day I am even more consciously aware of my relationships with others, how important they are, and the great value they hold in my life.

I believe in people. I greet each new relationship with faith and acceptance, and I consciously build the relationship toward trust and respect.

"Forgiveness is the answer to the child's dream of a miracle by which what is broken can be made whole again, what is soiled is again made clean." -- Dag Hammarskjold

<u>The Gift of Forgiveness</u>

Step Eight helps us identify the damage we have done and prepares us for Step Nine. Our continuing growth requires that we make amends, in order to reduce the likelihood of repeating our unhealthy patterns of behavior. A forgiving attitude will assist us with this work. If we do not accept and forgive ourselves, we cannot accept and forgive others. If we do not accept and forgive others as they are, we cannot make amends with dignity, self-respect and humility.

Making amends without extending forgiveness is meaningless and can lead us into further arguments or disputes. When looking at those we have harmed, we see that our ineffective behavior played a major part in sabotaging our lives and our relationships. For example:

- When we became angry, we often harmed ourselves more than others. This may have resulted in feelings of depression or self-pity.

- Persistent financial problems resulting from our irresponsible actions caused difficulty with our family and our creditors.

- When confronted with an issue about which we felt guilty, we lashed out at the other person rather than look honestly at ourselves.

- Frustrated by our lack of control, we behaved aggressively and intimidated those around us.

- Because of our indiscriminate sexual behavior, true intimacy was impossible to achieve or maintain.

- Our fear of abandonment sometimes destroyed our relationships, because we did not allow others to be themselves. We created dependency and tried to control their behavior in an effort to keep the relationship as we wanted it.

And forgive us our sins, for we also forgive everyone who is indebted to us. (Luke 11:14)

TODAY'S STEP: I ask God to free me from feelings of bitterness, resentment, anger, envy, and the desire for revenge in order that I receive the gift of forgiveness.

"Acceptance is not submission; it is acknowledgement of the facts of a situation. Then deciding what you're going to do about it." -- Kathleen Casey Theisen

Amends List Guidelines

The authors of **The 12 Steps for Adult Children: From Addictive and Other Dysfunctional Families,** list for us three categories in which we may have caused harm and for which we may want to make amends.

1. **MATERIAL ERRORS** – Actions which affected an individual in a tangible way.
   - Borrowing or spending extravagance; stinginess; spending in an attempt to buy friendship or love; withholding money in order to gratify ourselves.
   - Entering into agreements that are legally enforceable, cheating or refusing to abide by the terms.
   - Injuring or damaging persons or property as a result of our actions.

2. **MORAL ERRORS** – Inappropriate behavior in moral or ethical actions and

   conduct, including questions or rightness, fairness or equity. The principal issue is involving others in our wrong doing.

   - Setting a bad example for children, friends or anyone who looks to us for guidance.
   - Being preoccupied with selfish pursuits and using other people in the process.
   - Inflicting moral harm (e.g., sexual infidelity, broken promises, verbal abuse, lack of trust, lying).

3. **SPIRITUAL ERRORS** – "Acts of omission" as a result of neglecting our

   obligations to God, to ourselves, to family and to community.

   - Making no effort to fulfill our obligations and showing no gratitude toward others who have helped us.
   - Avoiding self-development (e.g., health, education, recreation, creativity).
   - Being inattentive to others in our lives by showing a lack of encouragement to them.

You have put gladness in my heart. . . . I will both lay me down in peace, and sleep: For You alone, O Lord, make me dwell in safety. (Psalm 4:7-8)

TODAY'S STEP: The Steps offer me a road map for living that leads to a spiritual awakening and beyond.

"Forgiving is not forgetting, it's letting go of the hurt." -- Mary McLeod Bethune

"Willingness Is The Key"

The technique of forgiveness is simple enough, and not very difficult to manage when you understand how. The only thing essential is **willingness** to forgive. Provided you desire to forgive the offender, the greater part of the work is already done.

People have traditionally had difficulty with forgiveness because they have been under the erroneous impression that to forgive a person means that you have to compel yourself to like him. People used to think when someone hurt them very much, it was their duty, as good Christians, to pump up, as it were, a feeling of liking for him; and since such a thing is utterly impossible, they suffered a great deal of distress, and ended, necessarily, with failure, and a resulting sense of sinfulness. We are not obliged to like anyone; but we are under a binding obligation to love everyone, love, or charity as the Bible calls it, meaning a vivid sense of good will.

The method of forgiving is this: Get by yourself and become quiet. Repeat any prayer that appeals to you, or read a chapter of the Bible. Then quietly say:

"I fully and freely forgive <u>X</u> (mentioning the name of the offender); I loose him/her and let him/her go. I completely forgive the whole business in question. As far as I am concerned, it is finished forever. I cast the burden of resentment upon the Christ within me. He/she is free now, and I am free too. I wish him/her well in every phase of his/her life. That incident is finished. The Christ Truth has set us both free. I thank God."

Afterward, whenever the memory of the offender or the offense happens to come into your mind, bless the offender briefly and dismiss the thought. Do this however many times the thought may come back. After a few days it will return less and less often, until you forget it altogether. The result of this exercise will be that very soon you will find yourself cleared of all resentment and condemnation, and the effect upon your happiness, your bodily health, and your general life will be nothing less than miraculous.

Put aside and rid myself of: anger, rage, bad feelings toward others, slander and abusive speech from my mouth. Put on my new self who is being renewed. (Colossians 3:8-10)

TODAY'S STEP: I ask God to free me from feelings of bitterness, resentment, anger, envy, and the desire for revenge in order that I receive the gift of forgiveness.

"Adversity is sometimes hard upon a man; but for one man who can stand prosperity, there are a hundred that will stand adversity." -- Thomas Carlyle, *The Hero as Man of Letters*

Great Dreams Can Turn into Riches

According to Dr. Napoleon Hill's classic book, *Think and Grow Rich,* we who are in the race for riches should be encouraged to know this changed world in which we live is demanding new ideas, new literature, new features for television, new ideas for movies. Behind all this demand for new and better things, there is one quality which one must possess to win, and that is **definiteness of purpose –** the knowledge of what one wants, and a burning desire to possess it.

A burning desire to be and to do is the starting point from which the dreamer must take off. There is, however, a difference between wishing for a thing and being ready to receive it. No one is ready for a thing until he believes he can acquire it. The state of mind must be belief, not mere hope or wish. Open-mindedness is essential for belief. Closed minds do not inspire faith, courage or belief.

Remember, no more effort is required to aim high in life, to demand abundance and prosperity, than is required to accept misery and poverty. A great poet had correctly stated this universal truth through these lines:

> I bargained with Life for a penny,
> And Life would pay no more,
> However, I begged at evening
> When I counted my scanty store;
>
> For Life is a just employer,
> He gives you what you ask,
> But once you have set the wages,
> Why, you must bear the task.
>
> I worked for a menial's hire,
> Only to learn, dismayed,
> That any wage I had asked of Life,
> Life would have paid.
>   (*My Wage,* by Jessie B. Rittenhouse)

Poor is he who works with a negligent hand, but the hand of the diligent makes one rich. (Proverbs 10:4)

TODAY'S STEP: I trust Truth, my instincts, and my ability to ground myself in reality.

"Failure is, in a sense, the highway to success, inasmuch as every discovery of what is false leads us to seek earnestly after what is true, and every fresh experience points out some form of error which we shall afterward carefully avoid." -- John Keats

<u>"Don't Quit 5 Minutes Before the Miracle Happens"</u>

<u>REMEMBER</u> – one day at a time is enough of a commitment! We do not need to overwhelm ourselves by thinking we will <u>NEVER</u> smoke again. Sometimes saying NEVER is self-defeating! If you need to, say, "I will not smoke for one minute, two minutes . . . three minutes . . . one hour," etc., just keep adding a little bit of time together and you'll make it through the day. Whatever it takes to keep from lighting that first cigarette!

After not smoking for some time you may begin to wonder if a cigarette will taste as good as you remember. <u>IT WOULD.</u> This phenomenon is called <u>EUPHORIC RECALL.</u> When you experience <u>EUPHORIC RECALL</u> it would be wise to also remember the reasons you quit in the first place: the hacking smoker cough, the tight chest, the sore throat, the awful taste in the mouth, the smell of stale smoke on your body and belongings, the cigarette burns in the furniture, on your clothing and your body; and the ultimate threat of impending cancer! <u>EUPHORIC RECALL</u> is your biggest <u>ENEMY!</u> Don't try to test waters!

As time accumulates, the pain of quitting lessens and lessens and soon I will be able to spend hours, days, and even weeks without <u>THINKING</u> about smoking!

When I get into my self-pity and begin to feel it's not fair I had to give up smoking and I think "Why me?" <u>I REMEMBER THIS: – NO ONE MADE ME QUIT – I CHOSE TO QUIT TO BE HEALTHIER! TO SMELL FRESH AND CLEAN! TO FEEL BETTER! TO LIVE LONGER!, ETC., ETC., ETC. THESE ARE ALL POSITIVE CHOICES – I AM GLAD I MADE THEM!</u>

Have I thought about how grateful I am that I stopped smoking <u>BEFORE</u> I got lung cancer or emphysema? <u>HOW GRATEFUL I AM THAT I AM STILL ALIVE?</u>

I like coming home to a house that doesn't stink from stale tobacco! I like not having that foul taste in my mouth! I like having clean windows in my car! I like not having to worry about offending others with my smoke! <u>NOT SMOKING IS SUCH A CLEAN THING TO DO!</u>

Cast your burden upon the Lord and He will sustain you; He will never allow the righteous to be shaken. (Psalm 55:22)

TODAY'S STEP: By calling on my Higher Power for help daily, I can turn my failures into an opportunity to learn and grow.

"If you have behaved badly, repent, make what amends you can and address yourself to the task of behaving better next time. On no account brood over wrongdoing. Rolling in the muck is not the best way of getting clean." -- Aldous Huxley

<u>Willing to Make Amends</u>

The Eighth Step is talking about a change of heart, a healing change. This attitude can begin a great chain of repair and healing in our relationships with others and ourselves. It means we become willing to let go of our hard-heartedness – one of the greatest blocks to our ability to give and receive love.

In the Eighth Step, we make a list of all people we have harmed, and we allow ourselves to experience a healing attitude toward them. It is an attitude of love.

We do not, in this Step, dash madly about and begin yelling, "Sorry!" We make our list not to feel guilty, but to facilitate healing. Before we actually make amends or begin to consider appropriate amends, we allow ourselves to change our attitude. That is where healing begins – within us. It can begin the process, before we ever open our mouths and say sorry.

How often have we, after we have been hurt, wished the person would simply die of a broken heart. How often are we involved in relationships tainted by unfinished business and bad feelings? Often?

Others do too. It is no secret. Healing begins with us. Our willingness to make amends may or may not benefit the other person; he or she may or may not be willing to put matters to rest. But we become healed. We become capable of love.

PRAY: God, I ask you to change my heart if hard-heartedness, defensiveness, guilt, or bitterness are present. Thank you, Lord for helping restore my health and my relationships.

Behold, I will bring health and healing, and I will heal you; and I will reveal to you an abundance of peace and truth. (Jeremiah 33:6)

TODAY'S STEP: I trust "The Program" works if I work it and I can be restored to wholeness with God's help.

"Happy the man, and happy he alone,
He, who can call to-day his own:
He who, secure within, can say:
'To-morrow, do thy worst, for I have liv'd today.'" -- Horace

The writer John Ruskin had on his desk a simple piece of stone on which was carved one word: **TODAY.** And while I haven't a piece of stone on my desk, I do have framed copies of the *Serenity Prayer* and a poem written by the famous Indian dramatist, Kalidasa:

Salutation to the Dawn

Look to this day!
For it is life, the very life of life.
In its brief course
Lie all the verities and realities of your existence:
The bliss of growth
The glory of action
The splendor of beauty,
For yesterday is but a dream
And tomorrow is only a vision,
But today well lived makes every yesterday a day
Of happiness
And every tomorrow a vision of hope.
Look well, therefore, to this day!
Such is the salutation to the dawn.

"Think," said Dante, "that this day will never dawn again." Life is slipping away with incredible speed. We are racing through space at the rate of nineteen miles per second. **Today** is our most precious possession. *It is our only sure possession!*

"How strange it is, our little procession of life!" wrote Stephen Leacock. "The child says, 'When I am a big boy.' But what is that? The big boy says, 'When I grow up.' And then, grown up, he says, 'When I get married.' But to be married, what is that after all? The thought changes to 'When I'm able to retire.' And then, when retirement comes, we look back over the landscape traversed; a cold wind seems to sweep over it; somehow we have missed it all, and it is gone. Life, we learn too late, is in the living, in the tissue of every day and hour."

So do not worry about tomorrow; for tomorrow will care for itself. Each day has enough trouble of its own. (Matthew 6:34)

TODAY'S STEP: I ask my Higher Power to help me let go of fear, doubt, and anxiety; and fill me with faith, trust and serenity.

"One receives only that which is given. The game of life is a game of boomerangs. Our thoughts, deeds, and words, return to us sooner or later, with astounding accuracy." -- Florence Scovel Shin

Tradition Eight

Members helping members is Al-Anon Twelfth-Step work in action. We are not experts, therefore non-professional. We talk from our own experiences, we share our joy and pain, we share our growth. A portion of our members may be employed as professionals; however, they come to Al-Anon because of their personal involvement with alcoholism. At their place of employment, they counsel; in Al-Anon they share their experience, strength, and hope.

Long-time members may feel they have grown to such an extent; they have the right to give advice. Aren't these people acting as Al-Anon professionals? Members can only give what they have received. Therefore, when we share, it is best to share only what we have experienced – from the "I" point of view. A Chairperson of one group, and long-time member, felt he had to give advice to each person who shared. Was it any wonder members became uncomfortable when their turn came around? They didn't want to be told what to do – they wanted to hear what others did, and choose for themselves.

We have members employed in Al-Anon service offices, e.g. Inter-Group, World Service Office, Literature Distribution Centers and Al-Anon Information Offices. They are paid workers, but by no means are they in authority. Their work in Al-Anon must not be confused with Twelfth-Step work, e.g. Alateen sponsoring, or Institutions work, etc.

Tradition Eight reminds us that our Twelve-Step work is always non-professional. We share our Recovery based on our experience, strength and hope; mindful not to tell others what to do. We only share what we have done, and let others choose their own plan of action.

For I am persuaded that neither death nor life, nor angels nor principalities . . . , nor things present nor things to come, . . . nor any other created thing, shall be able to separate us from the love of God. (Romans 8:38-39)

TODAY'S STEP: As I work the Steps, I grow in my capacity to be happy.

"There is a time in every man's education when he arrives at the conviction that envy is ignorance; that imitation is suicide; that he must take himself for better, for worse, as his portion; that though the wide universe is full of good, no kernel of nourishing corn can come to him but through his toil bestowed on that plot of ground which is given him to till. The power which resides in him is new in nature, and none but he knows what that is, which he can do, nor does he know until he has tried." -- Ralph Waldo Emerson, ***Self-Reliance***

I Promise Myself!

I promise myself:

To be so strong that nothing can disturb my peace of mind.

To talk health, happiness, and prosperity to every person I meet.

To make all my friends feel that there is something in them.

To look at the sunny side of everything and make my optimism come true.

To think only of the best, to work only for the best, and expect only the best.

To be just as enthusiastic about the success of others as I am bout my own.

To forget the mistakes of the past and press on to the greater achievements of the future.

To wear a cheerful countenance at all times and give every living creature I meet a smile.

To give so much time to the improvement of myself that I have no time to criticize others.

To be too large for worry, too noble for anger, too strong for fear, and too happy to permit the presence of trouble.

For our rejoicing is this, the testimony of our conscience, that in simplicity and godly sincerity . . . we have had our conversations in the world. (2 Corinthians 1:12)

TODAY'S STEP: I have faith that daily work on myself will result in my becoming the best person I can be.

"The most important thing in life is not to capitalize on our gains. Any fool can do that. The really important thing is to profit from your losses. That requires intelligence; and it makes the difference between a man of sense and a fool." -- William Bolitho

If It's Going To Be, It's Up To Me

The world doesn't give me a living –

If It's Going To Be, It's Up To Me

Society won't give you moral and ethical character –

If It's Going To Be, It's Up To Me

The university will not give you an education –

If It's Going To Be, It's Up To Me

Business doesn't owe me a job –

If It's Going To Be, It's Up To Me

Religious institutions will not save my soul –

If It's Going To Be, It's Up To Me

The minister who unites me in marriage to my spouse

won't give me a lifetime of happiness and harmony –

If It's Going To Be, It's Up To Me

The medical establishment can't give me good health –

If It's Going To Be, It's Up To Me

A new sunrise doesn't promise to give me a great day –

If It's Going To Be, It's Up To Me

I do not lose heart, but though my outer being is decaying, yet my inner being is being renewed day by day. My present troubles are small and won't last very long. (2 Corinthians 4:16-17)

TODAY'S STEP: I need to believe in myself and my dreams.

"The turbulent billows of the fretful surface leave the deep parts of the ocean undisturbed; and to him who has a hold on vaster and more permanent realities, the hourly vicissitudes of his personal destiny seem relatively insignificant things. The really religious person is accordingly unshaken and full of equanimity, and calmly ready for any duty that the day may bring forth." -- William James

<u>Six Ways to Prevent Fatigue and Worry</u>

One of England's most distinguished psychiatrists, J.A. Hadfield, said, "The greater part of fatigue which we suffer is of mental origin; in fact exhaustion of purely physical origin is rare." Here are some suggestions from Dale Carnegie's book ***How to Stop Worrying and Start Living*** to help us learn how to prevent fatigue and worry:

<u>**RULE 1**</u>: Rest before you get tired.

<u>**RULE 2**</u>: Learn to relax at work.

<u>**RULE 3**</u>: Learn to relax at home.

<u>**RULE 4**</u>: Apply these four good working habits:

- Clear your desk of all papers except those relating to the immediate problem at hand.

- Do things in the order of their importance.

- When you face a problem, solve it then and there if you have the facts necessary to make a decision.

- Learn to organize, deputize, and supervise.

<u>**RULE 5**</u>: To prevent worry and fatigue, put enthusiasm into your work.

<u>**RULE 6**</u>: Remember, no one was ever killed by lack of sleep. It is worrying about insomnia that does the damage – not the insomnia. If you can't sleep get up and work or read until you do feel sleepy. Exercise. Get yourself so physically tired you can't stay awake.

Anxiety in a man's heart weighs it down, But a good word makes it glad. (Proverbs 12:25)

TODAY'S STEP: I ask my Higher Power to help me let go of fear, doubt, and anxiety; and to fill me with faith, trust and serenity.

"Come to Me, all who are weary and heavy laden, and I will give you rest. Take my yoke upon you, and learn from Me, for I am gentle and humble in heart; and You shall find rest for your souls." -- Matthew 11:28,29 (NASB)

<u>The First Step to Healing</u>

In light of this promise in Matthew, it's fascinating to find that virtually everyone in the New Testament who desired healing came to Him. Either they came personally or a surrogate or an intercessor came on their behalf. Effort or action was required. They had to seek Him out. They had to find Him out. They had to find Him, and come to Him – and He never turned any away!

A leaper **came to Him**	Matthew 8:2
A centurion **came to Him**	Matthew 8:5
They brought to Him many	Matthew 8:16
They brought to Him a paralytic	Matthew 9:2
A woman suffering from a hemorrhage **came**	Matthew 9:20
Two blind men followed Him, **crying out**	Matthew 9:27
A man demon-possessed was **brought to Him**	Matthew 9:32
A Canaanite woman **came**	Matthew 15:22
Great multitudes **came, bringing** many others	Matthew 15:30
A man **came to Him** for his son	Matthew 17:14
Two blind men **cried out to Him**	Matthew 20:30

Shouldn't we also come to Him to be healed of our addictions and our emotional pain? Many who came to Him for healing were willing to pay the price. They were willing, in many cases, to walk a long journey to find Him in order that they might come to Him. Our work today is not as difficult. We already know where to find Him. We do not have to search for Him. **We only need come to Him!**

For my yoke is easy, and my burden is light. (Matthew 11:30)

TODAY'S STEP: I trust "The Program" works if I work it and that I can be restored to wholeness with God's help.

"No longer must we accumulate burdens of guilt or resentment that will become heavier and more potent over time. Each day, each new moment can be an opportunity to clear the air and start again, fresh and free . . . A part of me wants to cling to old resentments, but I know the more I forgive, the better my life works." -- *. . . In All Our Affairs*

"Drop the Rock"

Forgiveness is the key to loving yourself. If you can choose not to forgive and hold on to your pain, you can also choose to let go, for there are two sides to everything. Mary A. Dombroski, Ph.D., has developed a helpful acronym for the forgiveness process called **ADDS:**

A   **Awareness** means crossing the threshold of denial and acknowledging that he wrongs inflicted happened and that they hurt.

D   **Discovering** means sharing those feelings with others, for communicating them makes them real. You have been carrying the burden of your secret, and sharing that secret does away with it just as a sunrise does away with night. Once a secret is shared, it loses its power and becomes real.

D   **Decision** means a willingness to let go. Holding on to the discovery will give it power again. Detaching from it is a choice to make for health.

S   **Serenity** is the healing gift of forgiveness.

When people don't forgive, it's about false pride and being judgmental. Humility is about forgiving. It's learning to come to everyone with love, even people who have wronged you. It doesn't matter what people do. It's more important what you do.

Make a list of three people who have hurt you. Write each one a letter, describing in detail the harm they did to you and how it has affected your life. Describe the feelings you still carry about their deeds. Take each letter, crumble it in a ball, put it in a sink, and set fire to it. As it burns, say, "I forgive you." When the letters are nothing but ashes, dispose of them, clean the sink, and get on with the business of living.

Judge not, and ye shall not be judged. Condemn not, and ye shall not be condemned. Forgive, and ye shall be forgiven. (Luke 6:37)

TODAY'S STEP: I ask God to free me from feelings of bitterness, resentment, anger, envy, and the desire for revenge in order that I receive the gift of forgiveness.

"We cannot tell what may happen to us in the strange medley of life. But we can decide what happens in us – how we can take it, what to do with it – and that is what really counts in the end." -- Joseph Fort Newton

<u>Ten Points of a Positive Mental Attitude</u>

The following questions will help you to formulate thoughts for an effective life adjustment:

1. Check your personality temperature. Happiness is a by product, a result, of effective life adjustment. If you're not happy, what could you do to make your life more fun?
2. Do you have a zest for living? Can you be the developer of excitement and enthusiasm?
3. Are you socially adjusted? Do you like being with and sharing with others?
4. Do you have balance and unity? Balance is needed when you find yourself wrapping your life around one thing or one person. Unity is doing something or not doing something and then refusing to worry about it.
5. Can you live with each problem in your life as it arises? Do you worry about the future or the past? Of all the things you worried about last year, how many of them came true?
6. Do you have insight into your own conduct? Insight means you know the real underlying reasons for what you do.
7. Do you have a confidential relationship with some other person?
8. Do you have a sense of the ridiculous – of what the world does to you? Can you laugh at yourself? If you look to see who laughs and who doesn't, you need to work in this area of your mental attitude.
9. Are you engaged in satisfying work?
10. Do you know how to worry effectively? Overcome your worries by going to the proper people for help.

Positive self-esteem is the single most important quality in a salesperson, manager, leader, mother, father, or child. It is the feeling that I accept and believe in myself as a changing, imperfect, growing human being. Self-esteem is based on what you are going to do and what you feel you deserve. We see people holding back because they don't want the loneliness that comes with distancing from others who are jealous when you excel, The truth is we all want to belong and know we are enough.

Commit my works unto the Lord, and my thoughts shall be established. (Proverbs 16:3)

TODAY'S STEP: I accept who I am, where I am, and I continue to reach forward one day at a time.

"I cannot expect anyone to help me unless I am willing to share that I need help." -- *. . .
In All Our Affairs*

The Addictive Personality Profile

The following are characteristics of the addictive personality. Put a check by the ones with which you identify:

______ **Emotional Extremes.** You don't know anger, you know rage; you don't know   fear, you know panic; you don't know pleasure, you know euphoria. With   you it's all or nothing.

______ **Need for Intensity.** You don't relate to feelings, nor facts; you crave   excitement; you thrive on chaos.

______ **Need for Immediate Gratification.** You want what you want when you want it

and you want it now.

______ **Extreme Thinking.** You are either all wrong or you don't make mistakes. A

situation is either black or white, but never gray.

______ **Lack of Identity.** You need externals to feel alive. You must always be doing

something, and you over identify with whatever it is.

______ **Lack of Boundaries.** You don't know where you end and someone else begins.

______ **Lack of Moderation.** Whatever you do, you overdo. If something works, taking more of it will work better. You have a pattern of playing at cards for hours, or at sports until you drop from exhaustion.

______ **Over-Reaction.** You over-react to things outside of you and under-react to things inside of you.

______ **People Pleasing.** You are always looking for approval from others because you

can't give it to yourself.

______ **Low Self-Esteem.** You never feel you're good enough.

______ **Isolation.** You feel as if you don't belong anywhere.

______ **Judgmental Attitude.** You are constantly judging and defending both yourself and others.

______ **Need for Excitement.** If you create enough chaos in your life, you don't have to look at what's really going on.

______ **Poverty Mentality.** You worry there won't be enough of what you crave.

For God has not given me the spirit of fear; but of power, and of love, and of a sound mind. (2 Timothy 1:7)

TODAY'S STEP: I let go of denial and accept responsibility for myself and my life.

"The mind is its own place, and in itself can make a heaven of Hell, a hell of Heaven." -- John Milton

Dale Carnegie, the famous author of **How to Win Friends and Influence People,** also wrote **How to Stop Worrying and Start Living.** This book teaches us the mental attitudes we need to learn.

<u>Seven Ways to Peace and Happiness</u>

<u>RULE 1</u>: Let's fill our minds with thoughts of peace, courage, health, and hope, for "our life is what our thoughts make it."

<u>RULE 2</u>: Let's never try to get even with our enemies, because if we do we will hurt ourselves far more than we hurt them. Let's never waste a minute thinking about people we don't like.

<u>RULE 3</u>: A. Instead of worrying about ingratitude, let's expect it. Let's remember that Jesus healed ten lepers in one day – and only one thanked Him. Why should we expect more gratitude than Jesus got?
B. The only way to find happiness is not to expect gratitude – but to give for the joy of giving.
C. Gratitude is a "cultivated" trait; so if we want our children to be grateful, we must train them to be grateful.

<u>RULE 4</u>: Count your blessings – not your troubles!

<u>RULE 5</u>: Let's not imitate others. Let's find ourselves and be ourselves, for "envy is ignorance" and "imitation is suicide."

<u>RULE 6</u>: When fate hands us a lemon, let's make lemonade.

<u>RULE 7</u>: Let's forget our own unhappiness – by trying to create a little happiness for others.

Prove yourself doers of the word, and not merely hearers who delude ourselves. (James 1:22)

TODAY'S STEP: Instead of fretting about what I can't have or can't do, I'll take action to create something positive in my life today.

"I hope my achievements in life shall be these – that I will have fought for what was right and fair, that I will have risked for that which mattered, that I will have given help to those who were in need . . . that I will have left the earth a better place for what I've done and who I've been." -- C. Hoppe

Types of Twelve-Step Meetings

Twelve-Step meetings are divided into two primary types, open meetings and closed meetings, each having its own function within the fellowship (***Alcoholics Anonymous,*** 1993).

Open Meetings.   These meetings welcome any interested person.   Twelve-Step fellowships recognize that visitors may be motivated to attend an open meeting for a number of reasons. Individuals may feel a need to explore a personal drinking or drug problem, may be concerned about a friend or family member, or may simply be interested in learning about the 12-Step process. All are welcome at open meetings. The only obligation placed on attendance is that of honoring the anonymity of others by not disclosing names outside of the meeting.

Closed Meetings.   Depending on the specific fellowship involved, these meetings may be limited to alcoholics or addicts, those affected by another's drinking or drug use, or those who think they have a drinking or drug use problem. Closed meetings more surely safeguard member's anonymity and provide a more secure forum for the discussion of problems best understood by fellow members of a specific fellowship. The meetings are usually informal and encourage participation in the discussion. Newcomers and those who may be concerned about their anonymity within the community often find closed meetings particularly helpful.

Groups composed only of individuals with similar interests or backgrounds, such as health professionals, usually opt for a closed meeting format. By holding closed meetings, professionals can more freely discuss issues that would not be appropriate in a diverse group and can avoid encountering problems with doctor-patient or attorney-client relationships that might occur at open meetings. A number of professional self-help groups have been established in recent years, such as International Doctors in Alcoholics Anonymous.

Therefore accept one another, just as Christ also accepted me to the glory of God. (Romans 15:7)

TODAY'S STEP: When I rely on my Higher Power's help I can achieve.

"Daily vigilance will turn out to be a small price to pay for my peace of mind." --
The Dilemma of the Alcoholic Marriage

"Pass It On"

Within the two types of 12-Step meetings, there are several basic formats that meetings can take, although there are many variations in different areas of the U.S. and abroad.

Discussion meetings   These are the most common type of AA meetings, with other 12-Step fellowships usually following a similar format.   A member presides at a discussion meeting, opening with a topic involving Recovery.   Recurring themes include problems in maintaining abstinence; relationships; resentments; spirituality; and dealing with fear and anger.

Speaker meetings.   At these meetings, a member is asked to tell his or her story at the meeting. Although the speaker may talk for the entire meeting, many times a speaker's presentation will be limited to 20-30 minutes, followed by a discussion of a topic chosen by the speaker or a volunteer. The first time a member tells his/her story at a meeting is an important event and marks a positive growth experience.

Step meetings.   These meetings, which incorporate the Twelve Steps, provide a blueprint for developing individual spiritual growth within the fellowship. They usually begin by reading and discussing Step One at the first session and focusing on the following steps at subsequent meetings.

Book meetings.   These meetings are similar to Step meetings, but involve initial reading from AA's *"Big Book"* or other fellowship publications, such as ***Living Sober: Some Methods AA Members Have Used for Not Drinking*** or ***Came to Believe . . .: The Spiritual Adventure of AA as Experienced by Individual Members***. Passages are read and discussed as above.

Other meeting formats.   Some meetings adopt one particular format, which may be reflected in the meeting name, such as "12 and 12 Study," "Big Book Study," "Speaker's Meeting," or "Grapevine Discussion." Meetings may vary their format by holding 3 weeks of speaker-discussion meetings, then one Step meeting. There are no established rules on meeting format and meetings may vary among fellowships and groups.

. . . endeavoring to keep the unity of the Spirit in the bond of peace. (Ephesians 4:3)

TODAY'S STEP: I allow myself to feel my feelings without guilt or shame.

"If you are reluctant to ask the way, you will be lost." -- Malay Proverb

"Ninety and Ninety"
(90 Meetings in 90 Days)

The common wisdom of Twelve Step programs is that Newcomers should go to 90 meetings in 90 days to get started. The intensive and prolonged immersion in the 12-Step fellowship produced by attending meetings daily for three months provides the support, reorientation, and beginning behavioral changes that are necessary to break the grip of active addiction and to begin the process of Recovery.

Without intense and prolonged exposure, the behaviors, feelings, thoughts, and attitudes that provide the foundation for addictive behavior commonly persist, even if they are temporarily obscured under unusual circumstances or with great effort. The 90/90 prescription often initiates profound change in the addicted person. During this time, the alcoholic or addict has the opportunity to: (1) Meet new friends who are abstinent and supportive; (2) Learn to have fun without using alcohol or drugs; and, (3) Begin the quest to find a sponsor.

The peer support that is offered at 12-Step meetings is an important aspect of the program. Having a new social system to replace the former drug/alcohol or compulsive behavior involved life style strongly enhances Recovery. Addicts who can identify with other members of the fellowship in the quest of Recovery offer an acceptance, understanding, and empathy that is not available from the non-addicted.

Other 12-Step fellowships have borrowed the steps and traditions of AA and adapted them to their own specific problems. Narcotics Anonymous, in spite of its name, is somewhat more inclusive and welcomes individuals regardless of their drug of choice. Many other fellowships (including AA) believe their strength derives in part from the stronger identity and the validity of shared experience that the focus on alcoholism allows. However, in this age of dual addictions, most AA groups welcome to the fellowship people with other addictions, as long as they are or have been active alcoholics and currently have a desire not to drink alcohol.

Therefore encourage one another and build up one another . . . (1 Thessalonians 5:11)

TODAY'S STEP: I recognize and accept whatever feelings pass through me.

"No man can think clearly when his fists are clenched." -- George Jean Nathan

<u>"Anger Is But One Letter Away From Danger"</u>

Angry people aren't always able to see the fullness of their destructive behavior. This destructive behavior hurts them and it also hurts others. Anger without control is very damaging to relationships. Anger itself is not wrong, but expressing it in ways that damage relationships is wrong.

Inappropriate anger expressed to others cuts deeply. It hurts other's self-esteem. Inappropriate expression of anger is expressing the anger only for yourself. Appropriate expression of anger is expressing the anger for the benefit of yourself and the person(s) to whom you express it. You need to face the impact of your anger with others. You need to take responsibility for your behavior when you have expressed inappropriate anger.

Unbridled expression of anger is very damaging. Expressing your anger by raging at other people is rarely appropriate. When you do this, you stir up strife and broken relationships. If you desire to build relationships, you will express your anger in a way that will be best received by the other person.

For rageaholics it takes very little to provoke an unnecessary and unwarranted attack. Perhaps someone cuts you off on the highway, then your wife asks you to make a quick stop. Instead of raging at her, stop and think about what occurred. Recognize that you are angry at the man who just cut you off and that the stop she wants to make is a minor change in plans. Get things into perspective; then share your real anger with her. If you take the time to think when you feel rage about to flow, you may find many of the issues are really insignificant.

Before you speak is it:

> **T** rue ?
> **H** elpful ?
> **I** nspiring ?
> **N** ecessary ?
> **K** ind ?

Learn to control your anger. A big step toward controlling anger is to be slow in expressing it. Don't react in your anger. Stop and think about how to express your anger appropriately.

He who is slow to anger has great understanding, But he who is quick-tempered shows foolishness. (Proverbs 14:29)

TODAY'S STEP: I am seeking a saner approach to everything I encounter. The slogans are a valuable source of sanity in chaotic situations. If I am tempted to act out anger or frustration, I will remember to pause and "Think.

No Sorrow I Can't Heal
by Jo Winkowitsch

Like a child who scrapes her knee,
I sometimes limp to God for love.
It feels so safe in my Father's arms
As He lifts me up above.
But though I need such comfort
I know I often run away . . .
Causing untreated wounds to hinder
What I think and do and say . . .

It's easier to cover up my sores
So none can see them bleed.
But then I miss such opportunities
To show how God can meet each need.
I will not market misery,
Or flaunt it for selfish gain.
But I have to find the balance
As I allow God to heal the pain.

Most of us have scars of suffering
And a cross that we must bear . . .
God's children are never left alone –
His comfort's always there!
Christ remains the perfect Band-Aid . . .
For He sees pain's shape and length.
Any injury will not destroy us
If we trust God's power and strength.

As I work through years of denial . . .
Toward what God wants me to be,
I must deal with the rancid heartache
Of the little girl who hides in me.
Freedom from dreams that torment
Is part of His miraculous goal . . .
If I depend on Christ completely,
His love will medicate my soul.
When memories hit my heart with hurt,
Christ knows just how I feel.
And throughout my life He's been whispering . . .
"You have **no sorrow** I can't heal."

I am with you and will watch over you wherever you go . . . (Genesis 28:15)

TODAY'S STEP: I trust "The Program Works If I Work It" and I can be restored to wholeness with God's help.

"We acknowledge our faults in order to repair by our sincerity the damage they have done us in the eyes of others." -- La Rochefoucauld

"Easy Does It, But Do It"

By the time we reach this point in Recovery, we realize how important it is for us to let go of painful memories of our past and the circumstances surrounding them. Releasing the anger and resentment from our past opens the door to healing and to a new life for us, a life based on living one day at a time in harmony with ourselves and others.

Step Eight helps us identify the damage we have done and prepares us for Step Nine. Our continued growth requires that we make amends, in order to reduce the likelihood of repeating our unhealthy patterns of behavior. If we do not accept and forgive ourselves, we cannot accept and forgive others. If we do not accept and forgive others as they are, we cannot make amends. Making amends without extending forgiveness is meaningless and can lead us into further arguments or disputes. Our capacity to make amends must stem from a sincere desire to forgive and be forgiven.

When we look at those we have harmed, we see that our ineffective behavior played a major part in sabotaging our lives and our relationships. For example:

- When we became angry, we often harmed ourselves more than others. This may have resulted in feelings of depression or self-pity.
- Persistent financial problems resulting from our irresponsible actions caused difficulty with our family and our creditors.
- When confronted with an issue about which we felt guilty, we lashed out at the other person rather than look honestly at ourselves.
- Frustrated by our lack of control, we behaved aggressively and intimidated those around us.
- Because of our indiscriminate sexual behavior, true intimacy was impossible to achieve or maintain.

Forgive us our trespasses, as we forgive them that trespass against us. (Matthew 6:12)

TODAY'S STEP: I am seeking a saner approach to everything I encounter. The slogans are a valuable source of sanity in chaotic situations. If I am tempted to act out of anger or frustration, I will remember "Easy Does It", and "Think".

"Where there is an open mind, there will always be a frontier." -- Charles F. Kettering

<u>"Keep an Open Mind"</u>

God gives us everything we need and the strength, will, and courage to do whatever we want to do. That's the gift, but it always requires our active participation. And if God doesn't want us to have something we want, He stops us dead in our tracks. It happens every time! Sometimes it takes us a while to understand why we shouldn't have it. We must trust it's for our good or some other higher meaning that we may not understand at the time. Someday we will come to know it was in our best interest because God had a better plan in mind for us.

What do you want? If God wants you to have it, He will give you the gift necessary to achieve your goal.

The following visualization/meditation is designed to put you in a frame of mind to receive the kind of gift you need the most:

1. Sit comfortably, close your eyes, and relax

2. Breathe in and out ten times and focus on your breathing.

3. In your imagination you are walking along the beach. What do you see, feel, hear and smell?

4. Now sit down on the sand. Feel the water as it comes into the shore and then watch it go back out.

5. There is a gift here for you. You need to start digging in the sand until the gift appears.

6. When you have found your gift, look it over, touch it, listen to it, and smell it.

7. Place the gift in a safe place where you can enjoy it whenever you want to remember this special moment to nurture yourself.

God will keep me strong... He always does what he says he will do... He is the one who invited me into this wonderful friendship . . . (1 Corinthians 1: 8-9)

TODAY'S STEP: I move comfortably toward my wholeness, knowing my steps are guided by my Higher Power.

"No matter what the difficulty, no matter how unique we may feel, somewhere nearby are men and women with similar stories who have found help, comfort, and hope through Recovery in Al-Anon." -- *. . . In All Our Affairs*

<u>"We're all Here Because We're Not All There"</u>

The defensive roles in the following list are common among fearful people. The quotations are typical responses to help you identify them. Which roles do you play? What are the advantages of each? When do you find it necessary to assume the role? Examine the fear that motivates it. What would happen if you didn't need to play these roles?

1.	SUPERMAN/WONDER WOMAN	"I know what to do."
2.	PERFECT PETER	"Of course I always do it right.. What's the problem?"
3.	PLEASING POLLY	"I want to make you happy."
4.	BLAMING BETTY	"Why can't you do it right?"
5.	FIXING FANNY	"I'll take care of it."
6.	PAUL THE PROPHET	"It'll never work anyway."
7.	NEVER-MIND NELLY	"It doesn't matter."
8.	CHARLIE THE COMPUTER	"What do you want to do?
9.	OPPOSITE ORVILLE	"Be careful jogging. It could become an addiction."
10.	RUN-ABOUT RUTH	"I have to run."
11.	DEACON DAN	"I will tell you what is wrong with this country, etc., etc."
12.	LOGICAL LARRY	"It doesn't make sense."
13.	VICTIM VICKY	"I don't know why all these things happen to me."
14.	WONDERFUL WANDA	"Gosh, everything is great."
15.	CHIEF GURU	"Just stay calm."
16.	SLAVING SALLY	"I never have time for anything but work."
17.	MARGARET MARTYR	"I guess I deserve it."
18.	FUNNY FRANK	"Did you ever hear the story .
19.	PASSIVE PAM	"I don't know." "You decide."
20.	FRANTIC FRANNIE	"Oh, my God! What do we do now?"
21.	TERRIBLE TERRY	"This is the worst day I've ever had."
22.	CONTROLLING CARL	Do it this way"

For I the Lord thy God will hold thy right hand, saying unto you, Fear not; I will help you. (Isaiah 41:13)

TODAY'S STEP: My sense of humor helps me to carry – and to get – the message.

"Hell is made up of yearnings. The wicked don't roast on beds of nails; they sit on comfortable chairs and are tortured with yearnings." -- Issac Bashevis Singer

"Are You A Food Addict?

You have an important choice to make. More important than what is happening around you is what is happening inside you. Answer the following questions honestly with a "Yes" or "No".

1.   Have you had a weight problem for longer than five years?   ________
2.   Is there a history of obesity in your family?   ________
3.   Is food associated with good feelings in your family?   ________
4.   Does food make you feel good?   ________
5.   Do you ever get depressed about your weight?   ________
6.   Do you eat when you are not hungry?   ________
7.   Do you go on eating binges for no apparent reason?   ________
8.   Do you plan secret binges?   ________
9.   Have you ever tried to lose weight by severely restricting your food intake?   ________
10.   Do you ever self-induce vomiting?   ________
11.   Have you ever lost interest or pleasure in usual activities, or have you had a decrease in your sex drive because of your weight?   ________
12.   Do you feel depressed, guilty, or remorseful after overeating?   ________
13.   Do you avoid or withdraw from others due to your weight or food intake?   ________
14.   Have you ever lied about your weight?   ________
15.   Do you feel as if you won't be able to stop eating certain foods once you start?   ________
16.   Do you take things very personally?   ________
17.   Do you over commit yourself?   ________
18.   Do you have an intense fear of getting fat?   ________
19.   Do you lack confidence in yourself?   ________
20.   Do you ever feel like nothing you do matters?   ________

If you answered "Yes" to ten or more of the questions, you have an important choice to make. You can choose a new life for yourself, free of food addiction and depression. You can stop living to eat and start eating to live.

The Lord shall give me rest from my sorrow, and from my fear, and from the hard bondage where I was made to serve. (Isaiah 14:3)

TODAY'S STEP: Emotional health is from within not without.

"Every prison that men build is built with bricks of shame." Oscar Wilde, *The Ballad of Reading Gaol*

"Poor Me . . . Pour Me . . . Pour Me another Drink"

The fact is when something really bad happens, we all feel like victims. We all experience some sort of discomfort when we are in conflict. The victim option comes into play when we discount our own ability to resolve the conflict. Instead of focusing on what we can do for ourselves, we blame other people for not taking care of the problem for us. Check the following statements that sometimes fit your life pattern:

1. I can't cope with emotional pain.
2. Sometimes I am not appreciated.
3. I can't stand to be treated unjustly.
4. I judge my personal worth by comparing myself with other people.
5. Trust is difficult for me.
6. Sometimes I don't get the credit I deserve.
7. I can't function effectively under pressure.
8. I may try to control the feelings of others when I feel justified in doing so.
9. I believe in "Murphy's Law" -- If something bad can happen, it will.
10. Why does this have to happen to me?
11. I don't know where to begin.
12. Much of the time I feel like a victim.
13. Sometimes I don't care anyway.
14. I worry too much.
15. I numb out when things go wrong.
16. I repeat the same mistakes.
17. Forgiveness is hard.
18. I get depressed when things go wrong.
19. Under stressful conditions I try to escape.
20. Most of my bad feelings are caused by other people.
21. My anger sometimes turns into hate.
22. Sometimes I feel left out.
23. Most things can be categorized as right or wrong.
24. Over Committed.

If you checked six or more of the above as a reflection of your life, you may have an admission to make of dependence on an addictive agent or people. You are spending too much time in the victim role and you need to assume responsibility for your own emotional well-being. If you have switched from dependence on alcohol to food, you may have an addiction to sugar.

In the day when I cried out, You answered me, and made me bold with strength in my soul. (Psalm 138:3)

TODAY'S STEP: I face my problems squarely and without blame.

"A normal woman would not tolerate such a situation; these women need the role and so suffer it . . . ." -- M. L. Gaertner, *The Alcoholic Marriage*

<u>Alcohostages</u>

For anyone who has never been involved with an alcoholic, the fact that many women stay in such relationships must be somewhat puzzling. They are adults, after all, with freedom of choice. There are social services, self-help groups, an entire battery of apparent solutions. Why then continue on in a situation that is unfulfilling, unrewarding, hurtful, or humiliating? They do so for three reasons:

1.   Believe they have little or no choices; they feel trapped.

2.   Though there are reasonable options, they are unable to see them or they fear taking
a risk– they are stuck.

3.   Though there are reasonable options and they are aware of them and able to conceive of utilizing them, they choose to stay for numerous rational reasons of their own.

Not all hostages are taken by force or held at gunpoint. Many are held captive by circumstances, by their own beliefs and values, even by love. Wives of alcoholics are just such hostages – held captive by an emotional involvement with a fugitive from reality and responsibility.

What happens to these women is not unlike what happens to hostages taken under other conditions: Unable to mollify their captors, they attempt to adjust to the situation as best they can, the object being to survive. Rather than referring to them as enablers or any other negative term, these women should be seen as *"alcohostages"* -- hostages of an alcoholic and his disease.

Whatever their reasons for continuing in the relationship, these women are trapped in a no-win situation for which they receive criticism, blame, and judgment – when they really need help, support, and understanding.

Therefore you have no excuse, everyone of you who passes judgment, for in that which you judge another, you condemn yourself; for you who judge practice the same things. (Romans 2:1)

TODAY'S STEP: God help me believe in myself and help me let go of old beliefs and feelings that are hurting me.

"Alcoholism is not contagious, but Recovery is." -- Anonymous

"Bring the Body and the Mind Will Follow"

In the beginning, newly free from alcohol, some Newcomers go through what members call a "pink-cloud" experience. It may be merely a chemical change – sudden sobriety after years of heavy drinking – but the world can look absolutely marvelous. Gripped by gratitude and zeal, they often feel they have found the One Perfect Answer, the Magic Formula, or the Instant Fix. Older members see this state of exaltation as a possible danger sign, because it could lead to over-confidence and a "slip".

AA is not an Instant Answer. It is a process, a long-term and at times very difficult and frustrating process. The Twelve Steps are not a set of "musts" or rules, but a kind of road map. Simply stated the principles of "The Program" are:

- We admit we are licked and cannot get well on our own.

- We get honest with ourselves.

- We talk it out with somebody else.

- We try to make amends to people we have harmed.

- We pray to whatever greater Power we think there is, even as an experiment, or think of our AA group as our "Higher Power".

- We try to give of ourselves for our own sake and without duty to other alcoholics, with no thought of reward.

According to Damian McElrath, head of the Hazelden Rehabilitation Center near Center City, Minnesota, "The essence of AA is conversation, dialogue, one alcoholic talking with another in a meeting or over a cup of coffee elsewhere. The problem with the active alcoholic is that his life is a monologue – he connects with his addicted self, and that is all. Ninety percent of the Recovery process is through peers talking with one another. The beginning of all wisdom is self-knowledge. In AA, you connect first with yourself; then with another human being; and, then with your Higher Power. You can't say, "I love God and hate my brother."

But you, why do you judge your brother? Or you again, why do you regard your brother with contempt? For we will all stand before the judgment seat of God. (Romans 14:10)

TODAY'S STEP: As I work the Steps, I grow in my capacity to be happy.

"I must learn to give those I love the right to make their own mistakes and recognize them as theirs alone." -- *Al-Anon Faces Alcoholism*

"Be Part of the Solution, Not the Problem"

How does detachment work? How does it help you lose your fears of your alcoholic child or spouse? The general process goes something like this:

1. When you begin learning ways to stop focusing on the alcoholic in order to begin your healing process of seeing to your own needs, the alcoholic has radar and senses this switch in focus.

2. Much of the "games" stop then, because the alcoholic knows less attention will be paid to him or her.

3. By continuing to focus on yourself instead of the alcoholic, you get an even greater distance (detachment) from threats, and begin to lose your fears of them. You begin to see how *you* gave the alcoholic so much of his or her power. You can take it back!

4. Again, the alcoholic senses this. He or she begins to threaten even less.

5. You see that detachment works! You gain more confidence. Many of the illusions in your household are beginning to end.

6. You lose much of your preoccupation with the alcoholic. Your preoccupation was based on your needing to stop him or her from hurting you. You now see they are much less capable of hurting you than you thought. They've already done most of the damage they can do. But the game has been to keep up more of the same junk, to keep up the illusion that the alcoholic is powerful. This no longer works. You have learned to not look at him or her; to walk out of the room; out of the house – to not beg.

7. The alcoholic now stands alone with his or her disease. They've lost their audience, and therefore drop much of the bullying. You are not watching it.

8. The alcoholic can no longer get you to believe you are responsible for his or her drinking and for the craziness in the house.

9. The alcoholic has a chance to grow up and make a decision to get help.

10. You are free!!!

And be not drunk with wine, wherein is excess; but be filled with the Spirit. (Ephesians 5:18)

TODAY'S STEP: I avoid making excuses for my own or someone else's behavior.

"... someone suggested I stop concentrating on changing myself and think first about accepting myself. That gave me the boost I needed." -- *Alateen – A Day At A Time*

"Some of Us Are Sicker Than Others"

It may or may not be true that some alcoholics are sicker than others – many give it all they have and still fail to get well – but if there is one message in the Steps of AA that comes through loud and clear, it is this one – "If you want continuing sobriety, you must clean up your act and assume responsibility for your own actions – past, present, and future." Others can help, can explain, can lead the way, encourage the Newcomer, but ultimately, the individual alcoholic is responsible.

Eight Guidelines For Helping Alcoholics

1. Acquire proper attitudes. Too many members of AA seem to feel they can somehow absorb the burdens of others. It simply cannot be done. AA teaches alcoholics how to stay sober, and if they cannot or will not accept that, they simply cannot blame others.
2. Learn the disease through a knowledge if its symptoms. You can't help a person with alcoholism unless you see he or she has it.
3. Alcoholism is addiction to a drug. Will power is not enough; proper therapy is needed.
4. Confront the alcoholic with the fact of the disease, and offer a possible solution. Alcoholics never get well unless given a chance.
5. Make alcoholics responsible for their actions. Every time you pick up the consequence tab for the alcoholic, you have just paid for the next drunk.
6. Use all the alcoholism resources available. It is a complex illness; it needs a network of people to treat it.
7. Never give up hope; never be discouraged. Even if the alcoholic does not recover, at least you tried.
8. Alcoholism is a family disease; all family members are affected and all need treatment.

May God, who has loved me and given me eternal comfort and good hope by grace, comfort and strengthen my heart in every good work and word. **(2 Thessalonians 2: 16, 17)**

TODAY'S STEP: I let go of old ideas about myself and discover a new self through Recovery.

"Gratitude is not only the greatest of virtues, but the parent of all others." -- Cicero

"Try to Replace Guilt with Gratitude"

Often when we are having a difficult time and we are feeling sad we also start feeling guilty for not doing our best or for failing to live up-to our unrealistic expectations for ourselves. We also lose sight of feelings of gratitude in our lives. Our expectations of life can only ripen into true enjoyment when we apply gratitude. Without gratitude, we lose track of the goodness in our life.

When we take time for gratitude, we can perceive a better world around us; we can appreciate the miracles and gifts we have received; and we can be thankful for our relationship with our Higher Power. To help us develop an "Attitude of Gratitude" we can practice the following suggestions from Christian Larson:

1. Be so strong that nothing can disturb your peace of mind.

2. Talk health, happiness and prosperity.

3. Make your friends feel that there is something in them.

4. Look on the sunny side of everything.

5. Think only of the best.

6. Be just as enthusiastic about the success of others as you are about your own.

7. Forget the mistakes of the past and profit by them.

8. Wear a cheerful countenance and give a smile to everyone you meet.

9. Be too large for worry, too noble for anger, too strong for fear, and too happy to permit the presence of trouble.

I will bless the Lord at all times. His praise shall continually be in my mouth. (Psalm 34:1

TODAY'S STEP: I practice the discipline of H.O.W. – Honesty, Open-Mindedness and Willingness everyday.

<u>Step Nine</u>

<u>"Made direct amends to such people wherever possible, except when to do so would injure them or others."</u>

Step Nine is another action Step and requires us to confront issues from our past that may have been dormant for a long time. This Step clearly requires courage, as well as a renewed dedication to freeing ourselves from the guilt we feel about inflicting injuries upon others. The extraordinary life-restoring benefits we will receive greatly compensate for the risk of making amends.

The process of making amends should not be confused with making apologies. When we apologize, we express regrets for a fault or offense. An apology does not require action or imply a change in behavior. When we make an amend, we take action to improve, correct or alter that which we believe needs to be corrected. Apologies are sometimes appropriate, but apologies are not amends. We may discover in apologizing we are using excessive explanation to excuse our behavior rather than simple change. We can apologize a hundred times for being late for work, but this will not "mend" our tardiness.
Appearing on time is a change in behavior, and thus becomes an amend.

In reality, the Twelve Steps are intended to be repeated as we move toward our goal. Most of us need to repeat all or part of the Steps regularly, depending on our specific needs at a particular time throughout our course of Recovery. After the first or second time through, we may not need to repeat the Steps in order. As we grow spiritually we will be increasingly able to use them daily, as we journey toward further healing and a new life.

By repairing the damage we have done to others, we also will be overhauling our own lives. If we are through with our amends, we will find ourselves blessed with an amazing peaceful state of mind, free of guilt and resentment. We may feel satisfaction in knowing we have honestly done everything in our power to satisfy every material, moral and spiritual debt we have incurred – intentionally or unintentionally.

The importance of Step Nine to our Recovery process is obvious – it gives us a chance to put aside prior distractions and obsessions from our past, and to start living in the present. Since we have created and used this opportunity to repair past wrongs, we can now feel good about ourselves and our efforts to replace misery with serenity. The relief or joy we may give to others will never exceed the peace and increased self-esteem and acceptance we receive.

"Made direct amends to such people wherever possible, except when to do so would injure them or others."

Higher Power, I pray for the right attitude to make my amends, being ever mindful not to harm others in the process. I ask for Your guidance in making indirect amends. Most important, I will continue to make amends by staying abstinent, helping others, and growing in spiritual progress.

In this moment, I trust my Higher Power to guide me in making sincere and honest amends. In this moment, I experience my gratitude for the Twelve Steps of Recovery knowing that as I am willing to live this program, share the fellowship, and walk with God, I am free.

MEDITATIONS

Today I pray for total balance in every thought, word and deed. Help me, Father, to maintain this perfect balance; let no one upset the peace I find here with Thee this morning. Tranquility and peace are the result of temperance, and I pray for this total harmony in all that I may do this day. Speak my heart, dear Lord, and let me know if my actions offend thee. Purify my thoughts so that I do no one an injustice. Let the beauty of all Thy gifts to men inspire my soul, and may this day be filled and made complete by a contribution from me.

AFFIRMATIONS

I feel good about my self. And I experience fulfillment in all areas of my life.

I am aware of my self. I believe in my ability to express my self physically, spiritually, and emotionally – without reservation and without holding back.

I am warm, sincere, loving, considerate, and caring. These are qualities which I possess, and I find them also in others.

I view my self and my own intimacy with enthusiasm and with positive expectation. I believe in the best for my self. I am worth of the best and the best is what I get.

I like who I am, and I live every day in the freedom of my own self-acceptance , self-belief, and in the joy of expressing my self completely and fully.

"We have our own answers within ourselves and can find them with the help of our Al-Anon program and a Higher Power." -- **. . . In All Our Affairs**

The Specifics of Living Consciously

Living consciously entails:

> A mind that is active rather than passive.

> An intelligence that takes joy in its own function.

> Being "in the moment," without losing the wider context.

> Reaching out toward relevant facts rather than withdrawing from them.

> Being discerning to distinguish facts, interpretations, and emotions.

> Noticing and confronting my impulses to avoid or deny painful or threatening realities.

> Being concerned to know "where I am" relative to my various (personal and professional) goals and projects, and whether I am succeeding or failing.

> Searching for feedback from the environment to adjust or correct my course when necessary.

> Persevering in the attempt to understand in spite of difficulties.

> Being receptive to new knowledge and willing to reexamine old assumptions.

> Seeking always to expand awareness – a commitment to learning – therefore, a commitment to growth as a way of life.

> A concern to know not only external reality but also internal reality, the reality of my needs, feelings, aspirations, and motives, so I am not a stranger or a mystery to myself.

O Lord, I know that people's lives are not their own; it is not for them to direct their steps. (Jeremiah 10:23)

TODAY'S STEP: I accept who I am, where I am, and I continue to reach forward one day at a time.

"Nothing in the world can take the place of persistence. Talent will not; nothing is more common than unsuccessful men with talent. Genius will not; the world is full of educated derelicts. Persistence and determination alone are omnipotent. The slogan "press on" has solved and always will solve the problems of the human race." -- President Calvin Coolidge

Robert W. Service in his poem **"The Quitter"** sums up the spirit of persistence"

>It's easy to cry that you're beaten and die;
>
>It's easy to crawfish and crawl;
>
>But to fight and to fight
>
>When hope's out of sight
>
>Why, that's the best game of all.
>
>And though you come out of each grueling bout
>
>All broken and beaten and scarred –
>
>Just have one more try. It's dead easy to die;
>
>It's the keeping on living that's hard.

Why is persistence of such enormous importance? -- Because so little of consequence is achieved without it; and because lack of it leads so often to failure.

Dr. Norman Vincent Peale, in his book **Power Of The Plus Factor**, illustrates the importance of persistence by telling the story of an old rusty pickax stuck in a rocky wall of an unproductive mine, left there by a miner who had given up in disgust and walked away from it. Years later another miner idly swung his pick against the same wall and broke through into the fabulous Comstock lode. Untold wealth had been waiting for the first miner <u>if only</u> he had persisted a little longer. A few more swings of the pickax would have done it. But he gave up too soon . . . and never knew what that negative decision had cost him.

We can't afford to minimize the power of persistence. We need to just hang in there always, always. And never, never give up. Realization and achievement come <u>ONLY</u> to those who persist.

I sought the Lord, and He heard me, and delivered me from all my fears. (Psalm 34:4)

TODAY'S STEP: There are many things I can do to improve my life and further my Recovery, but I cannot heal myself. I need to continually ask God's help in becoming free of all that blocks me from my true self.

"The human spirit is so great a thing that no man can express it; could we rightly comprehend the mind of man nothing would be impossible to us upon the earth. Through faith the imagination is invigorated and completed, for it rarely happens that every doubt mars its perfection. Faith must strengthen the imagination, for faith establishes the will." -- Philippus Aureolus Paracelsus

YOU CAN HAVE ANYTHING YOU WANT – YOU JUST CAN'T HAVE EVERYTHING YOU WANT

According to John Roger & Peter McWilliams, authors of **You Can't Afford the Luxury of a Negative Thought,** to get what you want takes 10 simple steps and the willingness to "do whatever it takes." Consider applying below to your recovery:

1. Focus all your attention on what you want. Be interested in it. Be "obsessed" by it.

2. Visualize and imagine yourself doing or having whatever it is you desire.

3. Be enthusiastic about getting and having it.

4. Know exactly what you want. Write down a detailed description. Draw pictures. Make models.

5. Desire it above all else. Above everything else.

6. Have faith with involvement. Know you can have it, that it's already yours. Be involved with whatever you need to do to get it.

7. Do the work required. How do you know how much work is required? When you have it, that is enough. Until you've got it, it's not enough.

8. Give up all things opposing your goal.

9. Pretend you already have it. (Act as if)

10. Be thankful for what you already have.

. . . whose hope is the Lord . . . shall be like a tree planted by the waters, which spreads out its roots by the river . . . nor will cease from yielding fruit. (Jeremiah 17:7-8)

TODAY'S STEP: I am willing to turn my will and my life over to my Higher Power, to let go of willfulness, and to surrender myself to Recovery.

"All God wants of man is a peaceful heart." -- Meister Eckhart

Turn Setbacks into Comebacks

Dr. Norman Vincent Peale, *Power of the Plus Factor,* and Dr. Robert Schuller, *Tough Minded Faith for Tender Hearted People,* provide us with positive suggestions and steps to turn setbacks into comebacks through Faith.

Dr. Peale suggests we:

1. Always believe that with God's help you can ultimately turn any setback into a comeback.

2. Picture yourself as having a lot of rebound left in you.

3. Remind yourself that you are bigger than anything that can happen to you.

4. Never be afraid. Stand up to your fear with God. He will give you faith and faith is always bigger and stronger than fear.

5. Pray big, believe big, think big.

6. Always be helpful to others and you will have friends who will help you turn setbacks into comebacks.

Dr. Schuller shows us how to deal with obstacles:

"The way to tackle an impossible problem is to break it down and solve the several little problems one at a time."

- Part of the problem is a decision you need to make.
- Part of the problem is your lack of patience.
- Part of the problem is your negative attitude.
- Part of the problem is your preoccupation with yourself.

You can handle all of these parts of your problem with God's help — God doesn't know the meaning of *impossible.*

I can do all things through Christ who strengthens me. (Philippians 4:13)

TODAY'S STEP: I avoid making excuses for my own or someone else's behavior.

"To accuse others for one's misfortunes is a sign of want of education. To accuse oneself shows that one's education has begun. To accuse neither oneself nor others shows one's education is complete." -- Epictetus, ***Discourses,*** Book 1

<u>"Have A Good Day -- Unless You've Made Other Plans"</u>

Blaming our discomfort on outside events or people, can be a way to avoid facing the real cause – our own attitudes. We can see ourselves as a victim, or we can accept what is happening in our life and take responsibility for our response. We may be guided to take action or sit still, but when we listen to the guidance of our Higher Power we will no longer be the victim of circumstances.

The beliefs that become truth for us are those that French novelist, Andre Gide, described as allowing us to best use our strength and find the best means of putting our virtues into action. In other words, if we believe the unmanageability of our lives is caused by outside circumstances, we see ourselves as innocent victims. This belief blinds us to our own faults and we set up intricate defense mechanisms to prevent being exposed as weak and ineffectual.

We use denial as a typical defense tactic. We blame other people, places, and things for our failures. Often this denial is encouraged by significant others who buy into the myth because it explains why they remain in a relationship that is clearly dysfunctional.

Only by understanding the elaborate defense system our addictive behavior has set up are we able to concede our powerlessness and find the way out of the maze of our honest self-deception. In fact, we will find "honest self-deception", "failure is not final", and "surrendering to grow", will be recurring themes as we pursue our goal of Recovery.

Recovery is a much more complex process than we might have thought at the beginning. This is why it takes time and patience to really focus on our own responsibilities rather than complaining about the bad hand life has dealt us. When we finally treat ourselves with love and approval, then we will know we are recovering.

Be strong, and of a good courage; be not afraid, neither be thou dismayed. For the Lord your God is with you wherever you go. (Joshua 1:9)

TODAY'S STEP: I face my problems squarely and without blame.

"Do not look forward to the changes and chances of this life in fear; rather look to them with full hope that, as they arise, God, whose you are, will deliver you out of them. He has kept you hitherto, -- do you but hold fast to His dear hand, and He will lead you safely through all things; and, when you cannot stand, He will bear you in His arms. Do not look forward to what may happen tomorrow; the same everlasting Father who cares for you today, will take care of you tomorrow, and every day. Either He will shield you from suffering, or He will give you unfailing strength to bear it. Be at peace then, and put aside all anxious thoughts and imaginations." – Francis De Sales

Is there an area in your life that you treat as though it were too important to turn over to a Higher Power? Are your efforts to control that area making your life better and more manageable? Are you efforts doing any good at all? We can hold on to our will until the situation becomes so painful we are forced to submit, or we can put our energy where it can do us some good right now, and surrender to our Higher Power's care.

It's only when we let go and trust our Higher Power that our broken dreams can come true and our life can be fulfilled.

Broken Dreams

As children bring their broken toys
with tears for us to mend,
I brought my broken dreams to God
because He was my friend.
But then, instead of leaving Him
in peace to work alone,
I hung around and tried to help
with ways that were my own.
At last, I snatched them back and cried,
"How can you be so slow?"
"My child," God said,
"What could I do?
You never did let go,"

Author Unknown

Show Your marvelous loving kindness by Your right hand, O You who save those who trust *in You*. (Psalm 17:7)

TODAY'S STEP: I acknowledge my wants and needs, then turn them over to my Higher Power.

"The soul ceases to weary itself with planning and foreseeing, giving itself up to God's Holy Spirit within, and to the teachings of His providence without . . . He is not forever fretting as to his progress, or looking back to see how far he is getting on; rather he goes steadily and quietly on, and makes all the more progress because it is unconscious. So he never gets troubled and discouraged; if he falls he humbles himself, but gets up at once, and goes on with renewed earnestness." -- Jean Nicolas Grou

<u>Searching for Serenity</u>

The search is yours and mine. Each finds his way with help, but yet alone.

Serenity is the goal. It comes to those who learn to wait and grow; for each can learn to understand himself and say, "I've found a joy in being me, and knowing you; a knowledge of the depths I can descend, a chance to climb the heights above my head."

The way is not so easy all the time. Our feet will stumble often as we go. A friend may need to give some extra help, as we once gave to others when in the hour of fear.

This is no picnic path that we have found; but yet compared to other days and other times, it seems a better route.

We lost our way before, in fear, guilt, and resentments held too long. Self-pity had its way with us, we found the perfect alibi for all our faults.

We do not know what life may bring from day to day. Tomorrow is a task not yet begun, and we could fail to pass its test.

But this will wait, while in Today we do the best we can. Today we live, we seek to know, to give, to share, with You.
>Anonymous

Be complete, be of good comfort, be of one mind, live in peace; and the God of love and peace shall be with you. (2 Corinthians 13:11)

TODAY'S STEP: My reward for practicing the principles of "The Program" in all my affairs it the priceless gift of serenity.

"By putting off things beyond their proper times, one duty treads upon the heels of another, and all duties are felt as irksome obligations, -- a yoke beneath which we fret and lose our peace. In most cases the consequence of this is, that we have no time to do the work as it ought to be done. It is therefore done precipitately, with eagerness, with a greater desire simply to get it done, than to do it well, and with very little thought of God throughout." --F. W. Faber

<u>YESTERDAY, TODAY, TOMORROW</u>

There are two days in every week about which we should not worry, two days which should be kept free from fear and apprehension.

One of these days is *YESTERDAY* with its mistakes and cares, its faults and blunders, its aches and pains. *YESTERDAY* had passed forever beyond our control.

All the money in the world cannot bring back *YESTERDAY*. We cannot undo a single act we performed; we cannot erase a single word we said . . . *YESTERDAY* is gone.

The other day we should not worry about is *TOMORROW* with its possible adversaries, its burdens, its large and poor performance. *TOMORROW* is also beyond our immediate control.

TOMORROW's sun will rise, either in splendor or behind a mask of clouds – but it will rise. Until it does, we have no stake in *TOMORROW* for it is as yet unborn.

This leaves only one day . . . *TODAY* that drives people mad – it is remorse or bitterness for something which happened *YESTERDAY* and the dread of what *TOMORROW* may bring.

LET US, THEREFORE, LIVE BUT ONE DAY AT A TIME!

Anonymous

Every day will I bless Thee, and I will praise Thy name forever and ever. (Psalm 145:2)

TODAY'S STEP: I allow myself to recognize and accept whatever feelings pass through me.

"Committing yourself is a way of finding out who you are. A man finds his identity by identifying. A man's identity is not best thought of as the way in which he is separated from his fellows, but the way in which he is united with them." -- Robert Terwilliger

<u>Tradition Nine</u>

Our groups, as such, ought never be organized; but we may create service boards or committees directly responsible to those they serve.

Since 1960 Al-Anon groups have been helping families and friends of alcoholics – without rules or regulations. We are members helping members, no one having power over anyone else – and it works! At the group level, rotation of service positions gives everyone a chance to serve, and discourages dominance at the same time. A suggested meeting format to open and close the meeting serves as a guide, but can be changed according to group autonomy. Members contribute whatever they can afford to help cover group, Area and Al-Anon World Service Office expenses. By keeping things simple, groups can focus on our primary spiritual aim.

When it comes to creating service boards and committees within the Al-Anon structure, although organized to a degree, they are always " . . . directly responsible to those they serve." The spiritual principle of serving others is at the heart of Tradition Nine, as we put aside self-seeking motives and get involved with what is best for Al-Anon. Groups are directly responsible to members and Assemblies are directly responsible to groups in their Areas. The Al-Anon World Service Conference and World Service Office, linked to the groups Group Representatives, District Representatives, and World Service Delegates, are directly responsible to worldwide Al-Anon.

Problems arise when members keep service positions beyond a specified period of time, giving them a feeling of authority and self-importance. Groups do not benefit from self-centered actions on the part of its members. All members are responsible to carry out Al-Anon's mission – helping families and friends of alcoholics.

By this all will know that you are My disciples, if you love one another. (John-13:35)

TODAY'S STEP: With the help of a Higher Power, decision-making can be one of life's great adventures. Each crossroad brings a new challenge, and I am capable of dealing with whatever comes my way.

"In spite of illness, in spite even of the archenemy sorrow, one can remain alive long past the usual date of disintegration if one is unafraid of change, insatiable in intellectual curiosity, interested in big things, and happy in small ways."   -- Edith Wharton, *A Backward Glance*

<u>"Sick and Tired of Being Sick and Tired"</u>

The charter of the National Association for the Children of Alcoholics (NACOA) describes its twelve goals:

1. To increase public and professional awareness, understanding, and recognition of the needs of COAs of all ages.
2. To advocate accessible services addressing the unique problems arising from being the child of an alcoholic.
3. To protect the rights of children to live in a safe and healthy environment.
4. To involve the entire community, especially the schools, human services, mental health, medical, religious, and law-enforcement professionals.
5. To help existing alcoholism programs initiate primary and comprehensive services for COAs staffed by professionals specifically trained to meet the needs of COAs.
6. To support school-based programs which acknowledge and address the problems of COAs.
7. To create a network which will promote the exchange of information and resources.
8. To encourage clinical and biomedical research related to COA issues.
9. To advocate funding from public and private sources.
10. To encourage training for professionals in issues related to COAs.
11. To develop professional guidelines for those who work with COAs.
12. To offer support to professionals who are themselves COAs.

This is a faithful saying and worthy of all acceptance, that Christ Jesus came into the world to save sinners, of whom I am chief. However, for this reason I obtained mercy, that in me first Jesus Christ might show all longsuffering, as a pattern to those who are going to believe on Him for everlasting life. Now to the King eternal, immortal, invisible, to God who alone is wise, be honor and glory forever and ever. Amen. (1 Timothy 1:15-17)

TODAY'S STEP: I trust that "The Program" works if I work it and that I can be restored to wholeness with God's help.

<u>Walt Whitman *Leaves of Grass* (1855)</u>

I have said that the soul is not more than the body,
And I have said that the body is not more than the soul,
And nothing, not God, is greater to one than one's – self if,
And whoever walks a furlong without sympathy walks
     to his own funeral, dressed in his shroud.
And I or you pocket less of a dime may purchase the pick of the
     earth,

And to glance with an eye or show a bean in its pod
     confounds the learning of all times,
And there is no trade or employment but the young man following it may
     become a hero,
And there is no object so soft but it makes a hub for the wheeled
     universe,
And any man or woman shall stand cool and
     supercilious before a million universes.

And I call to mankind, Be not curious about God,
For I who am curious about each am not curious about God,
No array of terms can say how much I am at peace about
     God and about death.

I hear and behold God in every object, yet I understand
     God not in the least,
Nor do I understand who there can be more wonderful than myself.

Why should I wish to see God better than this day?
I see something of God each hour of the twenty-four,
     and each moment then,
In the faces of men and women I see God, and in my
     own face in the glass;
I find letters from God dropped in the street, and every
     one is signed by God's name,
And I leave them where they are, for I know that others
     Will punctually come forever and ever.

Because he has loved me, therefore will I deliver him: I will set him on high, because he has known my name. He shall call upon me, and I will answer him: I will be with him in trouble; I will deliver him, and honor him. (Psalm 91:14-15)

TODAY'S STEP: When faced with difficult or painful situations, I remember a loving God is always here for me, always available as a source of comfort, guidance and peace.

"Only in quiet waters things mirror themselves undistorted. Only in a quiet mind is adequate perception of the world." -- Hans Margolius

Trust is one of the variables that forms a measurable continuum and positive correlation with maturity. Immature persons trust only those people who make no mistakes. Juveniles trust a bit easier. However, they trust those people who think and as they do. They don't tolerate differences very well. Sometimes they "trust" too much and get taken advantage of over and over.

Adult-stage individuals trust because of their own personal resources. They can take care of themselves emotionally, so the behavior of others is less important. The very mature sometimes seem too trusting and accepting also, but they are capable of bouncing back when let down. They are not passive, but very accepting of reality – whatever happens.

Read the following statements and measure the degree of your progress in Recovery.

The Trust Thermometer

100%   I can take care of my emotional needs, so the behavior of other people seldom threatens me.

90%   When I have a feeling of mistrust, I view it as my problem to solve.

80%   I expect people to make mistakes and I can give them another chance.

70%   I trust most people until they let me down, then I write them off.

60%   I can be at ease with almost anyone as long as she or he approves of me.

50%   I feel safe only when I get special treatment from others.

40%   I have to know people well enough to know exactly what to expect from them.

30%   I have a select group of people who do things my way.

20%   I feel comfortable when others know exactly what I want and do it.

10%   I feel relaxed only when other people are perfect.

How excellent is thy loving kindness, O God! Therefore the children of men put their trust under the shadow of thy wings. (Psalm 36:7)

TODAY'S STEP: I trust God will bring out the best in me and others.

"The last of the human freedoms – to choose one's attitude in any given set of circumstances; to choose one's own way." -- Dr. Victor Frankl, *Man's Search for Meaning*

"Do It Sober"

In his book *Man's Search for Meaning,* Dr. Victor Frankl describes his experiences as s survivor of the Holocaust. He had **everything** and **everyone** in his life taken from him! But while he was in the concentration camp, he realized one essential truth: no matter **what** they put him through, he still had within him the power to **choose** how he was going to order his inner environment – his thoughts, his feelings, and his being.

No matter how much they took from him – which was every person and material thing he had – he still had his freedom to choose. It's a freedom we have, too. We can't always choose what happens to us, but we can **always** choose our reaction to it. We can choose not to live addicted, we can choose to **"Do It Sober"**.

We have this choice every day of our lives – we can take the path that leads to insanity and death [and remember, your next drunk/drug could be your last one] – or we can take the path that leads to a happy and useful life. We can make every day count, when we choose to **"Do It Sober"**.

We can think of time as a special kind of checking account. We have 24 hours to spend. By putting the principles of the program to work in our lives today, we can choose to use these hours to grow, enjoy, and improve. We have an opportunity to learn from our mistakes, since a brand new 24 hours can begin at any moment, if we choose to **"Do It Sober"**.

We can use this day to enrich our lives and improve our relationship with our Higher Power, other people, and ourselves. We can use each of the Twelve Steps to help us to pursue our goals regardless of our circumstances. We can use meetings, telephone calls and Recovery literature to apply the Steps to what is happening in our lives today. We can make a positive change – we can **"Do It Sober"**.

It was for freedom that Christ set us free; therefore keep standing firm and do not be subject again to a yoke of bondage. (Galatians 5:1)

TODAY'S STEP: With the help of a Higher Power, decision-making can be one of life's great adventures. Each crossroad brings a new challenge, and with God I am capable of dealing with whatever comes my way.

"The person . . . in the grip of an old distress says things that are not pertinent, does things that don't work, fails to cope with the situation, and endures terrible feelings that have nothing to do with the present." -- Harvey Jackins

"Nothing Is So Bad, Relapse Won't Make It Worse"

Cravings to use your drug of choice again will occur and tend to be strongest during early abstinence. They are triggered by people, places, things, feelings, and situations previously associated with your addiction – any reminders of it. The goal when you get a craving is to ride it out, and prevent it from leading to relapse. The following action plan will help you to short-circuit cravings:

1. **Leave** the situation in which the craving is occurring. Get away from the person, place, or thing causing it.
2. **Contact your sponsor or a member of your group** who understands addiction and can talk you through the craving. (Always have phone numbers with you.)
3. **Mentally detach** from the urge, and try to look at it as if you were an outside observer.
4. **Plan** what you will do in advance. Who can you call for help? How will you spend your time? Where will you go? What action steps will you take to help yourself?
5. **Get to a Twelve Step meeting** if possible, or read Recovery literature. Alternately, get involved in some other activity, e.g., exercise, walk, see a movie, etc.
6. **Think past the high** to what you'll get afterward if you give in and use. Focus on a negative memory or ugly reminder of your drug use, concentrate on the consequences and the losses – don't romanticize the high.
7. **Write it down.** It may be helpful to carry a small notebook and write down the date and circumstances of any cravings you get and what you did to cope with them.
8. **Use a relaxation exercise.** Cravings often have a physical component, including tensed muscles, increased heart rate, dry mouth, and sweating. Depending on the addiction, you may actually feel something in one particular part of your body: an overeater may feel his stomach in knots; a cocaine addict often gets a sensation of tenseness in her nose and throat. Relaxing your body can relieve these symptoms until they pass.

Take heed, and be quiet; fear not, neither be faint-hearted. (Isaiah 7:4)

TODAY'S STEP: Day by day, I entrust my problems to a power greater than myself.

"In fantasy and myth homecoming is a dramatic event: bands play, the fatted calf is killed, a banquet prepared, and there is rejoicing that the prodigal has returned. In reality, exile is frequently ended gradually, with no dramatic, external events to mark its passing. The haze in the air evaporates and the world comes into focus; seeking gives way to finding; anxiety to satisfaction. Nothing is changed and everything is changed." -- Sam Keen

"Utilize, Don't Analyze"

When I was a Newcomer in Al-Anon it was suggested I learn about the disease of alcoholism, and I became a voracious reader on the subject. As I read, I began to analyze everything: Was Al-Anon a philosophy or a philosophical system? What would be the logical outcome of believing in a Power greater than myself? What is a spiritual awakening and when could I expect to have one? What if I didn't?

These questions and many others like them kept my mind busy, but did not help me get better. Fortunately, I continued going to Al-Anon meetings, listening to others, talking to my sponsor, working the Steps and reading the Al-Anon approved literature. Gradually I began to catch on. When I stopped trying to analyze and explain everything and started living the principles, actually using them in my everyday situations, the Al-Anon program suddenly made sense – and I started to change.

It's very easy to fall into the "paralysis of analysis" trap and to get so caught up in our head games that we lose sight of our goal – we need to constantly remind ourselves it's a simple program. We need to frequently ask ourselves:

> Does analyzing my situation provide any useful insights, or is it
> an attempt to control the uncontrollable?

> Am I taking inventory or avoiding work that needs to be done by
> keeping my mind occupied?

Knowledge is power, but sometimes our thirst for knowledge can be an attempt to exercise power where we are powerless.

O the depth of the riches both of the wisdom and knowledge of God! How unsearchable are his judgments, and his ways past finding out! (Romans 11:33)

TODAY'S STEP: When I rely on my Higher Power's help I can make progress.

"If I can stop one heart from breaking, I shall not live in vain; if I can ease one life the aching, or cool one pain, or help one fainting robin into his nest again, I shall not live in vain." -- Emily Dickinson

Making Your First Amends

Certain guidelines can help when we plan to make amends.

1. Plan. Be sure of what you want to say. Be thorough in your preparation. Spend as much time as you need with your Higher Power, asking advice and listening to the response. Each amend will be different, based on the situation, so plan carefully each time.

2. Don't go into it with expectations about how the other person will respond. Simply be respectful and understand you must accept whatever happens. You don't have control over the outcome, only over your part in the process.

3. Ask permission first and be willing to accept the other's response. Some victims may not accept your amend and that's their right. We must not gain our peace of mind by being disrespectful.

4. Be careful to take the responsibility for what happened on your shoulders. Speak only of your part in the hurtful situation; don't comment on behavior of the other.
   If you have any remaining resentment or anger, the amend won't work.

5. Keep it simple.

6. Whatever the other's response, remain humble, without anger or resentment.

7. Be willing to forgive yourself and the other person, and when the amend has been made. Release your pain to your Higher Power.

Therefore, if you are offering your gift at the altar and there remember that your brother or sister has something against you, leave your gift there in front of the altar. First go and be reconciled to them; then come and offer your gift. (Matthew 5:23-25)

TODAY'S STEP: I understand the true nature of humility. I recognize the ability to develop and practice it is the basic foundation of the Twelve Steps.

"We move from being at the mercy of any problem that comes along to an inner certainty that no matter what happens in our lives, we will be able to face it, deal with it, and learn from it with the help of our Higher Power." -- *. . . In All Our Affairs*

The Stages of Recovery

Recovery Stage	Condition	Focus of Recovery	Approximate Duration
3	Human/Spiritual	Spirituality	Ongoing
2	Adult Child	AC Specific Full Recovery Program	3-5 years
1	Stage Zero	Basic Illness Full Recovery Program	½ to 3 years
0	Active Illness	Addiction, Compulsion, Disorder	Indefinite

Stage Zero is manifested by the presence of an active illness or disorder, such as an addiction, compulsion or another disorder. This active illness may be acute, recurring or chronic. Without Recovery, it may continue indefinitely. At Stage Zero, Recovery has not yet started.

At Stage One, Recovery begins. It involves participating in a full Recovery program to assist in healing the Stage Zero condition or conditions. (A partial Recovery program is less likely to be as successful as a full one.)

Stage Two involves healing Adult Child or co-dependence issues. Once a person has a stable and solid Stage One Recovery – one that has lasted for at least a year or longer – it may be time to consider looking into these issues. An Adult Child is anyone who grew up in an unhealthy, troubled or dysfunctional family.

Stage Three Recovery is spirituality and its incorporation into daily life. This is an ongoing process.

I am learning to be content in whatever situation I am. (Philippians 4:11)

TODAY'S STEP: God help me believe in myself, help me let go of old beliefs and feelings that are hurting me. I endeavor to live quietly and peacefully – to mind my own business.

"Children who are not loved in their very beginnings do not know how to love themselves. As adults, they have to learn to nourish, to mother their own lost child." -- Marion Woodman, ***Addiction to Perfection***

<u>I Am Me</u>

In the entire world, there is no one else exactly like me. Everything that comes out of me is authentically mine because I alone choose it. I own everything about me: my body, my feelings, my mouth, my voice, all my actions, whether they be to others or to myself. I own fantasies, my dreams, my hopes, my fears. I own all my triumphs and successes, all my failures and mistakes.

Because I own all of me, I can become intimately acquainted with me. By doing so, I can love me and be friendly with me in all my parts. I know there are aspects about myself that puzzle me, and other aspects I do not know, but as long as I am friendly and loving to myself, I can courageously and hopefully look for solutions to the puzzles and for ways to find out more about me.

However I look and sound, whatever I say and do, and whatever I think and feel at a given moment in time is authentically me. If later some parts of how I looked, sounded, thought, and felt turned out to be unfitting, I can discard that which is unfitting, keep the rest, and invent something new for what I discarded. I can see, hear, feel, think, say, and do.
I have the tools to survive, to be close to others, to be productive, and to make sense and order out of the world of people and things outside of me, and therefore I can engineer me.
I am me and I am O.K.
            -- Anonymous

I will give thanks to You, for I am fearfully and wonderfully made; marvelous are Your works, and my soul knows it very well. My frame was not hidden from You, When I was made in secret, *and* skillfully wrought in the depths of the earth; Your eyes have seen my unformed substance; and in Your book were all written The days that were ordained *for me*, When as yet there was not one of them. How precious also are Your thoughts to me, O God! How great is the sum of them! If I should count them, they would outnumber the sand. When I awake, I am still with You. (Psalm 139:14-19)

TODAY'S STEP: I accept who I am, where I am, and I continue to reach forward one day at a time.

"The child wants simple things. It wants to be listened to. It wants to be loved . . . . It may not even know the words, but **it wants its rights protected** and its self-respect unviolated. It needs you to be there." -- Ron Kurtz, ***Body-Centered Psychotherapy: The Haikomi Method***

Awakening the Inner Child

Many of us have shut the door on our childhood and don't want to think about it, much less recall any details. Yet inside our childhood memories lies a trapped "inner child" we may have abandoned.

We underestimate the importance of our child within, who was at one time so humble, teachable and trusting. Those child-like characteristics were the ones that Jesus said would make a person the "greatest in the kingdom of heaven" (Matthew 18:4).

One way to awaken this child within is to watch how children play. If you don't have children, go to a park and watch how simple, teachable and trusting they are.

We discover the child within ourselves by recalling our own childhood. What is your earliest positive memory? Your earliest negative one? Did you have a pet? What sounds do you remember?

Look at pictures of yourself as a child. What expression is on your face? Were you a happy child? What does it look like you were thinking? What did you like to do as a child?

It's important not to try to recall our childhoods in isolation. Show those childhood pictures to others, and tell them what you were like. They may identify with you and offer some sorely lacking affirmation and love for that child within. If your childhood was particularly painful, you may need a therapist to help you manage the fears that come with doing this.

As we value the child within, we regenerate this teachable, trusting part of ourselves. We find some of the best parts of ourselves that have been missing for a long time.

Except ye be converted, and become as little children, ye shall not enter into the kingdom of heaven. (Matthew 18:3)

TODAY'S STEP: How do I feel today? How am I doing? If I can answer those questions truthfully, I am more likely to pursue help and share the happy times with others as well.

"Everything an Indian does is in a circle, and that is because the power of the world always works in circles, and everything tries to be round. In the old days when we were a strong and happy people, all our power came to us from the sacred hoop of the nation, and so long as the hoop was unbroken the people flourished." -- Black Elk [Hehaka Sapa], ***Black Elk Speaks,Being the Life Story of a Holy Man of the Ogalala Sioux,*** as told through John G. Neihardt

<u>The Earth Is the Lord's</u>

Long before my people journeyed to this land your people were here, and you received from your elders an understanding of creation, and of the Mystery that surrounds us all that was deep, and rich and to be treasured.

We did not hear you when you shared your vision.

In our zeal to tell you of the good news of Jesus Christ we were closed to the value of your spirituality.

We confused western ways and culture with the depth and breadth and length and height of the gospel of Christ.

We imposed our civilization as a condition of accepting the Gospel.

We tried to make you like us and in so doing we helped to destroy the vision that made you what you were.

As a result you, and we, are poorer and the image of the Creator in us is twisted, blurred and we are not what we are meant by God to be.

We ask you to forgive us and we ask you to walk with us in the spirit of Christ so that our peoples may be blessed and God's creation healed.

Apology to Native Congregations – United Church of Canada, submitted by the United Church of Canada General Council to Native Elders and accepted by the Same on August 15, 1986.

That ye, being rooted and grounded in love, may be able to comprehend with all the saints what is the breadth, and length, and depth, and height; and to know the love of Christ, which surpasses knowledge, that you may be filled up to all the fullness of God. (Ephesians 3:17-19)

TODAY'S STEP: I search my own Truth, and I allow others to do the same.

"We have come to believe He would like us to keep our heads in the clouds with Him, but that our feet ought to be firmly planted on earth. That is where our fellow travelers are, and that is where our work must be done. These are the realities for us. We have found nothing incompatible between a powerful spiritual experience and a life of sane and happy usefulness." -- ***Alcoholic Anonymous, Big Book,*** p.130

<u>"Share Your Happiness"</u>

Lord help me today to:

- Mend a quarrel.
- Seek out a forgotten friend.
- Dismiss suspicion and replace it with trust.
- Write a friendly letter.
- Share a treasure.
- Give a soft answer.
- Encourage another.
- Manifest my loyalty in word and deed.
- Keep a promise.
- Find the time.
- Forego a grudge.
- Forgive an enemy.
- Listen.
- Acknowledge any wrong doing.
- Try to understand.
- Examine my demands on others.
- Think of someone else first.
- Be kind. Be gentle.
- Laugh a little.
- Smile more.
- Be happy.
- Show my gratitude.
- Welcome a stranger.
- Speak Your love. Speak it again. Live it again.
- LIFE IS A CELEBRATION !!!

Anonymous

You and your families will feast in the presence of the Lord your God, and you will rejoice in all you have accomplished because the Lord your God has blessed you. (Deuteronomy 12:7)

TODAY'S STEP: I search for my own Truth, and I allow others to do the same.

"God does not die on the day we cease to believe in a personal deity, but we die on the day when our lives cease to be illuminated by the steady radiance, renewed daily, of **a wonder**, the source of which is beyond all reason." -- Dag Hammarskjold

The Universal Prayer

Eternal Reality,
You are Everywhere.
You are Infinite Unity, Truth, and Love;
You permeate our souls,
Every corner of the Universe, and beyond.

To some of us, You are Father, Friend, or
     Partner,
To others, Higher Power, Higher Self, or
     Inner Self.
To many of us, You are all these and more.
You are within us and we within You.

We know You forgive our trespasses
If we forgive ourselves and Others.
We know You protect us from destructive
     temptation
If we continue to seek Your help and
     guidance.
If we but place our trust in You and try
     to do our best.

Give us this day knowledge of Your will
     for us and the power to carry it out.
For Yours is Infinite Power and Love,
Forever.

Author Unknown

That I may live a life worthy of the Lord and please Him in every way: bearing fruit in every good work, growing in the knowledge of God. (Colossians 1:10)

TODAY'S STEP: The Steps offer me a road map for living that leads to a spiritual awakening and beyond. I can't skip ahead to the end of the journey – which can at times be a tough one – but I can put one foot in front of the other and follow the directions I've been given, knowing that others who have gone before me have received more along the way than they had ever dreamed.

"We admitted we couldn't lick alcohol with our own remaining resources, and so we accepted the further fact that dependence upon a Higher Power (if only our AA group) could do this hitherto impossible job. The moment we were able to accept these facts fully our release from the alcohol compulsion had begun." -- ***As Bill Sees It***

"One Drink Is Too Many and A Thousand Not Enough"

When we think about having a drink, we're thinking of the kick we get out of drinking, the pleasure, the escape from boredom, the feeling of self-importance, and the companionship of other drinkers. What we don't think of is the let-down, the hangover, the remorse, the waste of money, and the facing of another day. In other words, when we think about that first drink, we're thinking of all the assets of drinking and none of the liabilities.

The reconstruction of our lives is the goal of Recovery – this we achieve by not taking that first drink, one day at a time. The spiritual life is not a theory; "it works, if we work it".

Step Two started us on our journey to develop a spiritual life; Step Nine allows us to move into the final phase. We can now begin to recognize that God works through us and for us. Proof comes to us when we realize God does for us what we could not do for ourselves – remove the gnawing compulsion to drink. We must continue to daily seek God's guidance. He grants us a daily reprieve and provides the power we need.

We must be willing to make amends to all the people we have harmed. We must do the best we can to repair the damage done in the past. When we make amends, when we say:
"I'm sorry," may or may not be impressed by our sincere desire to set right the wrong. Sometimes people we are making amends to admit their own faults, so feuds of long standing melt away. Our most ruthless creditors will sometimes surprise us. In general, we must be willing to do the right thing, no matter what the consequences may be for us.

Do not forget to do good and to share with others for with such sacrifices God is well pleased. (Hebrews 13:16)

TODAY'S STEP: Day by day, I entrust my problems to a power greater than myself.

"We ought daily or weekly to dedicate a little time to the reckoning up of the virtues of our belongings, -- wife, children, friends, -- and contemplating them then in a beautiful collection. And we should do so now, that we may not pardon and love in vain and too late, after the beloved one has been taken away from us to a better world." Jean Paul Richter

<u>Take Time</u>

Take time to think . . .
it is the source of power.

Take time to play . . .
it is the secret of perpetual youth.

Take time to read . . .
it is the fountain of wisdom.

Take time to pray . . .
it is the greatest power on earth.

Take time to love and be loved . . .
it is a God-given privilege.

Take time to be friendly . . .
it is the road to happiness.

Take time to laugh . . .
it is the music of the soul.

Take time to give . . .
it is too short a day to be selfish.

Take time to work . . .
it is the price of success.

Take time to do charity . . .
it is the key to heaven.

Anonymous

I have loved you with an everlasting love; therefore I have drawn you with loving kindness. (Jeremiah 31:3)

TODAY'S STEP: Day by day, I entrust my problems to a power greater than myself.

"The conditions of conquest are always easy. We have but to toil awhile, endure awhile, believe awhile, and never turn back." -- Simms

"Remember Your Last Drunk"

That's not a typographical error. The word is "drunk", not "drink", as you'll see.

"A drink" is a term which has awakened pleasurable echoes and anticipations in millions of people for years. Depending on our age, and on the circumstances which surrounded our first experiences with alcohol, we all have various memories and hopes (sometimes anxieties) aroused by the thought of a cool beer, a gin and tonic, a boilermaker, a Jell-O shot, a glass of wine, or whatever.

Repeatedly, in the early drinking of most people, the anticipations were fully met by the desired drink. And if that happened often enough, we naturally learned to think of "a drink" as a satisfying event – whether it gratified our thirst, graced a social occasion, relaxed us, stimulated us, or gave us any other kind of satisfaction we sought.

A searching, fearless look at our complete drinking record, however, shows that in the last years and months our drinking never created those perfect, magic moments again, no matter how often we tried for them. Instead over and over, we had no self-control, we wound up drinking more than that, and landed in some kind of trouble as a result. Maybe it was simply inner discontent, a sneaky feeling we were drinking too much, but sometimes it was marital squabbles, poor sleep, declining health, job problems, serious illness or accidents, or legal or financial worries.

Drinking for us no longer means music and gay laughter and flirtations. It means sickness and sorrow. An old-timer in AA once put it this way: "I know now that stopping in for a drink will never again be – for me – simply killing a few minutes and leaving a buck on the bar. In exchange for that drink, what I would plunk down now is my bank account, my family, our home, our car, my job, my sanity, and probably my life." He remembers his last drunk, not his first drink.

Remember not the sins of my youth, nor my transgressions; according to Thy mercy remember Thou me, for Thy goodness' sake, O Lord. (Psalm 25:7)

TODAY'S STEP: I am beginning to understand that surrender is not defeat and I welcome my powerlessness.

"The way of a superior man is threefold: virtuous, he is free from anxieties, wise, he is free from perplexities; bold, he is free from fear." -- Confucius

"Call Your Sponsor Before, Not After, You Take the First Drink"

At AA meetings, it is often recommended that Newcomers get a sponsor. One reason why it is a good idea to have a sponsor is that you have a friendly guide during those first days and weeks when "The Program" seems strange and new, before you feel you know your way around. Besides, a sponsor can spend more time with you, and give you far more individual attention, than a busy professional helper possibly could.

When you decide to ask someone to be your sponsor, you may find the following suggestions helpful:

A.   It's usually better if men sponsor men and women sponsor women.
         This helps avoid the possibility or romantic entanglements which might
         take the focus off ourselves and our ability to work the program.

B.   Whether or not we like what our sponsor suggests (and sponsors can only
         suggest; they cannot make anybody do anything, or actually prevent any
         action), the fact is the sponsor has been sober longer, knows pitfalls
         to avoid, and may be right.

C.   An AA sponsor is not a professional caseworker or counselor. A sponsor
         is not a medical expert, nor qualified to give religious, legal, domestic, or
         psychiatric advice, although a good sponsor is usually willing to discuss
         such matters confidentially, and often can suggest where the appropriate
         assistance can be obtained.

D.   Some people think it is a good idea to have more than one sponsor, so at
         least one is always likely to be available. This plan also has an additional
         advantage – three or four sponsors can provide a wider range of experience
         and knowledge than any one person alone. Bill W asked for help from different
         sponsors for different issues.

E.   You are under no obligation ever to repay your sponsor in any way for
         helping you. He or she does so because helping others helps us maintain
         our own sobriety.

The fear of the Lord is the beginning of knowledge: but fools despise wisdom and instruction. (Proverbs 1:7)

TODAY'S STEP: I have faith that daily work on myself will result in my becoming the best person I can be.

A Transpersonal Creed

I BELIEVE that the universe is spiritual as well as material, and that what happens to us is controlled by a combination of both physical and spiritual laws.

I AFFIRM that human beings are part of an integrated Order of life; that we have considerable potential to evolve toward higher levels of this Order; and that seeking to evolve toward this Order is one of the highest values of human life.

I MAINTAIN that there are higher spiritual beings and enlightened humans. Life and consciousness seek to evolve toward these higher, nonphysical manifestations, even though currently rooted in the physical. Like the rest of life, my life, and my consciousness share this purpose and destiny.

I BELIEVE that while some judgments, values, and moralities are subjective and personal, some are based on a valid intuition of higher possibilities. Satisfactory personal values and morality must be based on a continual dedication to understanding and living my and other's higher possibilities. Those who help me understand and develop these higher possibilities are my friends and teachers; those who hinder me should be helped as much as possible. Insofar as all Life may be one Being, in a real and transpersonal sense, we should seek to maximize our love of and minimize our harm to all Life.

I AFFIRM that churches or other transpersonally oriented activities may sometimes be useful for aiding my and other's spiritual evolution; that there are actions that are objectively wrong, which we should avoid committing once we understand their nature; that there is a real and objective sense in which harming others harms myself and Life; that
the universe is lawful on mental and transpersonal levels as well as physical levels, so all acts have consequences that must eventually be faced. Virtue for me is loving and helping myself and others, so I and Life may evolve.

I MAINTAIN that the death of the body may not be the death of the mind. While hope of an afterlife can be a rationalization for lack of evolutionary effort in this life, the probable reality of transpersonal values of existence not dependent on a physical body may mean that individual life is much greater than physical life.

Charles T. Tart, Open Mind, Discriminating Mind

To be spiritually minded is life and peace. (Romans 8:6)

TODAY'S STEP: I search for my own Truth, and I allow others to do the same.

"The life of every man is a diary in which he means to write one story, and writes another; and his humblest hour is when he compares the volume as it is with what he hoped to make it." -- James M. Barrie

"It's The First Drink That Gets You Drunk"

Expressions commonly heard in AA are "If you don't take that first drink, you can't get drunk" and "One drink is too many, but a thousand are not enough."

Many of us, when we first began to drink, never wanted or took more than one or two drinks. But as time went on, we increased the number. Then, in later years, we found ourselves drinking more and more, some of us getting and staying very drunk. Maybe our condition didn't always show in our speech or our gait, but by this time we were rarely sober.

If that bothered us too much, we would cut down, or try to limit ourselves to just one or two, or switch from hard liquor to beer or wine. At least, we tried to limit the amount we would drink or we tried to hide how much we drank.

But these measures got more and more difficult. Occasionally we even went on the wagon, and did not drink at all for a while. Eventually, we would go back to drinking – just one drink, until finally, we were right back where we had been – drinking alcoholically.

Such repeated experiences have forced us to this logically inescapable conclusion: If we do not take the first drink, we never get drunk. Therefore, instead of planning never to get drunk, or trying to limit the number of drinks or the amount of alcohol, we have learned to concentrate on avoiding only one drink: The first one.

Doctors who are experts on alcoholism tell us there is a sound medical foundation for avoiding the first drink. It is the first drink which triggers, immediately or some time later, the compulsion to drink more and more. Many of us have come to believe our alcoholism is an addiction to the drug alcohol; like addicts of any sort who want to maintain Recovery, we have to keep away from the first dose of the drug or behavior to which we are addicted.

Behold, we count them happy which endure. (James 5:11)

TODAY'S STEP: I have faith that daily work on myself will result in my becoming the best person I can be.

"Be such a man, and live such a life, that if every man were such as you, and every life like yours, this earth would be a God's Paradise." --Phillips Brooks

"Make Use of Telephone Therapy"

When we were first trying to achieve sobriety, many of us found ourselves taking a drink without planning to. Sometimes, it seemed to happen practically without our knowing it. There was no conscious decision to drink, and there was no real thought about possible consequences. We had not intended to set off an entire drinking episode.

Now we have learned that simply postponing that first drink, putting something else in its place, provides us with a chance to think about our drinking history, to think about the disease of alcoholism, and to think about the possible results of starting to drink.

Fortunately, we can do more than just think about it, and we do. We telephone someone. When we stopped drinking, we were told repeatedly to get AA people's telephone numbers, and instead of drinking, to call these people.

At first, we thought of telephoning a new acquaintance, someone we barely knew, seemed strange, and most of us were reluctant. But the AA's – those with more non-drinking days behind them than we had – kept suggesting it. They said they understood why we hesitated, because they had felt the same way. Nevertheless, they said, just try it, at least once. And so finally, thousands and thousands of us have. To our relief, it turned out to be an easy, pleasant experience. Best of all, it worked.

"Telephone therapy" works even when we don't know any individual to call. Since a number for AA is listed in practically every telephone directory in the United States and Canada (and in many other countries), it is easy to dial that number and instantly be in touch with someone who honestly understands, at gut level. It may be a person we have never met, but the same genuine empathy is there.

Your inner self, the unfading beauty of a gentle and quiet spirit, is of great worth in God's sight. (1 Peter 3:4)

TODAY'S STEP: With the help of a Higher Power, decision-making can be one of life's great adventures. Each crossroad brings a new challenge, and with God I am capable of dealing with whatever comes my way.

"It is said an Eastern monarch once charged his wise men to invent him a sentence, to be ever in view, and which should be true and appropriate in all times and situations. They presented him the words: 'And this, too, shall pass away.' How much it expresses! How chastening in the hour of pride! How consoling in the depths of affliction!" -- Abraham Lincoln, ***Address to the Wisconsin State Agricultural Society, Milwaukee (September 30, 1849)***

"Sober' N Crazy"

God, please direct my thinking, especially move it from self-pity, dishonest and self-seeking motives.

As I go through the day and face indecision, please give me inspiration, an intuitive thought, or a decision. Make me relax and take it easy; don't let me struggle. Let me rely upon Your inspiration, intuitive thoughts, and decision instead of my old ideas and old habits.

Show me all through the day what my next step is to be and give me whatever I need to take care of each problem. God, I ask You especially for freedom from self-will and I make no requests for myself only. But give me the knowledge of Your will for me and the power to carry it out in every contact during my day.

As I go through this day, let me pause when agitated or doubtful and ask You for the right thought or action. Let me constantly be reminded that I am no longer running the show, humbly saying many times each day, "Thy will be done" and agreeing that it is.

I will then be in much less danger of excitement, fear, anger, worry, self-pity, or foolish decisions. I will be more efficient. I won't be burning up energy foolishly as I was when trying to run life to suit myself. I will give You all the responsibility and all the praise.

When I receive help from God, as I understand Him, I can live my life one day at a time and handle any challenges that come my way. Only then can I live a life of victory over any addictive agent or behavior, in comfortable sobriety.

I have walked before You in truth and with a loyal heart, and have done what is good in Your sight. And the Lord said to Hezekiah, "I have heard your prayer . . . and I will add to your days fifteen years." (Isaiah 38:3-5)

TODAY'S STEP: I am beginning to understand that surrender is not defeat and I welcome my powerlessness.

Step Ten

"Continued to take personal inventory and, when we were wrong, promptly admitted it."

Our initial work with the Steps identifies the true nature of the ineffective and unhealthy behavior we have been using for most of our lives. We have examined our condition and
made restitution for our misdeeds wherever possible. For many of us, the Steps may be our first antidote for relieving the pain created by our addictive behavior. Our commitment to continue working the Steps acknowledges our intention to improve the quality of our lives and relationships through reliance on our Higher Power.

Step Ten requires that we continue to take personal inventory and, when wrong, promptly admit it. This is a critical part of our Recovery – we can no longer risk indulging in harmful attitudes and inappropriate behaviors. We must watch for signals that reactivate past resentments and fears or that suggest we are trying to manage our lives alone. When we see ineffective behaviors returning, we must stop ourselves and ask our Higher Power for help in removing them, then make amends promptly if harm has been done.

To effectively work Step Ten, we need to pay special attention to promptly admitting our wrongs. Delay in admitting them merely shows us how deeply ingrained some of our behavior patterns are. The sooner we are able to admit our wrongs, the sooner we can repair the harm done to ourselves and others. Vigilance in taking a daily inventory will help us develop a feeling of freedom, as we learn to promptly take care of things that bother us. Having taken an honest, in-depth look at ourselves, we are now ready to explore our relationship with our Higher Power and the community in Steps Eleven and Twelve.

Our commitment to completing the remaining Steps requires that we fully acknowledge our need for continued and ongoing spiritual development. Just as our bodies tell us when to eat or sleep, our spiritual nature tells us when we need nourishment. We recognize that diligence in taking care of ourselves spiritually, emotionally and physically is necessary. As we begin to appreciate the idea that we are whole and complete, we are able to see the long-range possibilities for our future security. With the help of our Higher Power, we slowly become more able to "Let Go and Let God." As we learn to do this, our stress level greatly diminishes and; as it becomes apparent that spiritual growth is a life-long process, we then understand our progress must be maintained daily. The routine practice of Step Ten helps us maintain our progress in Recovery.

TENTH STEP PRAYERS

"Continued to take personal inventory and, when we were wrong, promptly admitted it."

I pray I may continue:

To grow in understanding and effectiveness;
To take daily spot check inventories of myself;
To correct mistakes when I make them;
To take responsibility for my actions;
To be ever aware of my negative and self-defeating attitudes and behaviors;
To keep my willingness in check;
To always remember I need Your help;
To keep love and tolerance of others as my code;
And to continue in daily prayer how I can best serve You, my Higher Power.

In this moment, I live my life in a new way. As I continue to open my heart and mind, little by little, one day at a time, I reveal my True Self, mend my relationships, and touch God.

MEDITATIONS

I have lost sight of myself, dear Lord; I feel I have wandered far away from Thy heavenly love. I have been too concerned with myself and in my selfishness I forget to pray for those I love. Break down this facade, dear Father, and let me truly know myself. I am lost and full of false pride; take me unto Thy loving care, open my eyes and let me see the glory of truth. I feel afraid to let go and yet my need to return to Thee is much greater. Help me, Father, to come home and bless this new day with new life and hope. Let me start living again today.

AFFIRMATIONS

I am in control of my thoughts and my emotions. I control them – they do not control me.

I value my self, and I believe I deserve the best.

Although I make sure I do those things which expect the best of who I am, I do not need to live my life in a way that allows harmful emotions to get in my way.

I enjoy the deep, strong emotions I have within me. But I choose to turn those feeling and emotions into forces of good which work for me in my life.

" Out of the night that covers me, black as the pit from pole to pole, I thank whatever Gods may be for my unconquerable soul. In the fell clutch of circumstance I have not whinced nor cried aloud, under the bludgeoning of chance my head is bloody, but unbowed. Beyond this place of wrath and tears looms but the horror of the shade, and yet the menace of the years finds, and shall find me, unafraid. It matters not how strait the gate, how charged with punishments the scroll, I am the master of my fate, I am the captain of my soul." -- William Ernest Henley, *Invictus*

Live for Today

The language of Step Ten calls to mind Steps Four (made a searching and moral inventory of ourselves), Step Five (admitted to God, to ourselves, and to another human being the exact nature of our wrongs), Step Eight (made a list of persons we had harmed and became willing to make amends), and Step Nine (made direct amends to such people wherever possible, except when to do so would injure them or others).

If you have worked these Steps, you know the benefits they bring. You also know they required a great deal of soul-searching and risk-taking. As a result of this work, however, you are breaking free from the limiting influences of the past. Old feelings of guilt, shame, resentment, and fear have been relieved. The slate of emotional pain has been wiped clean, making it possible for new levels of peace and growth to develop.

Like Steps Four and Five, Step Ten calls for a daily inventory; like Steps Eight and Nine, Step Ten calls for making amends where necessary. In a sense then, Step Ten is a recapitulation of those four Steps, but on a daily basis, dealing with issues of that day <u>only</u> rather than with your whole life.

There are many ways to do a daily inventory. The first and best is to live each moment in awareness. Too many people go through life not quite awake and not quite asleep—just passing the time. As Thoreau wrote, most people lead lives of "quiet desperation." This attitude is the antithesis of Spiritual living! Old behaviors return quickly in such a state of mind.

Living in awareness calls for being present to what you are doing, to your inner life. Gently keep your attention in the now, on what you're doing, open to your feelings, willing to give of yourself as needed, and enjoying the sights and sounds around you. This is a difficult practice – the hardest you will ever do, but the healthiest and most likely to keep you from slipping back into old habits.

For the eyes of the LORD **move to and fro throughout the earth that He may strongly support those whose heart is completely His. (2 Chronicles 16:9)**

TODAY'S STEP: I have faith that daily work on myself will result in my becoming the **best** person I can be.

"Do not reject what is of Heaven, do not neglect what is of man, and you will be close to the attainment of Truth." -- Chuang Tu

True or False

The slogans and sayings we hear around AA are catchy reminders of some important tools. But like all statements, they can be interpreted in ways quite contrary to the original spirit. Here are some of the ways we can twist them around.

FIRST THINGS FIRST -- Don't bug me about getting a job. After all, I've stayed sober for five years, haven't I?

LIVE AND LET LIVE -- Let me alone. I'll do it my way.

BUT FOR THE GRACE OF GOD -- Maybe my luck will hold out one more time.

EASY DOES IT -- The Steps will take care of themselves if I don't bother with them.

LET GO AND LET GOD -- It's hardly worth making any effort.

SPIRITUAL PROGRESS RATHER THAN SPIRITUAL PERFECTION -- I'll grow up when I darned well please.

GOD GRANT ME THE SERENITY TO ACCEPT THE THINGS I CANNOT CHANGE – This is just the way I am. Everyone else needs to change.

THIS IS A SELFISH PROGRAM -- Twelfth-Stepping is fine for other people, but my sobriety comes first.

KEEP IT SIMPLE -- I have never read *The Big Book*. I don't want to get confused.
Unsigned, Pipeline, Fresno AA

The loving kindness of the Lord is from everlasting to everlasting to everlasting . . . . And His righteousness to children's children . . . And to those who remember His commandments to do them. (Psalm 103:17-18)

TODAY'S STEP: My sense of humor helps me carry – and get – the message.

"It is possible to fail in many ways . . . while to succeed is possible only in one way (for one is easy and the other difficult – to miss the mark easy, to hit it difficult). -- Aristotle, ***Nicomachean Ethics,*** Book 1 Chapter 6.

A Daily Inventory

Another way to work Step Ten is to take time for a daily examination of consciousness. Set aside fifteen to twenty minutes at the end of the day for prayer and review of the minutes at the end of the day. A suggested format is described below:

1. Take a few moments of quiet. Breathe deeply. Ask God to help you see yourself as you truly were during the day.

2. Look back over your day – not to see what you did wrong, but to honestly acknowledge what was going on with you and others.

3. Affirm the healthy things you recognize.

4. Admit to yourself and God the unhealthy things. Ask God's forgiveness, believe it is yours, then decide if you need to apologize or make amends.

5. Use creative visualization to grow stronger. Honestly acknowledge the troubling situations of the day. See and feel yourself acting honestly and lovingly in these situations. Ask God for the grace to help you act in this new way.

6. Close with simple awareness of the sights and sounds around you, grateful for the good things in your life.

This process can be undertaken as a daily journal exercise or by prayerfully reviewing your day in your own mind. If you commit to doing this for yourself daily you will experience tremendous spiritual rewards – you will (1) Grow in self-knowledge, (2) Find it easier to live in awareness, (3) Continue to break free from old reactions, and (4) Gain power to choose your response to situations.

Then your light will break out like the dawn, and your recovery will speedily spring forth. (Isaiah 58:8)

TODAY'S STEP: By calling on my Higher Power for help daily I can turn failure into success.

"Your circumstances may be uncongenial, but they shall not long remain so if you but perceive an Ideal and strive to reach it. You cannot travel **within** and stand still **without**." -- James Allen, *As A Man Thinketh*

Focusing On what's Right

Step Ten says: "Continued to take personal inventory and when we were wrong promptly admitted it." It does not suggest we ignore what is right in our life. It says we continue to take a personal inventory and keep the focus on ourselves.

When we take an inventory, we look at many things – we look for feelings that need our attention; we look for low self-esteem creeping back in; we look for old ways of thinking, feeling, and behaving; and we look for mistakes that need correcting. But a critical part of our inventory should also focus on what we're doing right and on all that is good around us.

Part of our codependency is an obsessive focus on what's wrong and what we might be doing wrong – real or imagined. In Recovery we're learning to focus on what's right.

Even on our worst days, we can find one thing we did right. We can find something to feel hopeful about. We can find something to look forward to. We can focus realistically on visions of what can be.

James Allen in his classic text, *As A Man Thinketh*, helps us realize the importance of pursuing our dreams. "And you, too, youthful reader, will realize the Vision (not the idle wish) of your heart, be it base or beautiful, or a mixture of both, for you will always gravitate toward that which you, secretly, most love . . . . The Vision that you glorify in your mind, the Ideal that you enthrone in your heart – this you will build your life by, this you will become."

Whatever is true, honest, right, pure, lovely or of good report. Anything of excellence or worthy of praise, let my mind dwell on these things. (Philippians 4:8)

TODAY'S STEP: I will let go of the negativity in my life. I will envision my Ideal and glorify the good in my life.

"The longest journey is the journey inwards of him who has chosen his destiny." -- Dag Hammarskjold

<u>Rejoice and Be Glad</u>

A review of the day's activities serves different and complementary purposes. It keeps us focused on today and prevents us from worrying about the future or living in the past. This inventory is much the same as our Step Four inventory, except we are concerned only with today. The review is brief and can be done just before going to sleep. Some things to consider are:

- If we are slipping back, trying to control and manipulate others, we need to recognize it, take steps to correct it, then ask our Higher Power for help.

- If we are comparing ourselves to others and feeling inferior, we need to reach out to supportive friends and examine our feelings, in order to renew our own sense of self-acceptance.

- If we are becoming obsessive or compulsive and not taking care of ourselves, we need to stop and ask our Higher Power for help, not only in determining the unmet needs we are trying to fulfill, but also how to meet these needs.

- If we are depressed, we need to discover the central issue causing us to feel withdrawn or sorry for ourselves.

- If we are withholding our feelings, becoming uncommunicative or giving in to other's wants and needs, we need to take the necessary risks and express our feelings assertively. Begin with "I" statements: "I feel <u>(mad, sad, glad, confused)</u>".

Today is the day the Lord has made; I will rejoice and be glad in it. (Psalm 118:24)

TODAY'S STEP: How do I feel today? How am I doing?   If I answer those questions truthfully, I am more likely to pursue the help I need and share the happy times with others as well.

"If I am under pressure and setting myself deadlines, I will stop for a few minutes and think of just this one day and what I can do with it." *-- One Day at a Time in Al-Anon*

"One Day at A Time"

We live in a society of instant gratification: instant coffee, instant breakfast, instant money from automatic teller machines – it's all around us! No wonder so many of us arrive at Al-Anon's doors looking for the instant answer to all our problems and expecting the "quick fix" to remedy all the years of living with and loving an alcoholic.

Al-Anon and all the other Twelve Step programs are "One day at a time" programs. Recovery is a process. It takes time to regain, reclaim, and recoup all that was lost while we tried on our own to cope with active drinking. Building trust takes time; there are no immediate, ready-made solutions. But the tools and principles of "The Program" – Steps, Traditions, slogans, meetings, sponsorship, service – lead us to the answers that are right for us.

We all have dark times in our lives, but the journey to better times is often what makes us happier, stronger people. When we stop expecting instant relief, we can come to believe where we are today is exactly where our Higher Power would have us be.

Al-Anon reminds us that we can only deal with "One day at a time." This allows us to be more realistic about what we can do to improve our situation. It gets rid of the constant urgency and fear of what tomorrow will bring. Today we can see that no problem will last forever. We don't have to feel that just because we don't solve a problem immediately, it will remain forever. Now we know everything passes eventually, the happy as well as the sad.

"Today is only a small manageable segment of time in which our difficulties need not overwhelm us. This lifts from our hearts and minds the heavy weight of both past and future."

The Lord, is the one who goes ahead of me. He will be with me, He will not leave me nor forsake me; do not fear nor be dismayed. (Deuteronomy 31:8)

TODAY'S STEP: I am not afraid because God is my courage and my strength; He helps me to face the Truth.

"I've heard people in Al-Anon say they got back their self-worth. I never had any in my life, so it was a whole new feeling to like the person called 'me'." -- *As We Understood*

I Am Really on The Path:

If I always look for the best in each person, situation, and thing.

If I resolutely turn my back on the past, good or bad, and live only in the present and future.

If I forgive everybody without exception, no matter what they may have done; and if I then forgive **MYSELF** wholeheartedly.

If I regard my job as sacred and do my day's work to the very best of my ability (whether I like it or not).

If I endeavor to make my life as much of service to others as possible, without interfering or fussing.

If I take every means to demonstrate a healthy body and harmonious surroundings for myself.

If I rigidly refrain from personal criticism, and neither speak nor listen to gossip.

If I devote at least a quarter of an hour a day to prayer and meditation.

If I train myself to give the first thought on waking to God.

If I specifically claim spiritual understanding for myself every day.

If I *PRACTICE* the Golden Rule of Jesus instead of merely admiring it. He said, **"In everything, treat people the same way you want them to treat you"** **(Matthew 7:12).** (The important point about the Golden Rule is I am to practice it whether the other fellow does so or not.) Taken from Emmet Fox, *Power Through Constructive Thinking*

TODAY'S STEP: I do not run myself, my circumstances, or my feelings. I am open to myself, others, my Higher Power, and to loving myself unconditionally.

"A man should never be ashamed to own he has been in the wrong, which is but saying, in other words, that he is wiser today than he was yesterday." -- Alexander Pope, ***Thoughts On Various Subjects***

In Al-Anon we learn to take down a rigid wall of seeming perfection, to honestly admit mistakes, and to open ourselves for growth. Step Ten helps us continue to take our personal inventory on a daily basis – we can look at ourselves and decide what improvements we can make, how can we grow today and whether there is something we can learn. The following is a suggested format to help us acknowledge our weaknesses, admit our mistakes and recognize our strengths:

<u>My Daily Moral Inventory</u>

<u>LIABILITIES</u>	<u>ASSETS</u>
Anger	Self-Control
Self-Pity	Self-Forgetfulness
Self-Justification	Integrity
Self-Importance	Modesty
Self-Condemnation	Self-Esteem
Dishonesty	Honesty
Impatience	Patience
Hate	Love
Resentment	Forgiveness
False Pride	Humility
Greed	Generosity
Laziness	Activity
Procrastination	Promptness
Negative Thinking	Positive Thinking
Criticizing	Look for the Good!
Fear	Faith

When I keep track of my inventory on a daily basis, I no longer have to fear that I will fall into denial. When I turn my inventory over to my Higher Power, I know I am moving toward freedom.

One thing have I desired of the Lord, that will I seek after; that I may dwell in the house of the Lord all the days of my life, to behold the beauty of the Lord, and to meditate in His temple. (Psalm 27:4)

TODAY'S STEP: As I work the Steps with God and my sponsor, I grow in my capacity to be happy.

"Don't aim at success – the more you aim at it and make it a target, the more you are going to miss it. For success, like happiness, cannot be pursued; it must ensue, and it only does so as the unintended side effect of one's personal dedication to a cause greater than oneself or as the by-product of one's surrender to a person other than oneself. Happiness must happen, and the same holds for success: you have to let it happen by not caring about it. I want you to listen to what your conscience commands you to do and go on to carry it out to the best of your knowledge. Then you will live to see that in the long run – in the long run, I say! -- success will follow you precisely because you had <u>forgotten</u> to think of it." -- Victor Frankl, ***Man's Search For Meaning***

<u>"Let Go, Let God"</u>

Higher Power, help me to understand:
To "let go" does not mean to stop caring, it
         means I can't do it for someone else.
To "let go" is not to enable, but to allow
         learning from natural consequences.
To "let go" is to admit powerlessness,
`   which means the outcome is not in my hands.
To "let go" is not to try to change or blame another,
         it's to make the most of myself.
To "let go" is not to care for, but to care about.
To "let go" is not to fix, but to be supportive.
To "let go" is not to judge, but to allow another
         to be a human being.
To "let go" is not to protect, to permit
         another to face reality.
To "let go" is not to deny, but to accept.
To "let go" is not to nag, scold or ague, but
         instead to search out my own shortcomings
         and correct them.
To "let go" is not to adjust everything to my desires, but
         to take each day as it comes and cherish myself
         in it.
Anonymous

For You love all these things that are, and hate nothing which You have made. For never would You have made any thing, if You had hated it. But You spare all. For they are Yours, O Lord, lover of souls. (Wisdom of Solomon 9:24-26)

TODAY'S STEP: I acknowledge my wants and needs, then turn them over to my Higher Power.

"Every morning compose your soul for a tranquil day, and all through it be careful often to recall your resolution, and bring yourself back to it, so to say. If something discomposes you, do not be upset, or troubled; but having discovered the fact, humble yourself gently before God, and try to bring your mind into a quite attitude. Say to yourself, 'Well, I have made a false step; now I must go more carefully and watchfully.' Do this each time, however frequently you fail. When you are at peace use it profitably, making constant acts of meekness, and seeking to be calm even in the most trifling things. Above all, do not be discouraged; be patient; wait; strive to attain a calm, gentle spirit." -- Francis De Sales

Tradition Ten

The Al-Anon Family Groups have no opinion on outside issues; hence our name ought never be drawn into public controversy.
Tradition Ten goes further than Tradition Six in confirming, once more, the purpose of all our Traditions – to keep ourselves, as a group and a fellowship, clear of anything not related to our program.

Those of us who are deeply concerned with other causes may be tempted to share them with the group, by bringing them up in group discussions or as topics for talks. But, within the fellowship, the one thing that has brought us together must remain our sole concern. If we fail in this, it could lead to controversy, not only within the group, but on the public level.

Tradition Ten suggests Al-Anon should not take a stand for or against public issues such as child abuse, politics, segregation, or any current social causes, however important they may be to members as individuals. Such involvement could lead Al-Anon into public controversy which might seriously affect our unity and continued growth.

We are a fellowship of many thousands; our members are of many races, religions, and nationalities and have a wide variety of viewpoints. Taking a position on any outside issue would surely divide us from within.

Applying this tradition personally, Tradition 10 helps me stay focused on my own attitudes and actions. This keeps me from giving unsolicited and unwanted opinions and advice to others. I detach from things that are not my business or responsibility. Distractions divert me from a manageable life. When I do not offer unsolicited opinions to others I avoid petty arguments, heated discussions and upsetting conversations. There is a difference conflict and controversy. I can turn a conflict into controversy when I fail to mind my own business. If I allow myself to go into controversy it is because I have failed to practice tradition 10. – *condensed from Al-Anon's "Reaching for Personal Freedom"*

That we may lead a quiet and peaceable life in all godliness and honesty. (1 Timothy 2:2)

TODAY'S STEP: I focus on the power available to me by learning to wait with a good attitude.

The Rosenburg Self-Esteem Scale*

On the 10 items below, indicate whether you strongly agree, agree, disagree, or strongly disagree with the statement.

		Strongly Agree	Agree	Disagree	Strongly Disagree
1.	On the whole I am satisfied with myself.	[ ]	[ ]	[ ]	[ ]
2.	At times I think I am no good at all.	[ ]	[ ]	[ ]	[ ]
3.	I feel I have a number of good qualities.	[ ]	[ ]	[ ]	[ ]
4.	I am able to do things as well as most other people.	[ ]	[ ]	[ ]	[ ]
5.	I feel I do not have much to be proud of.	[ ]	[ ]	[ ]	[ ]
6.	I certainly feel useless at times.	[ ]	[ ]	[ ]	[ ]
7.	I feel I'm a person of worth, at least on an equal plane with others.	[ ]	[ ]	[ ]	[ ]
8.	I wish I could have more respect for myself.	[ ]	[ ]	[ ]	[ ]
9.	All in all, I am inclined to feel I am a failure. [ ]	[ ]	[ ]	[ ]	
10.	I take a positive attitude toward myself.	[ ]	[ ]	[ ]	[ ]

SCORING: For items 1, 3, 4, 7, and 10 give yourself a score of 4 for each time you said "Strongly Agree", 3 for "Agree", 2 for "Disagree", and 1 for "Strongly Disagree". On items 2, 5, 6, 8, and 9, give yourself a score of 4 for each "Strongly Disagree", 3 for "Disagree", 2 for "Agree", and 1 for "Strongly Agree" answer.

Now total your scores. Scores on the **Rosenberg Self-Esteem Scale** can range from 10 to 40, where lower scores indicate poor or low self-esteem and higher scores, positive self-esteem. If your score is lower than 20, you are not feeling good enough about yourself and your negative self-esteem may be a significant causal factor of your problems – get help! [Reprinted with permission from Morris Rosenberg, Ph.D., ***Conceiving the Self.*** New York: Basic Books, 1979.]

So God created humans in his own image. He created us to be like himself. He created us male and female. (Genesis 1:27)

TODAY'S STEP: I have a positive attitude toward myself and others.

"We must alter our lives in order to alter our hearts, for it is impossible to live one way and pray another." -- William Law

Paradoxes of Prayer

I asked God for strength, that I might achieve
       I was made weak, that I might learn humbly to obey . . .
I asked for health, that I might do greater things
       I was given infirmity, that I might do better things . . .
I asked for riches, that I might be happy
       I was given poverty, that I might be wise . . .
I asked for power, that I might have the praise of men
       I was given weakness, that I might feel the need of God . . .
I asked for all things, that I might enjoy life
       I was given life, that I might enjoy all things . . .
I got nothing that I asked for – but everything I had hoped for
Almost despite myself, my unspoken prayers were
       answered
I am among all, most richly blessed!

Prayer of an unknown Confederate soldier

Like many people, I often prayed that someday I would win the lottery because then all my problems would be solved. Anything would be possible with that much money! But would it take away the effect of growing up in a dysfunctional family? Would it take away the pain of being in an unhealthy relationship? Could it guarantee happiness? Is money really what I want or need?

No, of course not. What I really wanted is to feel better, what I needed was a closer relationship with my Higher Power. Since there are difficulties with which I must live, the only real answer is to seek the serenity to accept the things I cannot change. Today, I know serenity is available to me free of charge when I go to12-Step meetings and apply the principles I learn there to my life.

Money won't buy serenity; in fact, it could create a whole new set of problems and decisions. As a member of a practicing 12-Step group who can rely on a Higher Power's help with any and every problem that comes along, today I am becoming more serene.

What does God really want from you? God wants you to respect him and do what he says. He wants you to love Him and to serve Him with all your heart and with all your soul. (Deuteronomy 10:12)

TODAY'S STEP: My reward for practicing the principles of "The Program" in all my affairs is the priceless gift of serenity.

"When one door closes another opens. But we often look so long and so regretfully upon the closed door that we fail to see the one that has opened for us."--Alexander Graham Bell

The Twelve Step process recognizes we must become as little children: Trusting and following the lead of those who have gone before us. When we do this, we begin to gain access to our inner wisdom. We become open to change.

After A While

By Veronica A. Shoffstall

After a while you learn
The subtle difference between
Holding a hand and chaining a soul
And you learn that love doesn't mean leaning
And company doesn't always mean security.
And you begin to learn
That kisses aren't contracts and
Presents aren't promises
And you begin to accept your defeats
With your head up and your eyes ahead
With the grace of a woman
Not the grief of a child
And you learn to build all your roads on today
Because tomorrow's ground is
Too uncertain for plans
And futures have a way
Of falling down in mid-flight.
After a while you learn
That even sunshine burns if you get too much
So you plant your own garden
And decorate your own soul
Instead of waiting for someone to bring you
flowers.
And you learn that you really can endure
That you really are strong
And you really do have worth
And you learn and you learn
With every good-bye you learn.

Why am I so sad? Why am I so upset? I tell myself, "Wait for God's help!" Hope in God; for I shall again praise him, my help and my God. (Psalm 42:11)

TODAY'S STEP: I avoid making excuses for my own or someone else's behavior.

"Each person should be able to leave an Al-Anon meeting secure in the knowledge that what he, or she, has shared will not be repeated." *Why Is Al-Anon Anonymous?*

"Respect the Anonymity of Others"

"<u>Anonymity</u> is the spiritual foundation of all our traditions, ever reminding us to place principles above personalities." *Tradition Twelve*

In taking our place among the thousands of anonymous individuals who make up the fellowship of the various Twelve Step groups we know we never again have to be alone. In order to not jeopardize this valuable resource, we must ensure that we never violate its most fundamental principle – "anonymity".

Where did the concept of anonymity come from? In *AA Comes of Age,* Bill W., AA's co-founder, states, "In the beginning anonymity was not born of confidence; it was the child of our early fears. Our first nameless groups of alcoholics were secret societies . . . although we were no longer drinking; we still thought we had to hide from public distrust and contempt."

Many of us resisted coming into a program because we didn't want anyone to know about our problems. We feared our boss or our friends would find out, or it would get back to our families. However, anonymity makes it possible to leave out not only our surnames, but all the labels and expectations with which we have been burdened outside "The Program". Through our commitment to anonymity we can put aside **what** we are and begin to know **who** we are.

"Our free expression – so important to our Recovery – rests on our sense of Security, knowing that what we share at our meetings will be held in strict confidence." *Al-Anon Spoken Here*

If we want the benefits "The Program" has to offer, we have an obligation to extend to others the same respect and courtesy that keeps us feeling safe, free from labels, and free to be ourselves. We can protect each others anonymity by practicing the wisdom in the following slogan, *"Whom you see here, what you hear here, when you leave here, let it stay here."*

GOD, help me control what I say, and guard my lips. (Psalm 141:3)

TODAY'S STEP: I trust God will bring out the best in me and others.

<u>Difficulties come into our lives when GOD is trying to: Teach Us, Lead Us, or Improve Us!</u>
– Nikhil Saluja

<u>Lead Me and Guide Me</u>

*A*lmighty God, I humbly pray,
*L*ead me and guide me through the day.
*C*ast out my selfishness and sin,
*O*pen my heart to let You in.
*H*elp me now as I blindly stray,
*O*ver the pitfalls along the way.
*L*et me have courage to face each task,
*I*nvest me with patience and love, I ask.
*C*are for me through each hour today,
*S*trengthen and guard me now, I pray.

*A*s I forgive, forgive me too,
*N*eeding Your mercy as I do.
*O*h, give me Your loving care,
*N*ever abandon me to despair.
*Y*esterday's wrongs I would seek to right,
*M*ake me more perfect in Your sight.
*O*h, teach me to live as best I can,
*U*se me to help my fellow man.
*S*ave me from acts of bitter shame,
        I humbly ask it in Your name. -- Anonymous

By the time we reach Al-Anon, many of us resent others whose lives appear less troubled, envying what we think they have. But in time we discover each of us is special. We have a unique set of skills, interests, and opportunities. We can be assured we have everything we need to do what we are here to do today. That doesn't mean we have everything we want, but we can trust our Higher Power has a better grasp of what's good for us than we do.

How much can God give us if we are not open to receive? When we hold onto a problem, a fear, or a resentment, we shut ourselves off to the help and guidance that is available to us. We need to loosen our grip, we need to "Let Go and Let God."

Obey my voice, and I will be your God, and ye shall be my people. And walk ye in all the ways that I have commanded you, that it may be well with you. (Jeremiah 7:23)

TODAY'S STEP: I move forward in confidence, knowing my steps are guided.

"If there be some weaker one, give me strength to help him on; if a blinder soul there be, let me guide him nearer Thee." -- J. G. Whittier

<u>My Medallion</u>

I always carry my medallion,
A simple reminder to me
Of the fact that I'm in Recovery
No matter where I may be.

This little chip is not magic
Nor is it a good luck charm
It isn't supposed to protect me
From every possible harm.

It's not meant for comparison,
Or for all the world to see,
It's simply an understanding
Between my Higher Power and me.

Whenever I doubt the cost
I paid for Recovery,
I look at my medallion
To remember what used to be.

It reminds me to be thankful
For my blessings day by day,
And to practice the principles
In all I do and say.

It's also a daily reminder
Of the peace and comfort I share
With all who work the Program
And show they really care.

So I carry my medallion
To remind no one but me
That the Promises will unfold
If I let God work for me.

Anonymous

As having nothing, and yet possessing all things. (2 Corinthians 6:10)

TODAY'S STEP: I understand the true nature of humility. I recognize that the ability to develop and practice it is the basic foundation of the Twelve Steps.

"All as God wills, who wisely heeds to give or to withhold; and knoweth more of all my needs than all my prayers have told." -- J. G. Whittier

The Beatitudes

Blessed are the poor in spirit: for theirs is the kingdom of heaven.

I am open and receptive to the inflow and outpouring of all there is in God.

Blessed are they that mourn: for they shall be comforted.

I am grateful for challenges that lead me beyond my extremity to God's opportunity.

Blessed are the meek: for they shall inherit the earth.

I am in tune with God – that which is God-inspired and God-directed shall prevail.

Blessed are they that hunger and thirst after righteousness for they shall be filled.

I seek with all my mind and heart, and I shall find.

Blessed are the merciful: for they shall obtain mercy.

I keep my thoughts centered upon only those things I want to see manifest in my life.

Blessed are the pure in heart: for they shall see God.

I see the world, not as it is, but as I Am, and I am in spiritual unity with God.

Blessed are the peacemakers: for they shall be called sons of God.

I am a child of God and I act like one. I am a radiating center of peace and love.

Blessed are they that have been persecuted for righteousness sake: for awareness theirs is the kingdom of heaven.

In my quest for truth I press on past my humanity to a deepening and an increasing releasement of my potential divinity.

Taken from *Discover the Power Within You* by Erick Butterworth, 1989, Harper & Row: San Francisco.

For You are great, and do wondrous things; You alone are God. Teach me Your way, O Lord; I will walk in Your truth. (Psalm 86:10-11)

TODAY'S STEP: I search for Truth, and I allow others to do the same.

"All things come round to him who will but wait." -- Longfellow, *Tales of a Wayside Inn, The Student's Tale*

The God Memorandum

Everyone longs to give themselves completely to someone; to have a deep, full relationship with another; to be loved thoroughly and exclusively. But God says, "No. Not until you are satisfied, fulfilled, and content with being loved by me alone; with giving yourself totally and unreservedly to me; to have an intensely personal and unique relationship with me alone. I love you, my child. Until you discover that only in me is your satisfaction to be found, you will not be capable of the perfect human relationship I have planned for you. You will never be united with another until you are united with me; exclusive of anyone or anything else exclusive of any other desires or longing. I want you to stop planning and stop wishing. Allow me to bring that person to you. You just keep watching me, expecting the greatest things. Keep listening and learning the things I tell you. You just wait; that's all."

"Don't be anxious, don't worry, don't look around at the things others have or what I've given them. Don't look at the things you think you want. You just keep looking up to me, for you will miss what I want to show you. When you are ready, I'll surprise you with a love more wonderful than you could dream of. You see, until you are ready, and until the one I have for you is ready – I am working even this minute to have you both ready at the same time – until you are both satisfied, exclusively with me and the life I have prepared for you, you will not be able to experience the love that exemplifies your relationship with me. This is perfect love."

"And dear one, I want you to have this wonderful love. I want you to see in the flesh a picture of your relationship with me, and enjoy materially and concretely, the everlasting union of beauty, perfection, and love I offer you with myself."

"Please know I love you utterly. Believe it and be satisfied."

You are precious in My sight . . . and I love you. (Isaiah 43:4)

TODAY'S STEP: I focus on the power available to me by learning to wait with a good attitude.

"Your ability to grow to your highest potential is directly related to your willingness to act in the face of imperfection. You will come to succeed not by finding a perfect moment, but by learning to see and use life's imperfections perfectly." – Melchor Lim

"Around The Program" or "In 'The Program?"

When Old-Timers in AA say they found "getting active" helpful in their Recovery from alcoholism, they usually mean getting active in and around AA.

As most AA meetings end, you'll generally notice some of those present start putting away the folding chairs, or emptying ashtrays, or carrying empty coffee cups to the kitchen. Join in. You may be surprised at the effect on your self of such seemingly little chores. You can help wash out the cups and coffeepot, put away literature, and sweep-up.

Helping out with these little physical tasks does not mean you become the group's janitor or custodian -- nothing of the sort. From years of doing it and seeing fellow members do it, we know practically every person happily recovered in AA has taken his or her turn at the K.P. or refreshment and clean-up detail. In fact, many of us began to feel comfortable around AA only when we began to help out.

As you stay around 12 Step groups and get more involved in "The Program," you'll hear the Secretary make announcements and see the Treasurer take charge of the contributions basket. Serving in one of those capacities, once you get a little accumulation of non-drinking time (about 90 days), is a good way to fill some of the time we used to spend on drinking.

When these "jobs" interest you, read a copy of the pamphlet "The AA Group." It explains what the group "Officers" do, how they are chosen, and what "Service Work" means in AA.

And in every work that he began in the service of the house of God, and in the law, and in the commandments, to seek his God, he did it with all his heart, and prospered. (2 Chronicles 31:21)

TODAY'S STEP: I am willing to turn my will and life over to my Higher Power, to let go of willfulness and to surrender myself to Recovery.

"Be patient toward all that is unsolved in your heart and try to love the questions themselves like locked rooms and like books that are written in a foreign tongue. Do not seek the answers . . . Live the questions." -- Rainer Maria Rilke

From Having the Answers to Living the Questions

To be on a quest is nothing more or less than to become an asker of questions. In the Grail legend, the classical tale of male heroism, we are told that when the Knights of the Round Table set out on their quest, each one entered the forest at the darkest place and forged a path where none had been before. The inner, psychological meaning of this myth is that full manhood is to be found only when we commit ourselves to a life of questioning.

What do I really want?
What brings me joy?
Who am I when I dream?
Why do I feel the way I do?
What do I fear?
Who had wounded me?
Where is my place?
Whom have I injured?
How do I deal with guilt?
How do I forgive?
Whom and what will I love?
How will I express my sexuality?
What is the source of my power?
My self-esteem?
What is sacred?
Worthy of respect?
Inviolable?
For what, or whom, would I sacrifice my time, my
    energy, my health, my life?
What have I sacrificed to win the approval of others?
    To become "successful"?
In what ways have I blinded myself, disowned my power,
    denied my potential?
In what measure are my "values" mere prejudices, my
    duties blind commitments to unexamined norms?
What can I do to lessen the quantity of evil in the world?
What myth have I been (unconsciously) living?

And now, Lord, for what do I wait? My hope is in you. (Psalm 39:7)

TODAY'S STEP: How do I feel today? How am I doing? If I can answer those questions truthfully, I am more likely to pursue the help I need and to share the happy times with others as well.

"Dare to be what you are meant to be and do what you are meant to do, and life will provide you the means to do it and be it." -- James Dillet Freeman

"Keep It Green"

We learn things by seeing and touching as well as hearing them; and reading about them reinforces the strength of such learning even further. There are several AA books, numerous pamphlets, and a monthly newsletter published by AA World Services, Inc. which are readily available to help us.

"Alcoholics Anonymous" – Commonly referred to as *"The Big Book",* this is the basic textbook of AA. The first eleven chapters were written by Bill W., co-founder of AA. Many other AA members stories are also included as well as several appendixes of additional material on the effects of alcoholism.

"Twelve Steps and Twelve Traditions" – AA fundamentals are discussed at even greater depth in this book, also written by Bill W. (It is sometimes nicknamed *"The Twelve and Twelve."*) Members who want to actively work the AA program of Recovery use it as a text, along with *"The Big Book".*

"Alcoholics Anonymous Comes of Age" – This brief history tells how the Fellowship started, and how it has grown.

"As Bill Sees It" – Is a reader of Bill W.'s thoughts, from his voluminous personal correspondence as well as other writings.

"Pass It On" – This biography of AA's co-founder is subtitled *"The Story of Bill Wilson and How the AA Message Reached the World."* It also traces the development of the Fellowship and includes thirty-nine photographs from AA's history.

"Came to Believe . . ." – Subtitled *"The Spiritual Adventure of AA as Experienced by Individual Members,"* this is a collection of 75 member's personal spiritual experiences with "a Power greater than ourselves."

"The AA Grapevine" – Every month, a fresh collection of AA thought and humor appears in this magazine. Almost all its articles, graphics, and cartoons are by AA members.

I myself always strive to have a conscience, without offending God or others. (Acts 24:16)

TODAY'S STEP: I practice the discipline of H.O.W. – Honesty, Open-mindedness and Willingness everyday. I presume goodwill in everyone. I don't apply my values to others.

"We all must recognize that it was the Christ within which made Jesus what He was; and our power now to help ourselves and to help others lies in our comprehending the Truth – for it is a Truth whether we realize it or not – that this same Christ lives within us that lived in Jesus. It is the part of Himself which God has put within us, which ever lives there, with an inexpressible love and desire to spring to the circumference of our being, or to our consciousness, and our sufficiency in all things." -- H. Emilie Cady, ***How I Used Truth***

"Take the Cotton Out Of Your Ears and Put It In Your Mouth"

The ideas that got so deeply embedded in our lives during drinking do not all disappear quickly, as if by magic, the moment we start -- "keeping the plug in the jug." Our days of wine and roses may be gone, but the malady lingers on.

So we have found it therapeutic to nip off many old ideas that start to sprout up again. And they do, over and over.

What we try to achieve is a feeling of being relaxed and freed from the bonds of our old thinking. Many of our former habits of thought, and the ideas they produced, limit our freedom. They just weigh us down and are of no use – so it turns out when we look them over with a fresh eye. We don't have to hang on to them any longer unless, upon examination, they prove valid and still truly fruitful.

We can now measure the present-day usefulness and truthfulness of a thought against a highly specific standard. We can say to ourselves, "Now, that is exactly what I used to think, in the drinking days. Does that kind of thinking help me stay sober? Is it good for me today?"

We have found that anybody who has trouble of any sort related to drinking may have the condition called "alcoholism." This illness strikes without regard for age, creed, sex, intelligence, ethnic background, emotional health, occupation, family situation, strong constitution, eating habits, social or economic status, or general character. It is not a question of how much or how you drink, or when, or why, but of how your drinking affects your life – what happens when you drink?

I listen carefully to what God is saying, for He speaks peace to his faithful people. But let them not return to their foolish ways. (Psalm 85:8)

TODAY'S STEP: I search for Truth, and I allow others to do the same.

"I try to hold fast to the truth that a full and thankful heart cannot entertain great conceits. When brimming with gratitude, one's heartbeat must surely result in outgoing love, the finest emotion that we can ever know." -- ***As Bill Sees It,*** p.37

Count Your Blessings, Not Just Your Errors

One of the most effective Recovery tools we can use is found in Step Ten – drawing up a daily **Gratitude List.** As ***The 12 x 12***, reminds us, " . . . inventory taking is not always done in red ink. It's a poor day indeed when we haven't done ***something*** right. As a matter of fact, the waking hours are usually well filled with things that are constructive. Good intentions, good thoughts, and good acts are there for us to see."

A **Gratitude List** can be made as we start our day or we may find it easier to do the inventory during the meditation that ends our day in the evening. Even if life hasn't been going very well, especially during the past twenty-four hours, we need to ask ourselves what we can do to get in touch with and affirm even our minor victories.

We need to develop the habit of seeing the good behind the things that may seem to be failures on the surface. The point is we are trying, and even if we failed we learned from the experience. ***The 12 x 12*** notes: "Even when we have tried hard and failed, we may chalk that up as one of the greatest credits of all. Under these conditions, the pains of failure are converted into assets. Out of them we have received the stimulation we need to go forward."

Another key part of a **Gratitude List** is "the basic blessings of life." If things haven't gone well today or even during the past week, we still have some underlying areas in which we can be grateful. These might include good health, a good job, a comfortable home, a loving spouse, and relatively obedient children.

The final area of a **Gratitude List** is "to value anything large or small that we have seen in our day that shows us how the grace of God is working in our lives." What things worked out that seemed to be beyond our human power to engineer? Are we aware of His guidance in our lives today?

In Him we live, and move, and have our being. (Acts 17:28)

TODAY'S STEP: I have courage to go forward; to meet the new day, to handle whatever confronts me. Peace is coupled with courage, now and forever.

"I hold a doctrine, to which I owe not much, indeed, but all the little I ever had, namely, that with ordinary talent and extraordinary perseverance, all things are attainable." -- T.F. Burton

<u>What Are The Twelve Steps?</u>

Steps One through Three are **surrender steps** – we surrender our addiction (and our efforts to control our addiction) and our lives to God.

Steps Four and Five are **spiritual and moral inventory steps** – we assess the damage of our addiction to ourselves and to others, and we think about our past, which may have laid the groundwork for our addiction.

Steps Six and Seven are the **miracle transformation steps** – we hand our character defects over to God's transforming touch.

Steps Eight and Nine are the **restitution steps** – we make amends, if we can, to those we have harmed and attempt to rebuild those critical, intimate relationships.

Steps Ten and Eleven are the **daily maintenance steps** – we continue to assess our lives (sorting through the distorted thinking and feeling patterns impairing our Recovery) and seek a daily walk with God, through prayer and meditation, so we can continue to know "His will for us" and "the power to carry that out."

Step Twelve is the **transcendence and evangelism step** – we realize we have had (and will continue to have) a spiritual experience and wish to share that experience with others.

As we take each Step, we come closer to a life of wholeness, a chosen life where:

- Our dependency doesn't make poor choices for us,
- Our own false identity doesn't make self-destructive choices,
- Others don't force their choices on us,
- And we don't surrender our choices to or for anyone.

For behold, the kingdom of God is within you. (Luke 17:21)

TODAY'S STEP: There are many things I can do to improve my life and to further my Recovery, but I cannot heal myself. I need to continually ask God's help in becoming free of all that blocks me from my true self.

"To live gloriously, we need hope, not security; the freedom not only to succeed, but to fail and come back. The tragedy of life lies not in failing to reach your goals, but having no hope and thus no goals to reach." -- Dr. Henry Viscardi, Founder, The National Center for Disabilities Services

Admitting Our Wrongs

Step Ten requires us to continue to take personal inventory and, when wrong, promptly admit it. The ongoing practice of Step Ten has many benefits; most importantly, it strengthens and maintains our Recovery. We find additional rewards in many areas, such as:

- **Relationship problems diminish.** Taking inventory and admitting our wrongs promptly dissolves many misunderstandings without further incident.

- **We learn to express ourselves,** rather than fear being "found out". We see, by being honest, we do not need to hide behind a false front.

- **We no longer have to pretend we are flawless** and, thus, can be candid about admitting our wrongs.

- **Through admitting our own wrongs, others may, in turn, become aware of the ineffectiveness of their own behavior.** We develop a true understanding of others and become capable of intimacy.

To effectively work Step Ten, we need to pay special attention to promptly admitting our wrongs. Delay in admitting them merely shows us how deeply ingrained some of our behavior patterns are. The sooner we are able to admit our wrongs, the sooner we can repair the harm done to ourselves and others. Vigilance in taking a daily inventory will help us develop a feeling of freedom, as we learn to promptly take care of things that bother us. Having taken an honest, in-depth look at ourselves, we are now ready to explore our relationship with our Higher Power and the community in Steps Eleven and Twelve.

I slip, but Your love supports me when doubts fill my mind. Your comfort delights my soul. (Psalm 94: 18-19)

TODAY'S STEP: How do I feel today? How am I doing? If I can answer those questions truthfully, I am more likely to pursue the help I need and to share the happy times with others as well.

"Problems will always be with us. The problem is not the problem; the problem is the way people cope. This is what destroys people, not the problem. Then when we learn to cope differently, we deal with the problem differently, and they become different." -- Virginia Satir

A Word to Drop: "Blame"

"To see how erratic emotions victimized us often
took a long time. We could perceive them quickly
in others, but only slowly in ourselves. First of all,
we had to admit that we had many of these defects,
even though such disclosures were painful and
humiliating. Where other people were concerned,
we had to drop the word 'blame' from our speech
and thought."

Twelve Steps and Twelve Traditions, p. 47

Often times we have such a desire for approval from people in powerful positions that we are willing to sacrifice ourselves, and others, to gain a foothold in the world. Invariably this will bring us to grief. However, in "The Program" we can find true friends who love, understand, and care to help us learn the truth about ourselves. With the help of the Twelve Steps, we are able to build a better life, free of guilt and the need for self-justification.

When we become willing to accept our own powerlessness, we begin to realize that blaming ourselves for all the trouble in our lives can be an ego trip back to hopelessness.

Blaming our discomfort on outside events can be a way to avoid facing the real cause – our own attitudes. We can see ourselves as a victim, or we can accept what is happening in our lives and take responsibility for our response. Asking for help and listening deeply to the messages inherent in the Steps and Traditions of "The Program" make it possible to change the attitudes which delay our Recovery.

Henry Ward Beecher noted, "God asks no man whether he will accept life. That is not the choice. You must take it. The only choice is how." We may be guided to take action or to sit still, but when we listen to the guidance of our Higher Power we will no longer be the victim of our circumstances.

It is good for me that I have been afflicted, that I might learn Thy statutes. (Psalm 119:71)

TODAY'S STEP: I face my problems squarely and without blame.

"If I am under pressure and setting myself deadlines, I will stop for a few minutes and think of just this one day and what I can do with it." -- ***One Day At A Time In Al-Anon***

God, Help Me Live Today

God, more than anything else in this world,
    I just don't want to be sick any more.
God, grant me the serenity to accept the things
    I cannot change (people, places, and things),
The courage to change the thing I can (my attitudes),
    And the common sense to know the difference.
God, help me please, stay clean and sober
    this day, even if it's in spite of myself.
Help me Lord, stay sensitive to my own needs,
    and the things that are good for me,
    the needs of others and the things that
    are good for them.
And if You please, Lord, free me enough,
    of the bondage of self that I may be of
    some useful value as a human being,
    whether I understand or not,
That I may carry my own keys, maintain my own
    integrity and live this day at peace with You,
    at peace with myself, and at peace with the
    world I live in, just for today.
God help me in this day, demonstrate that:
    It is good for me to love and to be loved.
    It is good for me to understand and to be
    understood.
    It is good for me to give and to receive.
    It is good for me to comfort and to allow
    myself to be comforted.
And it is obviously far better for me to be useful
    as a human being, than it is to be selfish.
God, help me please put one foot in front of the other,
    keep moving forward and do the best I can
    with what I have to work with today.
Accepting the results of whatever may or may not be.

Anonymous

Every good gift and every perfect gift is from above, and coming down from the Father. (James 1:17)

TODAY'S STEP: I focus on the power available to me by learning to wait with a good attitude.

"He whose heart is full of tenderness, and truth;
Who loves mankind more than he loves himself,
And cannot find room in his heart to hate,
May be another Christ. We all may be
The Saviors of the world, if we believe
In the Divinity which dwells in us
And worship it, and nail our grosser selves,
Our tempers, greed's, and our unworthy aims,
Upon the cross. Who giveth love to all,
Pays kindness for unkindness, smiles for frowns,
Lends new courage to each fainting heart,
And strengthens hope and scatters joy abroad,
He, too, is a Redeemer, Son of God."

Ella Wheeler Wilcox, ***Collected Poems of Ella Wheeler Wilcox***

Tony's Story

Sometimes the things we consider our greatest weakness prove to be our greatest strengths. They provide us with opportunities for growth we would never have had otherwise. All my life I prayed for courage, but it was through my shyness that I learned courage was already available to me.

For the longest time, I was hesitant about sharing at meetings. I sat there and kept my secrets to myself. However, I heard my own story so often I began to lose my fear. One night, when there were a particularly large number of long silences between speakers, it became obvious that my Higher Power was telling me it was my turn to share.

I said a quick prayer and asked for the courage to speak. Before I knew it I was saying, "Hi, my name is Tony and this is the first time I am sharing my story." I don't know what I said, but I do remember the encouragement the group gave me and the number of people who came up to me after the meeting to tell me they identified with what I said. I felt totally accepted and loved unconditionally.

If my fear of speaking had simply been removed, I might never have known I was capable of acting on my own. I didn't need enough strength to get up in front of a roomful of strangers; I only needed enough to keep me taking tiny steps. I had exactly enough strength and courage to reach my goal.

Be strong and let your heart take courage, All you who hope in the Lord. (Psalms 31:24)

TODAY'S STEP: I have courage to go forward; to meet the new day, to handle whatever confronts me. Peace is coupled with courage, now and forever.

"But it is from our twisted relations with family, friends, and society at large that many of us have suffered the most. We have been especially stupid and stubborn about them. The primary fact that we fail to recognize is our total inability to form a true partnership with another human being." -- ***Twelve Steps And Twelve Traditions***

Can these words apply to me, am I ***still*** unable to form a true partnership with another human being? What a terrible handicap that would be for me to carry into my Recovery! In my program I will meditate and pray to discover how I may be a trusted friend and sponsor.

The Fellowship Prayer

Dear Higher Power, I am grateful that:

> I am part of the Fellowship, one among
> > many, but I am one.
> I need to work the Steps for the development
> > of the buried life within me.
> Our Program may be human in its organization,
> > but it is Divine in its purpose.
> The purpose is to continue my spiritual awakening.
> Participating in the privileges of the movement,
> > I share in the responsibilities,
> > taking it upon myself to carry my fair share
> > of the load, not grudgingly, but joyfully.
> To the extent that I fail in my responsibilities,
> > The program fails. To the extent that I
> > succeed, the Program succeeds.
> I shall not wait to be drafted for service to
> > my fellow members. I shall volunteer.
> I shall be loyal in my attendance, generous in
> > my giving, kind in my criticism, creative
> > in my suggestions, loving in my attitudes.
> I shall give to the Program my interest, my
> > Enthusiasm, my devotion, most of all
> > . . . myself.

Anonymous

Finally, be of one mind, having compassion of one of another; love as brethren, be tenderhearted, be courteous. (1 Peter 3:8)

TODAY'S STEP: With the help of a Higher Power, decision-making can be one of life's great adventures. Each crossroad brings a new challenge, and with God I am capable of dealing with whatever comes my way.

"The immediate future of our race is indescribably hopeful. . . . In contact with the flux of cosmic consciousness all religions known and named today will be melted down. The human soul will be revolutionized. . . . The evidence of immortality will live in every heart as sight in every eye. Doubt of God and of eternal life will be as impossible as is now doubt of existence; the evidence of each will be the same. . . . Each soul will feel and know itself to be immortal, will feel and know that the entire universe with all its good and with all its beauty is for it and belongs to it forever." -- Richard Maurice Bucke, ***Cosmic Consciousness***

No Greater Power

To find direction and meaning I must tap into a Higher Power.
That power is God as I understand Him. I will start each day with
God and take Steps Three, Seven, and Eleven. There is no Greater
Power. And then I say:

Lord, I turn my life and my will over to You today.

I walk humbly with You and my fellow travelers.

You are giving me a grateful heart for my many blessings.

You are directing my thinking and separating me from
self-pity, dishonesty and self-seeking motives.

You are removing my resentments, fears and other
character defects that stand in my way.

You are giving me freedom from self-will.

Your will, Lord, not mine.

You will show me today what I can do to help someone
who is still hurting.

As I go today to do Your bidding,

You are helping me to become a better person.

Author Unknown

If I am suffering in the will of God, keep on doing what is right, and trust God who created me, for he will never fail me. (1 Peter 4:19)

TODAY'S STEP: Faith is recognizing the longer I suffer under trying circumstances, the more certain I am to appreciate my deliverance.

"We have found that God does not make too hard terms with those who seek Him. To us, the realm of spirit is broad, roomy, all inclusive, near exclusive or forbidding to those who earnestly seek. . . . Self-searching is the means by which we bring new vision, action, and grace to bear upon the dark and negative side of our natures. With it comes the development of that kind of humility that makes it possible for us to receive God's help." -- *As Bill Sees It*

Prayer for Healing

Higher Power,

You have told us to ask and we will receive, to seek and we will find, to knock and You will open the door to us.

I trust in Your love for me and in the healing power of Your compassion. I praise you and thank You for the mercy You have shown to me.

Higher Power, I am sorry for all my mistakes. I ask for Your help in removing the negative patterns of my life. I accept with all my heart Your forgiving love.

And I ask for the grace to be aware of the character defects that exist within myself. Let me not offend You by my weak human nature, or by my impatience, resentment, or neglect of people who are a part of my life. Rather, teach me the gift of understanding and the ability to forgive, just as You continue to forgive me.

I seek Your strength and Your peace so I may become Your instrument in sharing those gifts with others.

Guide me in my prayer that I might know what needs to be healed and how to ask You for that healing.

It is You, Higher Power, whom I seek. Please enter the door of my heart and fill me with the presence of Your Spirit now and forever.

I thank You, God, for loving me.

He heals the brokenhearted and binds up their wounds. He determines the number of the stars and calls them each by name. (Psalm 147:3-4)

TODAY'S STEP: I trust the Program works if I work it and I can be restored to wholeness with God's help.

Step Eleven

"Sought through prayer and meditation to improve our conscious contact with God as we understood God, praying only for knowledge of God's will for us and for the power to carry that out."

Step Eleven is a means to deepen our partnership with our Higher Power. Having developed a relationship in Steps Two and Three, we have relied upon it heavily as we worked the subsequent Steps. In many cases, it was the single source of courage and strength for achieving our level of progress in "The Program".

Our intention to do God's will can, at times, be compromised by the appearance of our old feelings and controlling attitudes. As we experience this struggle on a daily basis, the need for help from our Higher Power becomes clear. In Step Eleven, we focus on deepening with our Higher Power. It is mostly through our quiet moments of prayer and meditation that the presence and guidance of a Higher Power becomes clear to us. As our relationship with our Higher Power improves, we see how we can rely and depend upon that power for courage and strength in meeting life's challenges. We will experience a spiritual awakening when we are willing and able to acknowledge that a Higher Power can and will direct our lives.

Step Eleven requires that we improve our conscious contact with God, as we understand Him. To do this, we need to be consistent, patient and willing to practice. We have made contact with God in three of the earlier Steps. In Step Three we made a decision to turn our will and our lives over to God's care. In Step Five, we admitted our wrongs directly to God. In Step Seven, we humbly asked God to help us remove our shortcomings. Step Eleven gives us a means of strengthening that contact and enables us to bring our Higher Power into our daily lives. Now we can let go of our feelings of aloneness and alienation and enjoy the quality partnership that is truly life-giving and life-sustaining.

The means suggested for improving our conscious contact with our Higher Power are prayer and meditation. These are two channels through which we reach God – and experience God's reaching toward us. Prayer can mean focused thought, a talk directly with God or a request for guidance and knowledge of God's will in our affairs. Meditation is listening to God. Meditation techniques are designed to calm our minds and rid us of daily preoccupations and concerns, so we can hear God's guidance and will for our lives. We learn to ask that God's will for our lives be shown to us, trusting that our best interests will be served.

ELEVENTH STEP PRAYERS

"Sought through prayer and meditation to improve our conscious contact with God as we understood God, praying only for knowledge of God's will for us and for the power to carry that out."

Higher Power, as I understand You, I pray to keep my connection with You, I pray to keep my connection with You open and clear from confusion of daily life. Through my prayers and meditations I ask especially for freedom from self-will, rationalization, and wishful thinking. I pray for the guidance of correct thought and positive action. Your will, Higher Power, not mine, be done.

In this moment I quiet my thoughts and open my mind and heart to God's guidance for me. In this moment, I feel the gentle peace that conscious contact with God allows. If I am troubled and in doubt or joyful and serene, I turn to God. I know my path will be revealed and the way to my highest good be made known.

MEDITATIONS

I thank Thee, heavenly Father, for all Thy wondrous gifts: for the blessing of health Thou so generously bestoweth upon me; for my loved ones and the responsibilities I have toward them. Thank you, Father, for my home, and all my humble possessions. It is good to feel the life energies surging through my body and to know I am part of Thy Divine Plan. As I face this new day, let me be aware of all the blessings that surround me; may I take time to look at the flowers and to see Thy purpose in every little child. How merciful Thou art, dear Father, to be always with me, and each breath I take should be a constant reminder of Thy presence. How often I go through my day without speaking to Thee. Only when I am miserable and unhappy do I seem to acknowledge Thee. Let me take the time to count my blessings, and in the joy of this new day to thank Thee with my whole heart and soul. My every hope and desire is to know Thee better; please show me how.

AFFIRMATIONS

I have a good attitude about others and a good attitude about my self.

Because I have a good attitude about my self and my life, I create strong, positive feelings and emotions within me.

I think, act, and live in a way that brings me serenity.

"Peace I leave with you, my peace I give unto you . . . Let not your heart be troubled, neither let it be afraid." -- **John 14:27**

"Clean and Serene"

The greatest essential for successful living – the secret of healing ourselves and acquiring spiritual development – is that we first attain some degree of true peace of mind or serenity.

As long as there is fear, or resentment, or any trouble in our hearts it is not possible for us to attain very much.

According to Bill W., "In A.A. we have found that the actual good results of prayer are beyond question." They are matters of knowledge and experience. All those who have persisted have found:

1.   **Strength** not ordinarily their own;

2.   **Wisdom** beyond their usual capability; and,

3.   Peace of mind which can stand firm in the face of difficult circumstances. (***Twelve Steps and Twelve Traditions***, p. 104)

The Big Book suggests that upon awakening – we consider our plans for the day:

- We ask God to direct our thinking, especially that it be incongruent with self-pity, self-will, dishonesty and self-seeking motives.

- We ask that we be shown, all through the day, what our next step is to be; that we be given whatever we need to take care of our problems.

- During the day – we pause, when agitated or doubtful, and ask for the next right thought or action. We remind ourselves who is running the show by praying many times, "Thy will be done."

Agree with God, and be at peace; thereby good will come to you. (Job 22:21)

TODAY'S STEP: I will trust in my Higher Power. I will be still and know that God's will for me is peace of mind.

"He prayeth well who loveth well both man and bird and beast. He prayeth best who loveth best all things both great and small: For the dear God who loveth us, He made and loveth all." -- Samuel Taylor Coleridge, *The Rime of the Ancient Mariner*

The Power of Prayer

Prayer is the cornerstone upon which the Truth teaching rests because it is man's direct contact with God. Emmet Fox, *Stake Your Claim: Exploring the Gold Mine Within,*

Outlines for us the principles that make our prayers powerful:

1.   **Pray daily.** In prayer, as in other human activities, practice makes perfect. Praying daily brings increased ability to pray successfully.

2.   **Pray simply.** If your prayers are becoming literary masterpieces, to that extent they are lacking in power. Jesus told us to approach God with the simplicity of a little child.

3.   **Pray gently.** In prayer, effort defeats itself. Remember you are communing with God and He does not have to be forced into a decision.

4.   **Pray with faith.** Believe the prayer you are now making is being answered. Jesus told us to believe we have received and we shall receive.

5.   **Affirm you are good.** You do not have to beg God to do something. He has already provided for your good. It is your privilege, through prayer, to bring that good into your consciousness.

6.   **Give thanks.** Giving thanks for the good you expect from your prayer is really another indication of your faith in God and prayer. The high road to demonstration, is through praise and thanksgiving – "For Thine is the Kingdom, and the Power, and the Glory."

But now ask the beasts, and let them teach you; and the birds of the heavens, and let them tell you. Or speak to the earth, and let it teach you; and let the fish of the sea declare to you…That the hand of the LORD has done this. (Job 12:7-9)

TODAY'S STEP: I connect with my Higher Power daily through prayer and meditation in the morning and at night.

"As a matter of fact, prayer is the only real action in the full sense of the word, because prayer is the only thing that changes one's character. A change in character, or a change in soul, is a real change." -- Emmet Fox, *The Sermon on the Mount*

Prayer in Action

A --   Start your prayer by giving **A**doration to God for who He is. Rejoice in His wonderful attributes.

C --   Second, **C**onfess your weaknesses to God.

T --   Third, **T**hank God for what He has done in your life.

S --   Present your **S**upplications or requests to God.

Once we see prayer in terms of relationship, the traditional teachings about prayer and the message of Step Eleven begin to make sense. Consider the following disciplines and suggestions in terms of your growth in relationship with God, **"Draw near to God, and He will draw near to you."** (James 4:8)

Commitment. We make time for what is important to us. If growing in love and knowledge of God is important, our commitment to focus daily on that relationship is a must, ***Watch over your heart with all diligence, for from it flow the springs of life***. (Proverbs 4:23)

Time. It takes time to get in touch with our deeper feelings and thoughts. It is good to set aside at least 20-30 minutes daily to relate to God, **". . . in Thy presence is fullness and joy . . . ."** (Psalm 16:11)

Solitude. Husbands and wives do not want interruptions when they are sharing intimate matters. In the same vein, Jesus says, **"Go to your inner room, close the door, and pray to your Father in secret. And your Father who sees in secret will repay you."** (Matthew 6:6)

Silence . It is good to be with God in silence. This is contemplative prayer, and eventually this type of prayer will become the mainstay of our relationship. In loving silence, we come to know God's love for us; **"Be still, and know that I am God."** (Psalm 46:10)

He that dwells in the secret place of the most High shall abide under the shadow of the Almighty. (Psalm 91:1)

TODAY'S STEP: I will connect with my Higher Power daily through prayer and meditation in the morning and at night, and anytime in between.

"Man must evolve for all human conflict is a method which rejects revenge, aggression and retaliation. The foundation of such a method is love." -- Martin Luther King, Jr.

Reflections by Emmet Fox

To spend time in negative thinking is merely to

add disappointment to disappointment.

If you are not helping the other fellow, you are not helping yourself.

It is not the chosen who are saved, but those who choose God.

If you say one thing, and do another, you are not

living up to the highest you know.

Live one day at a time. To worry over tomorrow's

demands is to lose sight of today's blessings.

If you are minding somebody else's business, you

cannot be minding your own.

Rid your mind of the negative things so there

may be room for the positive.

If you fill your mind with resentment, criticism, and

anger, you will reap the reward.

There are a thousand good starters for one good
finisher.

If you have no sense of humor, the joy of the Lord

is not your strength.

To trust in God with one part of your mind and

harbor fear in the other part, is to be a house

divided against itself.

If you want to be on the spiritual path, you must

practice the Presence of God at all times.

Confess your trespasses to one another, and pray for one another, that you may be healed. The effective, fervent prayer of a righteous man can accomplish much. (James 5:16)

TODAY'S STEP: I ask God to free me from feelings of bitterness, resentment, anger, envy, and the desire for revenge in order that I receive the gift of forgiveness.

"Where there is charity and wisdom, there is neither fear nor ignorance. Where there is patience and humility, there is neither anger nor vexation. Where there is poverty and joy, there is neither greed nor avarice. Where there is peace and meditation, there is neither anxiety nor doubt." -- Saint Francis of Assissi, **The Counsels of the Holy Father Saint Francis, Admonition 27**

<u>Guidelines for Prayer and Meditation</u>

An overview of prayer and meditation for a given day may be outlined as follows:

>At the beginning of the day, review your priorities and:
>Ask your Higher Power for direction in your thoughts and actions.
>To keep you aware of self-pity, dishonesty or excessive self-interest.
>To provide the guidance needed to take care of any problems.
>Ask your Higher Power for freedom from self-will.
>
>During the day, in moments of indecision or fear:
>Ask your Higher Power for inspiration and guidance.
>Reflect on Step Three and turn it over.
>Relax and breathe deeply several times.
>Be aware of any desire to "be right".
>Pray to your Higher Power as often as necessary during the day.
>
>"Higher Power, please help me remove my__________ (feeling, obsession, addiction, etc.)."
>
>At the end of the day, review the events that happened and:
>Reflect on Step Ten and take a personal inventory.
>
>>Ask your Higher Power for guidance in taking corrective action where   necessary.
>>
>>Ask for knowledge of your Higher Power's will for you.
>>
>>Forgive yourself and ask your Higher Power to help you learn from your errors.
>>
>>Give thanks to your Higher Power for the guidance and blessings that were part of your day.

Now this is the confidence that I have in Him, that if I ask anything according to His will, He hears me. (1 John 5:14)

TODAY'S STEP: My life is brightened, my burdens lifted and my hopes become realities whenever I look to my Higher Power for inspiration.

"When I stopped dwelling on how things would work out, I was better able to pay attention to what I was doing." – *Living With Sobriety*

AA's View of Change

AA literature emphasizes the alcoholic's egocentricity, low frustration tolerance and demand for control. These are also some of the characteristics that have been found empirically to be descriptive of alcoholics. The AA book *Twelve Steps and Twelve Traditions* gives the following description of an alcoholic's personality:

"The chief activator of our defects had been self-centered fear –

primarily fear that we would lose something we already possessed

or would fail to get something we demanded. Living on a basis of

unsatisfied demands, we were in a state of continual disturbance

and frustration (p. 76) . . . . Our demand for emotional security, for

our own way, had constantly thrown us into unworkable relations

with other people. . . . Either we had tried to play God and dominate

those about us, or we had insisted on being over-dependent upon them,

being quite unable to see that our unreasonable demands had been the

cause." **(p. 115)**

The way in which AA suggests changing these personality characteristics, or "defects of character", is through the Twelve Steps. Steps 10, 11, and 12 are Called the "maintenance Steps" and are seen as the most important for spiritual growth and, therefore, for sobriety.

Only through an emphasis upon self-honesty, patience, tolerance, kindness and humility is spiritual growth begun. The pre-Recovery alcoholic is likened to a "tornado roaring through the lives of others" (Alcoholics Anonymous, 1976, p.82), but with Step 10 "we have entered the world of the Spirit . . . . And we have ceased fighting anything or anyone – even alcohol." (p.84)

Working the Twelve Steps helps us heal many old hurts and transform much darkness. Of all the Steps, however, Step Eleven is the most important for going deeper and deeper into the realization of our relationship with God. This realization is the source of our healing and inner freedom.

Clothe yourself with compassion, kindness, humility, gentleness and patience. (Colossians 3:12)

TODAY'S STEP: I visualize myself achieving my goal of changing for the better.

"No one is as capable of gratitude as one who has emerged from the kingdom of the night." -- St. Francis of Assisi

The Prayer of St. Francis

Lord, make me an instrument of Your peace!

Where there is hatred, let me sow love.

Where there is injury, pardon.

Where there is doubt, faith.

Where there is despair, hope.

Where there is darkness, light.

Where there is sadness, joy.

O Divine Master, grant that I may not so much seek

To be consoled as to console.

To be understood as to understand.

To be loved as to love.

For it is in giving that we receive.

It is in pardoning that we are pardoned.

It is in dying that we are born to eternal life.

In Step Eleven it is helpful to review portions of the prayer of St. Francis, and understand how aptly it reflects what we learned in preceding Steps:

"Where There Is Error, I May Bring Truth"

Step Nine taught us the very act of making amends to others involved an honest admission of our evasions and untruths. Now in working Step Eleven we ask for the power to carry out those principles.

"Where There Is Doubt, I May Bring Faith"

Step Three was the crucial turning point for us to release self-will and trust there was a power greater than ourselves. Step Eleven reinforces this trust as we willingly let that Higher Power guide us through the maze of Recovery.

Where There Is Despair, I May Bring Hope"

As we admitted and accepted our problem; released self-will; trusted our Higher Power; made reparation for misdeeds; and sincerely adopted the practice of prayer and meditation, we entered into the very essence of Step Eleven.

Give thanks in all circumstances. (1 Thessalonians 5:18)

TODAY'S STEP: Thank-fullness today will help me see the miracles at work in my life.

"I find the great thing in this world is not so much where we stand as in what direction we are moving." -- Oliver Wendell Holmes

"Think . . . Think . . . Think"

The following are some affirmations that may be appropriate for many Adult Children of Alcoholics (ACoA's). Choose only those that are meaningful to you, and feel free to make up your own. Remember to make them positive, brief, and in the present tense. For example, if you're working on having a specific behavior removed, instead of saying, "I don't ___________ anymore," affirm the positive behavior you want to replace it, or affirm that your Higher Power is now removing the behavior or underlying trait. As you say the affirmations, try to suspend your doubts, and for the moment, truly believe the affirmations.

- I always hear the voice of my Higher Power clearly and accurately and act on it appropriately.
- Every day I am getting better and better.
- I am now attracting healthy, loving relationships into my life.
- The light and love of God are now working in me and through me.
- I now let go of all my doubts, fears, and anxiety.
- I now forgive everyone in my life.
- I give freely of my time, talent and treasures.
- The world is a wonderful place to be.
- I love and care for myself.
- I forgive myself for all my past mistakes.
- I now relax and enjoy life.
- I am always relaxed and centered.
- I am now following the will of my Higher Power in all things.
- I am now guided by my Higher Power in everything I do.
- I accept and own all of my feelings.
- I now enjoy deep inner peace and serenity.
- God is with me, whatever I'm doing.
- I am now ready to accept happiness into my life.
- I am healthy and full of energy.
- I now look for the lesson in everything.
- I can now give and receive love freely.

This is a trustworthy saying...so that all who trust in God will devote themselves to doing good. (Titus 3:8)

TODAY'S STEP: Before I speak or write I ask myself: is it **T**rue, **H**elpful, **I**nspiring, **N**ecessary or **K**ind.

"Nothing can bring you peace but yourself." -- Ralph Waldo Emerson

Suggested Ways to Meditate

<u>Meditation One:</u> Sit comfortably in a chair or cross-legged on the floor with your back straight. Relax, close your eyes, and breathe deeply and slowly. Focus your attention on your breathe – coming in, going out, coming in, going out. As you inhale, silently count slowly to five, and as you exhale, count slowly to eight. Concentrate on your counting and breathing. When your mind wanders into other thoughts, gently return it to your breathing.

Do this as long as you feel comfortable and can keep focused on your breathing.

<u>Meditation Two:</u> Sit or lie comfortably with your back straight. Relax, close your eyes, and breathe deeply and slowly in a relaxed, natural way. In your mind, count slowly down from ten, relaxing your muscles beginning with your feet and moving up to the top of your head with each count. When you have counted down to one and your body is completely relaxed, let your thoughts drift lightly and don't grasp onto any idea or engage in any mental discussion. Remain quietly alert, but not holding onto any particular thoughts. Be calm and relaxed for a few minutes. Don't think about the past or the future. Feel where you are now.

<u>Meditation Three:</u> Sit or lie comfortably with your back straight. Relax, close your eyes, and breathe deeply and slowly. Focus your attention on your breathing. As you exhale, imagine you are releasing all your tension, anxiety, anger, fear, resentment, frustration, worry, self-hatred, self-pity . . . everything you don't want within you. If you like, you can picture grey clouds flowing out of you as you breathe. As you inhale, see yourself taking in hope, love, joy, relaxation, serenity, confidence, faith, energy, vitality, health, strength or any quality you want to have more of for your well-being. If you wish, you can see this as bright white light entering your body with every breath. Feel the positive qualities flowing in as you inhale and the negative feelings flowing out as you exhale.

A heart at peace gives life to the body. (Proverbs 14:30)

TODAY'S STEP: My life is brightened, my burdens lifted and my hopes become realities whenever I look to my Higher Power for inspiration.

And help me to resign
   Life, health, and comfort, to Thy will,
      And make Thy pleasure mine." -- William Cowper

A Loving Kindness Meditation*

This meditation may be practiced at any time, and takes only a few moments. It is based on the Buddhist practice of **metta**, which is used to send loving kindness to all beings who inhabit the earth. With this exercise, we will practice sending loving kindness to ourselves.

Sit comfortably in a chair or cross-legged on the floor with your back straight. Relax, close your eyes, and breathe deeply and slowly. Allow your awareness to rest in the breath, feeling the sensation of the rising and falling of each inhale and exhale. Use the breath to help you settle in your body, finding a place of belonging, a place you may rest inside.

Then gently say these words to yourself, or make a recording of these words and play them back:

May I dwell in the heart.

May I be healed.

May I be filled with love.

May I be free from suffering.

May I be happy.

May I be at peace.

Repeat each phrase slowly, using each breath to deepen the heart's ability to listen, to hear each word. Allow yourself to soften, to receive the nurture and the warmth of loving kindness. Cradling yourself in your own care, you may whisper these phrases again and again, until you begin to feel a genuine sense of mercy and love for yourself.

This meditation prayer of loving kindness can become a part of your daily practice. With it, you may cultivate an awareness of yourself as a child of creation, a precious being receiving the gifts of mercy and love. (*From **Legacy of the Heart: The Spiritual Advantages of a Painful Childhood***)

Because Thy loving-kindness is better than life, my lips shall praise Thee. (Psalm 63:3)

TODAY'S STEP: My life is brightened, my burdens lifted and my hopes become realities whenever I look to my Higher Power for inspiration.

"Since recovery from alcoholism is life itself to us, it is imperative that we preserve in full strength our means of survival." -- *Twelve Steps And Twelve Traditions*

Tradition Eleven

Our public relations policy is based on attraction rather than promotion; we need always maintain personal anonymity at the level of press, radio, TV and films. We need guard with special care the anonymity of all AA members.

The basic concept of humility is expressed in the Eleventh Tradition: It allows us to participate completely in the program in such a simple, yet profound, manner. It fulfills our need to be an integral part of a significant whole. Humility brings us closer to the actual spirit of togetherness and oneness, without which we could not stay sober. In remembering that every member is an example of sobriety, each one living the Eleventh Tradition, we are able to experience freedom because each one of us is anonymous.

It is essential for our personal survival and that of the Fellowship that we not use any 12 Step program to put ourselves in the limelight. Since pride is one of our most dangerous shortcomings, practicing humility is one of the best ways to overcome it. The Fellowship of 12 Step programs gains worldwide recognition by its various methods of publicizing its principles and its work, not by its individual members advertising themselves. The attraction created by our changing attitudes and our altruism contributes much more to the welfare of 12 step groups than self-promotion.

Attraction is the main force in the Fellowship of 12 Step groups. The miracle of continuous sobriety of those who struggle with addictions within 12 Step groups confirms this fact every day. It would be harmful if the Fellowship promoted itself by publicizing, through the media of radio and TV, the sobriety of well-known public personalities who became members of AA. If these personalities happened to have slips, outsiders would think our movement is not strong and they might question the veracity of the miracle of the century. 12 Step Groups are not anonymous, but members practice anonymity.

Living Tradition 11:

When I "promote" I am trying to force a solution of my own choosing on someone else. It provokes resistance and conflict. Trying to persuade (manipulate) someone into following my advice makes attraction impossible. I have to let go entirely of trying to "help" someone else. Holding on to the delusion that I can offer a solution to someone else obstructs my spiritual growth.

But the meek shall inherit the earth; and shall delight themselves in the abundance of peace. (Psalm 37:11)

TODAY'S STEP: I understand the true nature of humility. I recognize the ability to develop and practice it is the basic foundation of the Twelve Steps.

"Make me patient, kind, and gentle, Day by day;
Teach me how to live more nearly as I pray." *-- Sharpe's Magazine*

Powerful Prayers

The Bible is a treasure house of prayers and meditation. Select those that cover your need at the moment. (For additional help with topical issues go to page 411 **Where to Turn for Help**)

I and my Father are one. If I take the wings of the morning, and dwell in the uttermost parts of the sea; even there shall Thy hand lead me, and Thy right hand shall hold me. (John 10:30, Psalms 139:9-10)

When my soul fainted within me I remembered the Lord: And my prayer came in unto Thee. I will fear no evil: For Thou art with me. He is my refuge and my fortress: My God; in Him will I trust. I will rejoice in Thy salvation. By my God I can leap over a wall. (Jonah 2:7, Psalms 23:3, Psalms 91:2, 2 Samuel 22:30)

God is not the Author of confusion, but of peace. I will go before thee, and make the crooked places straight: I will break in pieces the gates of brass, and cut through the bars in iron. A thousand shall fall at thy side, and ten thousand at thy right hand; but it shall not come near thee. (1 Corinthians 14:33, Isaiah 45:2, Psalms 91:7)

I will restore health unto thee, and I will heal thee of thy wounds. God is the health of my countenance. (Jeremiah 30:17, Psalms 42:11)

Let every soul be subject to the higher powers. There is no power but of God. God is love. God is the strength of my heart. God is my strength and power, and He makes my way perfect. He guides my way in perfectness. (Rom 13:1, I John 4:16, 2 Samuel 22:33)

The Lord shall give that which is good, and our land shall yield her increase. Our sufficiency is of God. Riches and honor are with me; enduring wealth and righteousness. (Psalm 85:12, 2 Corinthians 3:5, Proverbs 8:18)

My heart is glad and my glory rejoices... I will praise the Lord *all my life; I will sing praises to my God as long as I live... (Psalm 16:9, Psalms 146:2)*

In all my **ways acknowledge Him, and He shall direct** my **paths. (Proverbs 3:6)**

TODAY'S STEP: I connect with my Higher Power through prayer and meditation in the morning and at night.

"Oh for a closer walk with God, a calm and heavenly frame; a light to shine upon the road that leads me to the Lamb!" -- William Cowper

<u>Walking Meditation</u>

You may do this meditation inside or outdoors. Begin by finding a place to stand quietly, centering your attention in the body. After a moment, begin walking very slowly, at a fraction of your normal walking speed. Allow each step to take a few seconds. Find a comfortable pace, not so slow that you feel off-balance, yet not so fast that it is difficult to focus your attention on each step. The object is not to get somewhere, but to observe what it feels like to be walking.

Let yourself become aware of three distinct movements contained in each step you take. The first movement occurs when you lift your foot up from the earth. As your foot rises off the ground, note silently to yourself, "lifting". The second movement is "moving", when you move your foot through the air as you step forward. Again, as it happens, note "moving". Last, as you place your foot on the ground and complete the step, note "placing".

As you walk slowly forward, allow your eyes to rest on a spot a few feet ahead of you. The object is not to look from side to side as you would when you took a stroll in the park. The point of this meditation is to experience the many sensations that arise when you simply use your body to walk, one step at a time. Walking mindfully straight ahead, after about fifteen feet you may slowly turn around, noting "turning", and return back to your original point. If the mind wanders, gently return your attention to the sensations of lifting, moving, and placing. You may repeat this cycle as many times as you like.

Be aware of the unique qualities of each movement. Feel the simplicity of each action as you lift, move, and place your foot on the ground. Feel the sensations that arise with each movement. What do you notice? Do this exercise for fifteen minutes. Notice what happens to the quality of your concentration. Later, you may extend the practice to 30 minutes or more.

My mouth will speak wisdom, and the meditation of my heart will be understanding. (Psalm 49:3)

TODAY'S STEP: My life is brightened, my burdens lifted and my hopes become realities whenever I look to my Higher Power for inspiration.

"To be upset over what you don't have is to waste what you do have." -- Ken S. Keys, Jr.

A Gratefulness Meditation

At the end of the day, take a few moments to recall all the pleasant people and events that occurred, noting also those that were uncomfortable or difficult. Close your eyes and allow the significant events to arise one by one. Let yourself give thanks for whatever gifts may have touched your life today. Silently name any gratefulness you may feel for each person or event, taking the time to let your heart open and receive the gift of that experience. Giving thanks for each gift, allow each image to arise and fade away until you feel complete.

Next, begin to recall any unpleasant experiences from the day. Focus your attention on one particularly painful encounter or event. Now, try to touch that memory with gratefulness. What do you notice as you practice giving thanks for something painful? What emotions arise? Does it make you soft or angry? Does it feel easy or hard? Stay with one image, repeatedly giving thanks that this person or event was a part of your day. Be thankful for whatever teaching they brought, whatever they helped you notice about yourself. One by one, touch each painful memory with some gratefulness.

Finally, give thanks for your life. Take a moment to explicitly name all the qualities of your life for which you are grateful. Practice naming thankfulness for your breath, your body, the people who care for you, your spouse, lover, or children, for the colors of the day, for your home, for your food. Reviewing as many gifts as come to mind, speak a word of silent thanksgiving for everything you have and for all you have become.

Notice what happens in your body as you practice giving thanks. What emotions arise? What do you notice about how you perceive your life? Using this practice of gratefulness, we can begin to dispel habitual feeling of expectation and disappointment and open the door to happiness and joy.

Because the Lord is my Shepard, I have everything I need. (Psalm 23:1)

TODAY'S STEP: My life is brightened, my burdens lifted and my hopes become realities whenever I look to my Higher Power for inspiration.

"Life, for all its agonies . . . is exciting and beautiful, amusing and artful and endearing . . . and whatever is to come after it – we shall not have this life again." – Rose Macaulay

<u>DESIDERATA</u>

Go placidly amid the noise and haste, and remember what peace there may be in silence. As far as possible, without surrender, be on good terms with all persons. Speak your truth quietly and clearly; and listen to others, even the dull and ignorant; they too have their story.

Avoid loud and aggressive persons; they are vexations to the spirit. If you compare yourself with others, you may become vain and bitter; for always there will be greater and lesser persons than yourself. Enjoy your achievements as well as your plans.

Keep interested in your own career, however humble; it is a real possession in the changing fortunes of the time. Exercise caution in your business affairs; for the world is full of trickery. But let this not blind you to what virtue there is; many persons strive for high ideals; and everywhere life is full of heroism.

Be yourself. Especially, do not feign affection. Neither be cynical about love; for in the face of all aridity and disenchantment it is perennial as the grass.

Take kindly the counsel of the years, gracefully surrendering the things of youth. Nurture strength of spirit to shield you in sudden misfortune. But do not distress yourself with imaginings. Many fears are born of fatigue and loneliness. Beyond a wholesome discipline, be gentle with yourself.

You are a child of the universe, no less than the trees and the stars; you have a right to be here. And whether or not it is clear to you, no doubt the universe is unfolding as it should.

Therefore be at peace with God, whatever you conceive Him to be, and whatever your labors and aspiration, in the noisy confusion of life, keep peace with your soul.

With all its sham, drudgery, and broken dreams, it is still a beautiful world. Strive to be happy.

Anonymous

Wisdom is the principal thing; therefore get wisdom; and with all thy getting, get understanding. (Proverbs 4:7)

TODAY'S STEP: As I work the Steps, I grow in my capacity to be happy.

"Once we learn to let go of the problem . . . the loving concern and help of the other members will provide strong support to help us understand what the Al-Anon program can do for us." – ***This Is Al-Anon***

<u>Touching the Pain of Others</u>

We are never alone in our suffering. The pain of being human is shared by all who live. In this meditation, we use our own pain to make contact with the simultaneous suffering of all other beings.

Find a comfortable sitting position. Gently close your eyes and allow your attention to rest on the breath. Slowly become aware of the sensations of breathing, noting "rising, falling" with each inhale and exhale. Take a few moments with this practice to center yourself in your body.

After awhile bring your attention to your heart, noticing any sensations in the area of the chest. Going deeper, become aware of any places within where there is sadness, grief, or loss. Allow the images to arise one after another, feeling the depth of your sadness. Acknowledge to yourself that all your friends, your children, and your family will die some day; feel the place that knows you, too will die one day, and perhaps leave so much undone. Become aware of all the things left unspoken, all the love you didn't get or give, all the hurts and disappointments that have touched your life. Feel the depth of your sorrows.

After awhile, allow images of others who are in pain to arise. Begin with people close to you who are suffering illness, loss, or physical or emotional discomfort. Become aware of the nature of their pain, the sadness and grief they feel deep within. Feel how their pain is a mirror of the sorrows you carry within yourself. Feel how the pain connects you: feel also how touching this pain together, with mindful attention, opens a door to a mutual love and intimacy. Observe how birth, suffering, illness, and death touch each one of us who lives on the earth. This is the pain we all share, in which we all partake, the pain of being human that touches our common bodies, hearts and minds.

Do not fear any of those things which you are about to suffer... you may be tested, and you will have tribulations... Be faithful until death, and I will give you the crown of life. (Revelations 2:10)

TODAY'S STEP: My life is brightened, my burdens lifted and my hopes become realities whenever I look to my Higher Power for inspiration.

"Life is not a cup to be drained, but a measure to be filled." -- Anonymous

Cultivating a Sense of Abundance

The experience of scarcity and abundance is influenced by what we feel is "enough" in any given moment. When we become trapped in "wanting", we find ourselves propelled into fear and scarcity, and we desperately look for that person or thing that is going to make everything work for us. If only we had the right job, the right relationship, more money, more time, less pain . . . then we would be okay.

The "wanting mind" brings us much suffering; it is a self-perpetuating habit preventing us from experiencing the fullness of where we are and what we have in this moment, driving us to grab desperately for something else, something different. It teaches us when we are here and now, we are somehow incomplete, and what we already have could never be enough. We are cut off from the abundance of now.

In this meditation, as we mindfully investigate our wants and desires, the way we constitute what is "enough" begins to shift. When we observe the endless play of desires without identifying with them, we may begin to sense a whole new inner spirit of freedom, and the experience of abundance becomes available to us.

For approximately ten minutes, sit comfortably in a meditation posture. Let your mind be blank like a clear sky, and wait carefully for each want, each desire as it arises. They may appear as pictures, words, feelings, or sensations in your body. When a desire arises, make a silent mental note of it "wanting to move, to eat, to sleep, to scratch, etc."

With the inhalation, experience the fullness and completeness of this moment. With the exhale, allow the word "enough" to flow out with the breath. Take several moments to use the breath as a tool to explore what the sensation of "enough" feels like in your body. As we expand and deepen our ability to cultivate a sense of "enough", we may find a reservoir of nurture and peace open within us, bringing a sense of abundance. All we need is here, now. Enough.

Be careful for nothing; but in everything by prayer and supplication with thanksgiving let your requests be made known unto God. (Philippians 4:6)

TODAY'S STEP: My life is brightened, my burdens lifted and my hopes become realities whenever I look to my Higher Power for inspiration.

"Peace of mind depends on recognizing our own shortcomings. An honest personal inventory helps us recognize the faults that so often increase confusion and despair." -- *This Is Al-Anon*

"Let It Begin with Me"

Al-Anon says, "Let it begin with me."   When we identify something we dislike in another, we can look for similar traits within ourselves and begin to change them. By changing ourselves, we truly can change the world around us.

We can easily itemize our loved one's limitations. Hours pass while we list the ways in which *they* could stand to change. But not one thing will ever improve as a result of our mental criticism. All it does is keep our mind on someone other than ourselves. Instead of admitting our powerlessness over another person's choices and attitudes, we delude with illusions of power. In the end we may become more bitter, more hopeless, and more frustrated. And nothing about our situation, or the other person, has changed.

What would happen if we took our list of criticisms and applied it, gently, to ourselves? We may complain about our loved one's verbal abuse – after all, we don't speak to him/her that way. However, at the level of thought, we may be just as abusive – only we manifest it differently, internally, with harmful words we don't say out loud.

Responding in kind to behavior directed at us is a character defect which leads to reacting to insults with more insults and to rudeness with rudeness. We may never have thought to act any other way until we started our Twelve Step work. We are powerless over other people's attitudes, but we don't have to permit them to goad us into lowering our own standards. To the best of our ability, we can choose to treat everyone with kindness.

"Let it begin with me" means not having to accept unacceptable behavior. We can begin by refusing to accept it from ourselves. We can choose to behave courteously and with integrity.

Mercy, peace, and love be multiplied to you. (Jude 1:2)

TODAY'S STEP: There are so many ways in which I can improve the quality of my life. Instead of fretting about what I can't have or can't do, I'll take action to create something positive in my life today.

"Prayer should be the key of the day and the lock of the night." -- Old Proverb

Parts of Prayer

F   **FAITH**: the foundation of all prayer.

A   **ADORATION**: your expression of love to the Lord.

C   **CONFESSION**: your admission of agreement with the Lord.

T   **THANKSGIVING**: your expression of praise and appreciation for *who* He is more than for *what* He has done for you.

S   **SUPPLICATIONS**: your requests you bring to the Lord for yourself and others.

FACTS is a good formula for our prayer. Each part does not necessarily have to be present each time we pray, but it will help us on those days when we feel "dried up."

The Psalms also provide excellent guidelines for our prayers. In Psalm 31:3, for example, we pick up two ideas that are perfectly appropriate for prayer.

> **Thou art my rock and my fortress; therefore for Thy name's sake lead me, and guide me.**

As we face decisions or clouds of uncertainty, we ask Him to lead and guide us. We might want to begin our prayer by using this verse and telling the Lord how it applies to our needs today.

Another valuable example of a short prayer is made by the Syrophenician woman in **Matthew 15:25. She came "and worshipped him, saying, 'Lord, help me.'"** It is no doubt the shortest prayer in the Bible. The woman had a serious problem: She couldn't stand to live with her daughter. She came to the Lord asking for mercy and pity because of her daughter, and left acknowledging there were problems in her own life that needed to be addressed. When she prayed, "Lord, help me," and was willing to admit her part of the problem, "her daughter was made whole from that very hour".

TODAY'S STEP: I connect with my Higher Power daily through prayer and meditation in the morning and at night, and anytime in between.

"Though no one can go back and make a brand new start, anyone can start from now and make a brand new end." -- *As We Understood . . .*

<u>"Keep It Simple"</u>

The purpose of the Eleventh Step it to reaffirm for us, each day, the first three Steps of "The Program" – (1) To admit our powerlessness, (2) To recognize a healing Power outside of ourselves, and (3) To turn our wills and our lives over to the care of that Power, which has given us the strength to turn our lives around. Now we have to keep it that way. This Step is our chance to develop an ever deepening awareness of our Higher Power and the peace that comes with that relationship. <u>It 's a daily recommitment to our spirituality.</u>

Step Eleven works in tandem with the Tenth Step. As we make a commitment to carry out both our spot check and daily inventories, we use conscious contact with our Higher Power to help and sustain us. And, like the inventories of Step Ten, daily meditation and prayer keeps "The Program" in our consciousness and keeps it growing. We may feel a letdown when we have passed through the initial excitement and dedication to our new way of life – the Eleventh Step helps us deal with that.

It's like love. First there is the romantic attraction, thrilling in its newness and possibility. Then this passes, and we are ready to begin to learn to deeply love, to become completely involved and intimate with our loved one, in good times and in bad. Living within the belief system of the Twelve Steps is the process of love, love for the very deepest and most important part of ourselves: Our spiritual core.

Seeking guidance toward spiritual wellness is challenging and may continue to cause us problems. It's so easy to fall back into rigidly trying to manage our lives and asking our Higher Power to support us in our will. Again and again we need to give up our attempts to control, accept our powerlessness, and seek guidance – it's our way to the spiritual health we're looking for. Controlling keeps us focused outward, watching ourselves managing others. Step Eleven helps us increase our inward focus, and that focus becomes clearer through our Higher Power. It encourages our spirits to take root in the fertile soil of our internal relationship and become strong.

I have taught thee in the way of wisdom; I have led thee in right paths. (Proverbs 4:11)

TODAY'S STEP: I move forward in confidence, knowing my steps are guided.

"Learn to be as an angel, who could descend among the miseries of Bethesda without losing his heavenly purity or his perfect happiness. Gain healing from troubled waters. Make up your mind to the prospect of sustaining a certain measure of pain and trouble in your passage through life. By the blessing of God this will prepare you for it; it will make you thoughtful and resigned without interfering with your cheerfulness." -- J. H. Newman

Sobriety Prayer

If I speak in the tongues of men and even of angels, but have no sobriety, I am a noisy gong or a clanging cymbal. And if I have prophetic powers, and understand all mysteries and all knowledge, and if I have all faith, so as to move mountains, but have not sobriety, I am nothing. If I give away all that I have, and if I deliver my body to be burned, but have not sobriety, I gain nothing.

When I am sober, I am patient and kind. When I am sober, I am not jealous nor boastful, nor arrogant or rude. When I am sober, I do not insist on my own way. When I am sober, I am not irritable or resentful. I do not rejoice at wrong as I used to do, but rejoice in what is right.

When I am sober, I can bear all things, believe in all things, hope all things, and endure all things.

Sobriety never ends and never fails.

When I was using, I spoke like an arrogant child, thought like a stubborn child, and reasoned like a rebellious child. When I chose sobriety for my life, I gave up my childish ways.

So faith, hope, love and sobriety abide, but for me, the most important has to be sobriety, for without it, I cannot have the other three, nor can I ever have the serenity I yearn to possess.

Let the words of my mouth, and the meditation of my heart, be acceptable in Thy sight, O Lord, my strength, and my redeemer. (Psalm 19:14)

TODAY'S STEP: My reward for practicing the principles of "The Program" in all my affairs is the priceless gift of serenity.

"If we stand in the openings of the present moment, with all the length and breadth of our faculties unselfishly adjusted to what it reveals, we are in the best condition to receive what God is always ready to communicate." -- T. C. Upham

<u>The Gratitude Prayer</u> [Unknown]

O God,

> I want to thank You for bringing me this far along the road to Recovery.
>
> It is good to be able to get my feet on the floor again.
>
> It is good to be able to do at least some things for myself again.
>
> It is best of all just to have the joy of feeling well again.

O God,

> Keep me grateful; grateful to all the people who helped me back to health;
>
> Grateful to You for the way in which You have brought me through it all.

O God,

> Still give me patience.
>
> Help me not to be in too big a hurry to do too much.
>
> Help me to keep on doing what I'm told to do.
>
> Help me to be so obedient to those who know what is best for me, that very soon I shall be on the top of the world and on the top of my job again.

I can say what the psalmist said (Psalm 40: 1-3):

"I waited patiently for the Lord;

He inclined to me and heard my cry.

He took me from a fearful pit, and from the miry clay,

And on a rock He set my feet, establishing my way."

And He hath put a new song in my mouth, even praise unto our God: Many shall see it, and fear, and shall trust in the Lord. (Psalm 40:3)

TODAY'S STEP: I trust God will bring out the best in me and others.

"He whose heart is full of tenderness, and truth;
Who loves mankind more than he loves himself,
And cannot find room in his heart to hate,
May be another Christ. We all may be
The Saviors of the world, if we believe
In the Divinity which dwells in us
And worship it, and nail our grosser selves,
Our tempers, greed's, and our unworthy aims,
Upon the cross. Who giveth love to all,
Pays kindness for unkindness, smiles for frowns,
Lends new courage to each fainting heart,
And strengthens hope and scatters joy abroad,
He, too, is a Redeemer, Son of God."
 -- Ella Wheeler Wilcox, ***Collected Poems of Ella Wheeler Wilcox***

Tough Minded Faith for Tender Hearted People

In his book ***Tough Minded Faith For Tender Hearted People***, Dr. Robert Schuller encourages us to exercise our growing faith daily by using the following declarations:

"I'm on the right road. I am walking the walk of faith. I have made
   the decision to follow the Lord."

"I have given my life to God and He is in control of it."

"The God who has command over my life is protecting me from hidden
   shoals that could sink the ship of my soul and spirit."

"God is opening doors that will surprise me with new opportunities."

"God is closing doors that I want to go through because He knows
   they will lead to my failure and destruction.

Thank you, Father for assuring me of success on my walk of faith. I know I'm on the right road. Thank You for opening and closing doors, thereby guiding me on my daily walk.

So we are always confident; . . . for we walk by faith, not by sight. (2 Corinthians 5:6-7)

TODAY'S STEP: The Steps offer me a road map for living that leads to a spiritual awakening and beyond. I can't skip ahead to the end of the journey – which can at times be a hard one – but I can put one foot in front of the other and follow the directions I've been given, knowing that others who have gone before me have received more along the way than they had ever dreamed.

"I am not the brood of the dust and sod,
Nor a shuttled thread in the look of fate;
But the child divine of the living God,
With eternity for my life's estate.
I am not the sport of a cosmic night,
Nor a thing of chance that has grown to man;
But a deathless soul on my upward flight,
And my Father's heir in His wondrous plan.

As I weigh the suns on the rim of space,
Who can care to doubt of my destiny?
Who can fence my feet within time and place,
As I search the worlds of infinity?
I am man: the son of the Most High;
am man, and one with the Life divine;
I am Lord of earth, and of sea and sky;
And behold! The powers of heave are mine.

I am man the chosen, and man the free,
And it matters not what I may have been;
For I walk erect through eternity
To the far-off goal that is yet unseen.
With unswerving faith in the coming Day,
I have turned my course from the things of time,
And with Jesus, my brother, to point the way,
I have found my place in the Life sublime."
-- Alva Romanes, *Weekly Unity*

"Help Is Only a Phone Call Away"

Sometimes we become so busy staring at our problems we miss the guidance we've been given. When we become willing to let go of the need to do it ourselves, we can listen to others and receive direction from our Higher Power. We can become better able to move beyond our problems and start solving them if we can:

1. Accept that help often comes in unexpected forms;
2. Let go of it long enough to reach out for help; and,
3. Understand we need the help, support, and guidance we receive from our Higher Power and our Twelve Step friends.

For all who are led by the Spirit of God are children of God. So you have not received a spirit that makes you fearful slaves. Instead, you received God's Spirit when he adopted you as his own children. Now we call him, "Abba, Father." (Romans 8:14-15)

TODAY'S STEP: I move forward in confidence, knowing my steps are guided.

"Man's self is not yet man,
Nor shall I deem his object saved, his end attained,
His genuine strength put fairly forth,
While only here and there a star dispels the darkness,
Here and there a towering mind o'erlooks its prostrate
Fellows. When the host is out at once,
To the despair of night:
When all mankind alike is perfected,
Equal in full-blown power, -- then, not till then I say,
Begins man's general infancy."

Robert Browning, *Paracelsus*

<u>"Am I Willing?"</u>

Dear Higher Power, help me:

To forget what I have done for other people, and to remember what other people have done for me.

To ignore what the world owes me, and to think what I owe the world.

To put my rights in the background, and my duties in the middle distance, and my chances to do a little more than my duty in the foreground.

To see that my fellow members are just as real as I am, and try to look behind their faces to their hearts, hungry for joy as mine is.

To own that probably the only good reason for my existence is not what I can get out of life, but what I can give to life.

To close my book of complaints against the management of the universe and look for a place where I can sow a few seeds of happiness – am I willing to do these things even for a day?

Then I have a good chance of staying with "The Program".

(Author Unknown)

And everyone who thus hopes in him purifies himself as he is pure. (1 John 3:3)

TODAY'S STEP: I am willing to turn my will and life over to my Higher Power, to let go of willfulness and to surrender myself to Recovery.

"It is said that nature abhors a vacuum; I tell you God abhors a vacuum and cannot abide a vacuum anywhere on earth. So, empty yourself of self and automatically fill with God."
– Meister Eckhart

The Process of Spiritual Growth

Believing is the beginning of each thing that we accomplish in our lives. To be successful, believing must become strong enough to incite a decision, <u>which is a choice of a course of action.</u> Once this decision is made and it has become strong enough, it will bring about results. Once the results are plain and clear, we grow in conviction, trust, confidence and hope in God. Faith grows as the result of actions.

The Twelve Steps are based on this plan. These are the principles by which humankind has succeeded or failed.

The Twelve Steps:

Step 1:   **Willingness** to change

Step 2:   **Believe** we can change.

Step 3:   **Decision** to change.

Step 4:   **Inventory** to change.

Step 5:   **Actions** to change.

Step 6:   **Actions** to change.

Step 7:   **Actions** to change.

Step 8:   **Actions** to change.

Step 9:   **Actions** to change.

Step 10:   **Actions** to change.

Step 11:   **Actions** to change.

Step 12:   **Changed.**

We can see faith comes as a result of a complete process. This is why Step 12 is the conclusion, and we should not expect this result (faith) in Step 2. Many people fail because they are expecting faith before they make a decision to take any action and get results. We cannot begin with faith; we can only believe in the beginning. But this is all we need to get us started. (Adapted with permission from ***Recovery Dynamics,*** 2nd Edition, Little Rock, Arkansas: Kelly Foundation, 1989.)

Tell those rich in this world's wealth to quit being so full of themselves and so obsessed with money, which is here today and gone tomorrow. Tell them to go after God, who piles on all the riches we could ever manage—to do good, to be rich in helping others, to be extravagantly generous. If they do that, they'll build a treasury that will last, gaining life that is truly life. (1 Timothy 6:17-19)

TODAY'S STEP: When I rely on my Higher Power's help I can achieve.

"There are only two ways to live your life. One is as though nothing is a miracle. The other is as though everything is a miracle." — Albert Einstein

The Way of Self-Knowledge

Devote one short hour every day to serve your Maker and your Lord,

Do worship, meditate or pray or sow some seeds of Good abroad.

Do something, in His name, to show that you are mindful of the debt

Which children to their parents owe for all the gifts they freely get.

Do something noble, something fine that has no color of the self,

Nor shade of ego, me or mine, no thought of honor, fame or self.

Do something good to benefit the humble crowds surrounding you,

Whose minds not yet by Wisdom lit cannot decide what they should do.
--Gopi Krishna

The Way is toward the "relationship that has no end" between our own soul and God. One begins it in silence and solitude. In silence and solitude we find "peace with God." We find a deeper and subtler way of communicating with the divine by listening in silence. We are healed in silence.

It is in solitude the word is passed to us, the message is given. We become conscious of all things, see divinity in all beings, even the unseemly. And from this place, intuition, our inner wisdom, is fine tuned.

I don't think the way you think. The way you work isn't the way I work. God's Decree. For as the sky soars high above earth, so the way I work surpasses the way you work, and the way I think is beyond the way you think. Just as rain and snow descend from the skies and don't go back until they've watered the earth, Doing their work of making things grow and blossom, producing seed for farmers and food for the hungry, So will the words that come out of my mouth not come back empty-handed. They'll do the work I sent them to do, they'll complete the assignment I gave them. (Isaiah 55:11)

TODAY'S STEP: I have faith that daily work on myself will result in my becoming the best person I can be.

"The feelings of release, of yielding or letting go, when we acknowledged that no change in others can be forced, helped to loosen the suffocating grip of our destructive emotions: guilt, fear, self-pity, resentment." -- *Al-Anon's Twelve Steps & Twelve Traditions*

What Is Guilt?

We need a clarification about guilt because we spend a great deal of our time wallowing in it and don't seem to be able to find our way out of it. There is no one who has not or is not now struggling with guilt as a major issue in life.

- Guilt is the experience of having separated ourselves from God and thereby having attacked God.

- Guilt is the psychological experience of the belief in sin, the experience of having done something wrong.

- Guilt is self-hatred, a feeling of inferiority and incompleteness.

- Guilt is manifest in our sense of failure, apathy, and despair.

- Guilt is a sense of shame about our bodies.

- Guilt is always disruptive.

- Guilt is more than merely not of God. It is the symbol of attack on God.

The ultimate source of our guilt is the belief we have rebelled against God. Believing we have done something wrong and harmful to God, we inevitably believe we will be punished for our sins. Because we fear God, when we are anxious and need help we do not turn to God, we turn to the ego instead. The ego, fearing God, makes the experience of God's love inaccessible and reinforces our experience of separation and fear. In truth, we cannot separate ourselves from God, like the prodigal son, we can return home anytime.

Those who obey God's commandments remain in fellowship with him, and he with them. And we know he lives in us because the Spirit he gave us lives in us. (1 John 3:24)

TODAY'S STEP: I avoid making excuses for my own or someone else's behavior.

"We perceive that only through utter defeat are we able to take our first steps toward liberation and strength." -- *Twelve Steps And Twelve Traditions*

Five Uses of Adversity That Really Work

It may be difficult to believe we can learn from adversity, yet it is our best teacher. Think what it can do for us if we let it.

- **It can open our eyes.** It can force us to look at our life and our lifestyle, to let go of old, inappropriate hopes, fruitless love affairs, dependencies which hold us back, self-deception which feeds our ego, but does nothing else.

- **It can make us grow in ways we never knew.** Storms demand more alertness from us than sunshine does. From somewhere deep inside we can find more patience, more endurance, more courage, more concentration – when we are sure there are no resources left, we find even more.

- **It can give us the precious gift of compassion.** Nobody helps the homeless as much as those who have known homelessness; nobody knows pain so well as someone who has suffered. Adversity gives us the rare gift of empathy.

- **It can teach us a universal truth: Life is not fair.** People die before they should; lovers who belong together quarrel and part; a conglomerate seizes a company and we lose our job; someone else gets the lead in the school play. When we are very young we believe life will be trouble-free and justice always will triumph – the quicker we learn that isn't so, the easier time we will have.

- **If we are very thoughtful it can lead us to God.** Good fortune rarely does that. It is human nature to believe when we lose anything that someone else had a hand in our misfortune. We may blame a Higher Power – when we do we are at the same time acknowledging Him! A strange spiritual dynamic gets set in motion: After blaming God, we can begin appealing to Him for help out of adversity – and with that we find our hope. (Taken from *The Power of Hope* by Maurice Lamm)

He grants the desires of those who revere Him; He hears their cries for help and will save them. (Psalm 145:19)

TODAY'S STEP: God will strengthen me when life gets tough.

"A most beneficial exercise in secret prayer before the Father, is to write things down so that I see exactly what I think and want to say. Only those who have tried these ways know the ineffable benefit of such times in secret." -- Oswald Chambers

Benefits of Written Prayer

The idea of writing prayers is not new. It is, in fact, scriptural. We have an excellent example in the Bible of written prayers. If David hadn't written his pleas, hurts, and rejoicings to the Lord, we would not have the Psalms.

When we quietly take time to write our prayers to the Lord, we are also led to hear His word. And when He speaks to us, we can immediately record in our prayer book what He has said to us. He directed Jeremiah: **"Write thee all the words that I have spoken unto thee in a boo**k" (Jeremiah 30:2). The blessings of written prayers are as follows:

1. It Prepares Us to Hear the Voice of the Lord.

2. It Enables Us to Fulfill Scripture in Our Lives.

3. It Fixes Our Focus on Him.

4. It Encourages Daily Discipline.

5. It Establishes a Communion With God.

6. It Lifts Us Out of Loneliness.

7. It Strengthens Us Against Attacks.

8. It Allows God to Control Our Emotions.

9. It is the Key to Our Healing and Maturing Process.

10. It Deepens Love and Commitment to the Lord.

11. It Keeps Us Alert in Prayer.

12. It Refocuses What We Want From God.

Here's what I want you to do: Find a quiet, secluded place so you won't be tempted to role-play before God. Just be there as simply and honestly as you can manage. The focus will shift from you to God, and you will begin to sense his grace. (Matthew 6:6)

TODAY'S STEP: I connect with my Higher Power daily through prayer and meditation in the morning and at night.

Step Twelve

"Having had a spiritual awakening as the result of these steps, we tried to carry this message to others and to practice these principles in all our affairs."

The Twelfth Step is the goal we were seeking when we began our journey toward healing and Recovery. As we worked our way through the Steps, personal intuition told us there was hope for us when we completed the cycle of this process. No mystery surrounds the Twelve Steps when we realize they really work for those who are willing to risk self-discovery through surrender to a Higher Power. If we have practiced the other eleven Steps to the best of our ability, we will receive all of the gifts that result from our surrendering to a Higher Power and can pass them on to others.

Spiritual growth is an ongoing process – it may have begun early in the Steps, but it will continue for the rest of our lives. Spiritual growth is not a distinct event with a clear beginning and ending; it is continuing evolution of becoming more compassionate, loving, caring and content. Our relationships with our families improve as we draw closer, yet we recognize each other's need for independence. We rarely have unrealistic expectations of ourselves, and we accept others as they are, not as we might want them to be.

Because we know "The Program" works, and it is working for us, we are ready to share it with others. The message we carry to those who are in bondage, as we once were, is a liberating one. Sharing the message strengthens our own Recovery and advances our spiritual growth. In return, the new strengths and insights we receive help us continue our growth in heart, mind and spirit. Our ability to effect change convinces others of the value of the Steps and, in this way, "The Program" grows and prospers.

There is no specific way to "carry this message to others" besides telling our stories as honestly as we can – by explaining what our lives were like, what happened to us as a result of the Steps and how our lives have changed. This is one time when truly being ourselves is the gift we give to others. It can happen anywhere – when we are called upon to do volunteer work, share in meetings, and interact with co-workers and family members. Sharing our story with others often helps them recognize their own needs and teaches us more about humility and honesty. As we share our experience, strength and hope with newcomers, we can inspire them to solve their own problems, look at themselves honestly and stop blaming others for their pain. The process is gradual, regenerative and never-ending.

"Having had a spiritual awakening as the result of these steps, we tried to carry this message to others and to practice these principles in all our affairs."

My spiritual awakening continues to unfold. The help I have received I shall pass on and give to others, both in and out of the Fellowship. For this opportunity I am grateful.

I pray most humbly to continue walking day by day on the road of spiritual progress. I pray for the inner strength and wisdom to practice the principles of this way of life in all I do and say. I need You, my friends, and "The Program" every hour of every day. This is a better way to live.

I dedicate myself to the love and care of my Higher Power. All healing work is the result of my partnership with my Higher Power. I am committed to surrendering all concerns, from the largest to the smallest, to my Higher Power. I accept that my self-will no longer needs to control my beliefs, thoughts or actions. Each day, I give thanks for the part of me that is being healed. I cooperate with this healing by agreeing to face my discomfort, knowing my Higher Power is there. I know my healing is a source of joy and serenity to me. I am ever-open for the opportunity to spread the truth and the joy of my Recovery.

MEDITATIONS

Thank you, Father, for the awakening I feel inside me; how fortunate I am to be a child of God. Thou hast known my torment and struggle, and when I was in the darkness of despondency Thou did show me the way. How grateful I am to know Thy love; in Christ all things are possible. There is so much I must learn and accomplish; help me to completely restore my soul with Thy love. May this day be filled with continued joy of the spirit; how glad I am to be alive! May every thought and action glorify thy Holy Name.

AFFIRMATIONS

I have learned the skill of creating those emotions that give me peace of mind, improve my physical health, and improve my relationships with those around me – each day, at all times, and in all situations.

I have **faith**, I have **courage**, and I have **belief** – in my self and in the best possible outcome of any problem I face.

"A strong body and a bright, happy or serene countenance can only result from the fine admittance of thoughts of joy and goodwill and serenity into the mind." -- James Allen, ***As A Man Thinketh***

We've come a long way. And we still have a long way to go. But what a way! The freedom we now enjoy will be triply enhanced when we have finished Step Twelve – the ultimate Step in decisiveness and resolve – for its benefits are without number.

Our sense of self-worth is propelling us into the awakening that Step Twelve promises. By now, of course, we understand there is no uniformity in the awakening process. Some of us experience a spiritual conversion that dispels all doubt. Others benefit by an educational process allowing us to view spirituality in a new and comfortable light. But no matter how it comes to us, the experience is so profound it releases us from the bondage of self.

Ten Steps to Serenity

1. BEGIN EACH DAY CHEERFULLY AND UNHURRIEDLY.

2. IF YOU FEEL SAD, TRY TO ACT HAPPY AND SMILE.

3. CALMLY ACCEPT THE DIFFICULT.

4. AVOID NEGATIVE AND USELESS WORRIES.

5. SUBSTITUTE POSITIVE THOUGHTS AND EMOTIONS.

6. "DO WHAT YOU'RE DOING," THAT IS, THROW YOURSELF INTO THE TASKS OF LIFE.

7. HAND NOBODY THE RIGHT TO DEPRESS YOU EMOTIONALLY.

8. FOLLOW A MORAL CODE YOU BELIEVE IN.

9. CULTIVATE A SENSE OF HUMOR AND PROPORTION.

10. MEDITATE DAILY OR RECREATE REASONABLY OFTEN.

Great peace have they which love thy law; and nothing shall offend them. (Psalm 119:165)

TODAY'S STEP: My reward for practicing the principles of "The Program" in all my affairs is the priceless gift of serenity.

"You are as young as your faith, as old as your doubt; as young as your self-confidence, as old as your fear, as young as your hope, as old as your despair." -- General Douglas MacArthur

"God Is Never Late"

Youth is not a time of life. It is a state of mind. Nobody grows old by merely living a number of years. People grow old only by deserting their ideals. Years wrinkle skin, but to give up enthusiasm wrinkles the soul. Worry, doubt, self-distrust, fear and despair – these are the long, long years that bow the head and turn the growing spirit back to dust.

When you feel so depressed you think you can't make it through the day and you are ready to give up, do you ever honestly ask God for his help? Do you ever consider saying, "Help me, Lord"?

Perhaps you wouldn't dream of praying this way, of really opening up to the Lord and sharing with him your darker side – the strong negative thoughts and emotions, the desperate quality of your existence. However, the truth is you feel very alone, exhausted from the stresses in your life. You want to keep hoping, but you feel defeated.

When you pray, you needn't pretend everything is fine. Why not be honest with the Lord? He knows you are suffering. Tell God exactly how you feel. Say, "Lord, I'm sad." "Lord, I'm hurting." "Lord, I'm so lonely." Then ask God to help.

You don't have to hide your feelings of doubt and worry from God or omit talking about your struggles. Don't feel you always have to be on top of things or always feeling good. God loves you just as you are at each moment – whether you are happy or sad, enthusiastic or exhausted.

It's essential to tell God in all honesty you need help. Saying, "Lord, I love you; help me," is a simple, yet profound prayer. God wants to help you, you need only ask.

Let the wicked forsake his way, and the unrighteous man his thoughts; and let him return unto the Lord, and he will have mercy upon him. (Isaiah 55:7)

TODAY'S STEP: I will ask my Higher Power to help me let go of fear, doubt, and confusion and fill me with faith, trust and serenity.

"Our birth is but a sleep and a forgetting,
The soul that rises with us, our life's Star,
Hath had elsewhere its setting,
And cometh from afar;
Not in entire forgetfulness,
And not in utter darkness,
But trailing clouds of glory, do we come,
From God, who is our home."
                    -- William Wordsworth, ***Ode, Intimations of Immortality***

<u>"If God Seems Far Away, Who Moved?"</u>

When you are up against a very difficult problem, you may feel you are fighting alone. You call out to the Lord, but God remains silent. You ask for comfort, but you are not comforted. You feel abandoned, even rejected.

God never abandons you. After creating you, God keeps you in existence and promises you everlasting life. Consider the relationship between parents and children: Parents do not abandon children who are in trouble. Even if they are separated by long distances, they still care. So it is with the Lord. He never leaves you completely alone. While dying on the Cross, Jesus knew the terrible loneliness that comes when God seems far away. He felt the emptiness, the sadness. But this did not stop him from carrying out his mission, from facing his trials, and from emerging victorious. That God is with you at **<u>all</u>** times can be seen from the following ***Footprints*** story:

> "One night a man had a dream and in his dream he reviewed the footsteps he had taken in his life. He noticed that all over the mountains and difficult places that he had traveled there was one set of footprints; but over the plains and down the hills, there were two sets of footprints, as if someone had walked by his side. He turned to Christ and said, "There is something I don't understand. Why is it that down the hill and over the smooth and easy places you have walked by my side; but, here over the tough and difficult places I have walked alone, for I see in those areas only one set of footprints."

Christ turned to the man and said, "It is that while your life was easy I walked along your side, but here, where the walking was hard and the paths were difficult, was the time you needed Me most, and that is why I carried you,"

. . . I trust in the mercy of the Lord forever and ever. (Psalm 52:8)

TODAY'S STEP: I will consciously let go and let God.

"God loves you! He has a plan for your life. He has given you talents. Develop them! He has given you some gift. Discover it! He is giving you opportunities. Seize them! God is willing to provide you with all you need! This is your inheritance. No man can take that from you! You can never lose what you choose to give away." -- Dr. Robert F. Schuller

Love Is the Key

According to Emmet Fox, in **Power Through Constructive Thinking,** LOVE is by far the most important thing of all. It is the Golden Gate of Paradise. Pray for the understanding of love, and meditate upon it daily, it casts out fear. It is the fulfilling of the Law. It covers a multitude of sins. Love is absolutely invincible.

There is no fear in love; but perfect love casts out fear, because fear involves torment. But he who fears has not been made perfect in love. (1 John 4:18)

Love Conquers All

There is no difficulty that enough love will not conquer; no door that enough love will not open; no gulf that enough love will not bridge; no wall that enough love will not throw down; no sin that enough love will not redeem.

Jesus said: A new commandment I give unto you, That ye love one another; as I have loved you . . . By this shall all men know that ye are my disciples, if ye have love one to another. (John 13:34, 35)

Love Is Enough

It makes no difference how deeply seated the trouble, how hopeless the outlook, how muddled the tangle, how great the mistake; a sufficient realization of love will dissolve it all. If only you could love enough you would be the happiest and most powerful being in the world.

Beloved, let us love one another, for love is of God; and everyone who loves is born of God and knows God. He who does not love does not know God, for God is love. (1 John 4: 7-8)

We love Him, because he first loved us. (1 John 4:19)

TODAY'S STEP: I create a healthy atmosphere of love and nurturing around and within me. I accept the love and support of my sponsor and my group.

"There is a principle which is a bar against all information, which is proof against all arguments and which can not fail to keep a man in everlasting ignorance – that principle is contempt prior to investigation." -- Herbert Spencer

<u>"Mind Your Own Business"</u>

"I've chosen my epitaph," said an Al-Anon friend at our regular Wednesday night meeting. "I want it to read, 'She's finally minding her own business.'"

We laugh, enjoying some relief in discussing the lighter side of a serious subject – the constant struggle to recognize and remove our defects of character. Laughter makes our frailties seem easier bear, and we can now more readily forgive ourselves for our imperfections. What a change from the days when we hid in shame from our flaws or used them to beat ourselves over the head!

When we have practiced the Twelve Steps for some time we can finally begin to acquire wisdom enough to try less, accept more, and let go of our impatience, self-criticism, and self-hatred. We can take a deep breath and say, "Help me, Higher Power. Help me remember the purpose of making mistakes is to prepare myself to make more; help me remember when I'm no longer making mistakes I'll be out of this world."

In a way, no matter how long we are in "The Program," we will always be *beginners*. There will always be some new challenge to face because life is ever-changing and so are we. Because of this constant change, every tiny little action we take involves some risk of making a mistake. It takes courage to participate in life. Today we can applaud ourselves for trying.

Because we have experienced a spiritual awakening, we can affirm without reservation that no matter what happens to us we can "live joyfully in a sorrowful world."

If any of you lacks wisdom, let him ask of God, who gives to all liberally and without reproach, and it will be given to him. [6] But let him ask in faith, with no doubting, for he who doubts is like a wave of the sea driven and tossed by the wind. For let not that man suppose that he will receive anything from the Lord. (James 1:5-7)

TODAY'S STEP: My sense of humor helps me to carry – and to get the message.

"When anyone, anywhere, reaches out for help, I want the hand of AA always to be there. And for that: I am responsible." -- Declaration of the 30th Anniversary International Convention Of Alcoholics Anonymous, 1965

The Promises of Recovery

If we are painstaking about this phase of our development, we will be amazed before we are half way through:

1. We are going to know a new freedom and a new happiness.

2. We will not regret the past nor wish to shut the door on it.

3. We will comprehend the word serenity.

4. We will know peace.

5. No matter how far down the scale we have gone, we will see how our experience can benefit others.

6. The feeling of uselessness and self-pity will disappear.

7. We will lose interest in selfish things and gain interest in our fellows.

8. Self-seeking will slip away.

9. Our whole attitude and outlook upon life will change.

10. Fear of people and economic security will leave us.

11. We will intuitively know how to handle situations which used to baffle us.

12. We will suddenly realize that God is doing for us what we could not do for ourselves.

"Are these extravagant promises? We think not. They are being fulfilled among us – sometimes quickly, sometimes slowly. They will always materialize if we work for them." (Adapted and reprinted from pages 83 and 84 of *Alcoholics Anonymous, The Big Book*)

Surely goodness and mercy shall follow me, all the days of my life. (Psalm 23:6)

TODAY'S STEP: I do not run myself, my circumstances, or my feelings.

"Not all of me will die, not all of me
Pass hence to unrelieved oblivion;
Some quintessential spark must needs break free
And soar and seek and touch at last the sun.
Else were the very breath of life a liar,
Which hath thereof, since my first sentient hour,
Instinctive been a certitude, a star,
A motive unto action, and a power.
How otherwise could viewless poesy
Prick me to render things invisible
Half glimpsed through magic phrases, how and why
Urge me unresting, bind me with a spell even,
To echo forth, tho' faint, scarce audible,
The ultimate music of the heart of heaven?" -- Horace, *Odes*

When . . .

When your knees are knocking together, and you do
not know which way to turn – **give thanks for God and His goodness.**

When your coffers are empty and prosperity seems out of the question –
give thanks for God's abundance.

When you want peace of mind – **get away from things, dwell upon the
Presence of God instead.**

When your health is under par – **speak the healing Word as Jesus did.**

When you need inspiration – **browse through the Bible.**

When your faith is low – **remember the words of Jesus, believe
you have received and you shall receive.**

When the situation seems to need a miracle – **remember nothing is
too difficult for God, and He is performing miracles every day.**

Always "make a joyful noise unto the Lord." Go to Him with praise and thanksgiving – this is the most powerful prayer. Taken from Emett Fox's book, *Stake Your Claim: Exploring the Gold Mine Within.*

I am the resurrection and the life. He who believes in Me, though he may die, he shall live. And whoever lives and believes in Me shall never die. Do you believe this? (John 11:25-26)

TODAY'S STEP: I need to believe in myself and my dreams.

"Look to this day, for it is the very life of life. In its brief course lie all the verities and realities of your existence." -- Ervin Seale, *Take Off From Within*

Daily Living

Step Twelve calls for "practicing these principles in all our affairs." In other words, what we learned in the Steps must be brought into our daily lives and become a way of life for us. Daily life is not a thing apart from the spiritual journey; the two must become one and the same.

The following four principles are the foundation for ongoing growth and joined with a life of prayer and service they will take us all the way on our spiritual journey:

1. **Honesty, especially emotional honesty with self, God, and others, is the cornerstone.** Without honesty, a moral life, much less a spiritual life, is not possible.

2. **Awareness, being here-now, resisting useless and negative preoccupation.** Do what you're doing and nothing else.

3. **Surrender, letting go of things you cannot control – in yourself, other people, and the world.** Entrust these to the care of God, and then do what is yours to do in serenity and trust.

4. **Forgiveness, letting go of hurts others have caused you, letting go of self-hatred.** Realize God has let go of all this and you cannot really live unless you let go, too. It is God's will that you live this moment awake, and to do this, you must let go of the past.

The spirit of outreach is undoubtedly one of the reasons for the success of the Twelve Step movement. From the beginning, Bill W. and Dr. Bob, cofounders of Alcoholics Anonymous, discovered "you can't give what you don't have, but you can't keep what you don't share." They learned helping other alcoholics find sobriety helped them stay sober, too.

I have come that you might have life, and that you might have it more abundantly. (John 10:10)

TODAY'S STEP: I trust truth, my instincts, and my ability to ground myself in reality.

"Spiritual love is born of sorrow . . . . For men love one another with a spiritual love only when they have suffered the same sorrow together, when through long days they have ploughed the stony ground buried beneath the common yoke of a common grief. It is then they know one another and feel one another in their common anguish, and so thus they pity one another and love one another. For to love is to pity; and if bodies are united by pleasure, souls are united by pain. . . . To love with the spirit is to pity, and he who pities most loves most." -- Miguel de Unamuno, ***The Tragic Sense of Life***

<u>Show Me Thy Face</u>

Show me Thy face – one transient gleam
Of loveliness divine,
And I shall never think or dream
Of other love than Thine;
All other light will darken quite,
All lower glories wane,
The beautiful of earth will scarce
Seem beautiful again.

Show me Thy face – I shall forget
The weary days of yore;
The fretting thoughts of vain regret
Shall hurt my soul no more;
All doubts and fears for future years
In quiet trust subside,
And naught but blest content and calm
Within my breast reside.

Show me Thy face – the heaviest cross
Will then seem light to bear;
There will be gain in every loss
And peace with every care.
With such light feet the years will fleet,
Life seems as brief as blest;
Till I have laid my burden down
And entered into rest. – Hymnal 1921

The Lord your God in your midst, the Mighty One, will save; He will rejoice over you with gladness, He will quiet you in His love, He will rejoice over you with singing. (Zephaniah 3:17)

TODAY'S STEP: I create a healthy atmosphere of love and nurturing around and within me. I accept the love and support of my sponsor and my group.

"To free oneself is nothing, the really arduous task is to know what to do with one's freedom." -- Andre Gide

"Having Had a Spiritual Awakening"

The Twelfth Step completes the climb of this particular mountain. Remembering the milestones in this adventure brings to mind the pain and joy we have experienced while accomplishing our objective. Our experiences have been unique and individual to each of us. We now realize that all the events of our lives have pulled together to show us our connection to God and creation. Our spiritual awakening has changed us, so now we have the capacity to live our lives as an expression of God's will.

Step Twelve requires that we be instrumental in helping others receive the message of Recovery. Many of us were introduced to "The Program" by someone who was working the Twelfth Step. Now we have the opportunity to promote our own growth by helping others.   Our willingness to share our commitment to Recovery and our growing awareness of God's presence in our lives keeps us ever-vigilant for ways to share our new confidence. "The Program" calls us to take responsibility for the daily living of our values.

We are reminded by this Step that we have not yet completed our journey to wholeness. To continue our process of growth, we must be aware we have just begun to learn the principles that will enhance our walk with God. Each of the Twelve Steps is a vital part of fulfilling God's plan for us. When our daily challenges distract us and separate us from God, we can use the Steps as tools God has given us for coping with our problems.

Taken from Friends in Recovery, ***The Twelve Steps for Christians***

PRAYER: Lord, thank you for leading me onto this path of Recovery. Empower me not only to stay on that path, but to share the message with others.

I pray that you may be active in sharing your faith, so that you will have a full understanding of every good thing we have in Christ. Your love has given me great joy and encouragement, because you, brother have refreshed the hearts of the saints. (Philemon 1:6-8)

TODAY'S STEP: I let consequences and responsibility fall where they belong.

"The greatest gift that can come to anybody is a spiritual awakening." -- Bill W., December 1957 *Grapevine*

"Expect a Miracle"

Whether we know it or not, we've undergone a number of spiritual experiences as we worked the previous Eleven Steps. These have all led to the spiritual awakening promised in Step Twelve.

Although many of us do not feel we've truly arrived at this stage, the promise of the Step is at work within us. It might not happen right this moment, but the seeds have been planted and are germinating in our subconscious. For those of us who are discouraged by a lack of concrete evidence, we suggest reaffirming the Third Step commitment to turn our lives and wills over to the Higher Power we've chosen as our guide.

Even though we now have irrefutable evidence of the dramatic changes in our lives, we may still find it difficult to dismiss those old ideas of doom and gloom and believe it's possible to rid ourselves of the negative conditions we have created. Some of us find it hard to believe that having screwed up so badly, we're truly on the right track at last.

But, believe it we must, for by applying the lessons of the Twelfth Step, we become not only increasingly comfortable with ourselves, but also with our fellows. Perhaps one of the most conclusive pieces of evidence that we have achieved a spiritual awakening occurs when we try to help someone whose disorder is much like our own. In communicating with a newcomer, we often find ourselves verbalizing beliefs and assurances we sometimes didn't know we possessed. As we share what we used to be like, what happened and what we're like now, our own doubts diminish. Our progress is clearer to us. The therapeutic value of such action not only touches the newcomer, but also reinforces our own resolve to cling to the principles we're pursuing. And the amazing thing about action of this kind is, whether or not our prospect is receptive, we have intensified our own commitment to a far greater degree.

The LORD bless you and keep you; The LORD make His face shine upon you, and be gracious to you; The LORD lift up His countenance upon you, and give you peace. (Numbers 6:24-26)

TODAY'S STEP: Faith is recognizing the longer I suffer under trying circumstances, the more certain I am to appreciate my deliverance.

"Resolve to perform what you ought. Perform without fail what you resolve." --
Benjamin Franklin

<u>Tradition Twelve</u>

Anonymity is the spiritual foundation of all our Traditions, ever reminding us to place principles above personalities.

In Al-Anon, one of our greatest gifts is the privilege of helping others find their way out of darkness into light. We help others, and keep ourselves open to being helped. There is no room in this important purpose for self-glorification and pride, and much room for gratitude, humility and willingness to serve.

The same theme runs through our Steps as well, beginning with the word "powerless" in the First Step. The power we have comes from a Higher Power and not from our own wisdom and virtue. This is directly stated when we are reminded to place principles above personalities.

The Twelfth Tradition reaffirms the principles of all our Traditions. When we act and think as a member of Al-Anon, we are able once more to see our perception and will alone do not determine the reality of a situation.

When we subordinate our will to the spiritual strength of the group, unity adds to the healing process. When we do not emphasize our uniqueness, we gain strength from being part of a group conscience which flows from a power greater than ours alone. When we leave our other affiliations outside Al-Anon's doors and recognize the common problem that brings us together, we often feel for the first time in our lives we are where we belong.

Through this sense of belonging, when we stop holding ourselves aloof, comes a realization that the material values that ruled our lives before Al-Anon, are no longer important. Principles are everything. Accepting this idea may not be easy since it requires true humility. Eventually we realize, with a sense of discovery, that this Tradition has within it the basis for change that can lead to solutions of personal, family and group problems. Our spiritual growth through humility has its roots in the principle of anonymity.

Before honor is humility. (Proverbs 15:33)

TODAY'S STEP: I practice the discipline of H.O.W. – Honesty, Open-Mindedness and Willingness everyday.

"It is good to have an end to journey towards; but it is the journey that matters in the end." -- Ursula LeGuin

"Remember Happiness And Serenity Are an Inside Job"

Our inner growth has profound effects on our outer lives. Many of our relationships may have improved since we began working the Twelve Steps. We may have seen dramatic, positive changes occur, and we feel healthier than before. Even things we seemingly have nothing to do with may improve tremendously. We may seem to have better "luck" now attracting harmonious relationships and beneficial events into our lives. These outward signs reflect our spiritual awakening and our Higher Power's influence in our lives,

We can continue in this positive way of living as long as we care for ourselves and remain open to our Higher Power's help. We've gained, through the Twelve Steps, a spiritual connectedness that will help us cope with problems in a healthy, adult fashion. We can continue to care for ourselves by eliminating unnecessary anxiety from our lives, eating properly, sleeping enough, and exercising regularly. Also important is getting medical and dental care, praying and meditating, continuing to take inventories and dealing with our errors promptly, and reading inspiring literature. Other self-care exercises include sharing our stories with other people, accepting help from others, and helping others whenever we can. We can now give ourselves what we need for true well-being. If we remember to put our spiritual growth first, everything else will naturally follow.

We started this journey with the understanding that even positive change can be frightening. We now know it can also be rewarding. The changes we've made through taking the Twelve Steps in spite of our fears have led us to a spiritual awakening. We have begun, through these Steps, to recognize our self-worth. We're all a part of humanity, a part of the universe, a part of God. Our Recovery and continued growth contributes to the whole of life.

I pray that out of His glorious riches He may strengthen me with power through His Spirit in my inner being. . . **Now to Him that is able to do immeasurably more than all that I ask, think or imagine, according to His power that works in me, to Him be glory, throughout all ages, forever and ever. (Ephesians 3:16, 20-21)**

TODAY'S STEP: When I rely on my Higher Power's help I can achieve.

"To be truly rich, a person must acknowledge that money is a sacred trust from God to be employed wisely and not wasted." -- Glenn Bland, *Legend Of The Golden Scrolls*

The *Legend Of The Golden Scrolls* focuses on a young man's search for the secrets of building wealth. He is guided by the wisdom contained in six ancient scrolls, which explain how to:

- Properly think about money;
- Begin creating wealth today, regardless of current financial conditions;
- Effectively manage and increase income dramatically; and,
- Protect what you have earned while conquering debt.

The principles and laws of building wealth are summarized in the following rules:

"My Goals for Building Wealth"

1. Measure every decision by the standards of the Holy Scriptures.

2. Study the Holy Scriptures to learn about skillful living and success.

3. Form the habit of praying and seeking God's guidance about everything.

4. Seek employment in the path of opportunity and growth.

5. Render more and better service than my competition.

6. Eliminate my personal debts within the next 24 months.

7. Save a minimum of one-tenth of all that I earn.

8. Give a minimum of one-tenth of all that I earn.

9. Seek wise counsel regarding the best way to invest my savings.

10. Take the right steps to protect my future earning power.

11. Show proper respect for money, so I may manage it wisely.

12. Follow a detailed budgetary plan all the days of my life.

Blessed be the Lord, who daily loads me with benefits. (Psalm 68:19)

TODAY'S STEP: I trust truth, my instincts, and my ability to ground myself in reality.

"Deep into that darkness peering, long I stood
        there wondering, fearing,
Doubting, dreaming dreams no mortal ever dared
        to dream before." -- Edgar Allen Poe, *The Raven*

To Achieve Your Dreams Remember Your ABC's

Avoid negative sources, people, places, things and habits.
Believe in yourself.
Consider things from every angle.
Don't give up and don't give in.
Enjoy life today, yesterday is gone, and tomorrow may never come.
Family and friends are hidden treasures, seek them and enjoy their riches.
Give more than you planned to.
Hang on to your dreams.
Ignore those who try to discourage you.
Just do it.
Keep trying no matter how hard it seems, it will get easier.
Love yourself first and most.
Make it happen.
Open your eyes and see things as they really are.
Practice makes perfect.
Quitters never win and winners never quit.
Read, study and learn about everything important in your life.
Stop procrastinating.
Take control of your own destiny.
Understand yourself in order to better understand others.
Visualize it.
Want it more than anything.
Accelerate your efforts.
You are unique of all God's creations, nothing can replace YOU.
Zero in on your target and go for it!

Anonymous

Ask, and it will be given to you; seek, and you will find; knock, and it will be opened to you. For everyone who asks receives, and he who seeks finds, and to him who knocks it will be opened. Or what man is there among you who, if his son asks for bread, will give him a stone? Or if he asks for a fish, will he give him a serpent? If you then, being evil, know how to give good gifts to your children, how much more will your Father who is in heaven give good things to those who ask Him! (Matthew 7:7-11)

TODAY'S STEP: I move confidently toward wholeness, knowing my steps are guided by my Higher Power.

"God is in all things as being, as activity, as power, but He is procreative in the soul alone; for though every creature is a vestige of God, the soul is the natural image of God . . . Such perfection as enters the soul, whether it be divine light, grace, or bliss, must needs enter the soul in this birth and no other wise. Do but foster this birth in thee and thou wilt experience all good and all comfort, all happiness, all being, and all truth. What comes to thee therein brings the true being and stability; and whatsoever thou mayest seek or grasp without it perishes, take it how thou wilt." -- Meister Eckhart, ***Sermons and Collations***

<u>"You Can't Give Away What You Don't Have"</u>

I'd read the Twelfth Step many times before I heard it. But there it was: "Having had a spiritual awakening as the result of these Steps . . ."   What a promise! If I worked the Steps, I'd have a spiritual awakening! There was hope, even for me!

Now that's not why I first came to Al-Anon. Like many, I came to find out how to make someone stop drinking. It was much later when I realized that my life was missing a sense of direction only a Higher Power could provide.

Those wonderful Twelfth Step words gave me the encouragement I needed to begin at the beginning. Slowly, sometimes painfully, I realized what a wonderful gift the Al-Anon program was. It gave me an understanding of this disease, the tools to change my life, the courage to use them, and a place to talk about my secrets and to hear others share theirs. I wanted my family and friends to have all of these things as well.

The Twelfth Step says to carry the message to others, so I began my "promoting". I dragged people to meetings, I preached what I'd learned to anyone who would listen – and I made a fool of myself!

Then I read the Twelfth Step again. This time I noticed the part about practicing these principles in all my affairs. Slowly I came to understand that in living these principles I could carry the message by example, by attraction.

By this I know that I abide in Him, and He in me, because He has given me of His Spirit… Whoever confesses that Jesus is the Son of God, God abides in him, and he in God. (1 John 4:13,15)

TODAY'S STEP: I let consequences and responsibility fall where they belong.

"The obvious lesson . . . is that the first step to the knowledge of the highest divine symbol of the wonder and mystery of life is in the recognition of the monstrous nature of life and its glory in that character: the realization that this is just how it is and that it cannot and will not be changed. Those who think – and their name is legion – that they know how the universe could be better than it is, how it would have been created had they created it, without pain, without sorrow, without time, without life, are unfit for illumination. Or those who think – as do many – 'Let me first correct society, then get around to myself' are barred from even the outer gate of the mansion of God's peace. All societies are evil, sorrowful, inequitable; and so they will always be. If you really want to help this world, what you will have to teach is how to live in it. And that no one who has not himself learned how to live in it in the joyful sorrow and sorrowful joy of the knowledge of life as it is." -- Joseph Campbell*, Myths To Live By*

<u>The Man (Woman) In the Glass</u>

When you get what you want in your struggle for self. And the world makes you king (queen) for a day. Just go to a mirror and look at yourself – and see what THAT man (woman) has to say.

For it isn't your father or mother or wife whose judgment you must pass – the person whose verdict counts most in your life is the one staring back from the glass.

Some people may think you a straight-shooting chum and call you a wonderful guy (gal) – but the man (woman) in the glass says you're only a bum if you can't look him (her) straight in the eye.

He (she)'s the one to please, never mind all the rest. He (she)'s with you clear up to the end. You've passed your most difficult test – if the man (woman) in the glass is your friend.

You may fool the whole world down the pathway of years and get pats on the back as you pass. But your final reward will be heartaches and tears – if you've cheated the man (woman) in the glass.

When you can look at yesterday without regret, and at tomorrow without fear, you're on your way to living in today. Today counts, make the most of it!

For if anyone only listens to the Word without obeying it *and* being a doer of it, he is like a man who looks carefully at his [own] natural face in a mirror. (James 1:23)

TODAY'S STEP: I pray that my Higher Power gives me the courage and strength to recognize the Truth about myself and help me accept that I am powerless.

"The interchange between sponsor and sponsored is a form of communication that will nourish both of you." -- *Sponsorship – What It's All About*

Twelve Steps of a Sponsor

1. I will not help you stay and wallow in limbo.

2. I will help you grow, to become more productive, by your own definition.

3. I will help you become more autonomous, more loving of yourself, more free to continue becoming the authority of your own living.

4. I can't give you dreams or "fix you."

5. I can't give you growth, or grow for you. You must grow yourself, by facing reality, grim as it may be at times.

6. I can't take away your loneliness or pain.

7. I can't sense your world for you, evaluate your goals, or tell you what is best for you in your world.

8. I can't convince you of the crucial choice of choosing the scary uncertainty of growing over the safe misery of not growing.

9. I want to be with you and know you as a rich and growing friend, yet I can't get close to you when you choose not to grow.

10. When I begin to care for you out of pity, when I begin to lose trust in you, then I am toxic, bad and inhibiting for you, and you for me.

11. You must know – my help is conditional. I will be with you, hang in there with you, as long as I continue to get even the slightest hints that you are trying to grow.

12. If you can accept all of this, then perhaps we can help each other to become what God meant us to be . . . mature adults, leaving childishness forever to little children. -- Anonymous

When I was a child, I spoke as a child, I understood as a child, I thought as a child: but when I became a man, I put away childish things. (1 Corinthians 13:11)

TODAY'S STEP: I let go of old ideas about myself and discover a new self through Recovery.

"Within the fellowship, the one thing that has brought us together must remain our sole concern." -- Al-Anon's Twelve Steps & Twelve Traditions

Questions and Answers on Sponsorship

The Twelfth Step encourages members to carry the message of Recovery to others.

Individuals in the fellowship work this step in different ways, including making visits

to an addicted person who has asked for help. This outreach activity encourages Recovering individuals to redirect their focus to helping others as a way of helping themselves.

A larger Twelfth Step commitment to help other addicts is to become a sponsor. AA, NA, and Al-Anon all have pamphlets that discuss the role and responsibilities of sponsorship. Newcomers to 12-Step programs benefit from the support and guidance of a sponsor. A sponsor, a 12-Step member in stable Recovery, develops a personal relationship with a newer member and guides that individual in working the Twelve Steps. In the words of John Chappel, quoting a common AA description, a sponsor is "someone who sees through you and still sees you through."

The sponsorship role is unwritten and informal. An AA pamphlet, "**Questions and Answers on Sponsorship**," provides general suggestions and guidelines for developing sponsor relationships. These suggestions include the sponsor having maintained abstinence for at least one year and being the same sex as the person sponsored. Beyond these guidelines, the decision to connect with a particular sponsor is a personal one, with the main goal of the sponsor being able to help the newcomer "work 'The Program'", to stay sober "one day at a time" and grow in sobriety through the fellowship and the Twelve Steps.

Helping other alcoholics and addicts become abstinent and stay clean and sober is not an act of altruism, but is a vital part of a personal program of Recovery. This discovery, initially made by Bill Wilson, AA's cofounder, is one of the many unique features of the Twelve Step process of Recovery. Sponsorship is one of the ways this process is expressed
in these programs.

A man who has friends must himself be friendly, but there is a friend who sticks closer than a brother. (Proverbs 18:24)

TODAY'S STEP: If I want to become skillful at applying "The Program" to my life, I need to do more than go to an occasional meeting. I must make a commitment and practice, practice, practice.

"Service gladly rendered, obligations squarely met, troubles well accepted or solved with God's help, the knowledge that at home or in the world outside we are partners in a common effort, the fact that in God's sight all human beings are important, the proof that love freely given brings a full return, the certainty that we are no longer isolated and alone in self-constructed prisons, the surety that we can fit and belong in God's scheme of things – these are the satisfactions of right living for which no pomp and circumstance, no heap of material possessions, could possibly be substitutes." -- Bill W., Twelve Steps and Twelve Traditions, p.124.

<u>"Before You Say: I Can't . . . Say: I'll Try"</u>

The hardest part of Recovery is it requires us to be **totally committed** to change. We may be intrigued by the idea of Recovery. We may be inspired by stories about Recovery. We may be convinced of our need for Recovery. These and many other cognitive processes are relatively easy for us. But the *doing* of Recovery is hard because it means we have to change. And change and commitment are difficult for us.

We resist change. We are angry we have to change. We feel shame that we need to change. And we are afraid we will not be able to change. We know there will be moments when we'll find ourselves saying, "I can't do it." "It's too hard."

But change is also the most exhilarating part of Recovery. We don't have to live in bondage to our addictions. We don't have to run in fear from relationships. We don't have to live as if we were responsible for the world. We can learn Serenity. We can find Freedom. We can experience Love.

Change is the most difficult and the most wonderful part of the Recovery process. It engages us in a major internal battle. It is not a comfortable battle. But our capacity to change is the key to our hope. We can change if we are "totally committed" to change.

God has given us the ability to change and grow. He calls us to change. He gives us the perspectives and disciplines and encouragement we need. And, as we allow and invite him, God himself works within us to strengthen us, heal us and make us new.

And the work of righteousness shall be peace; and the effect of righteousness quietness and assurance forever. (Isaiah 32:17)

TODAY'S STEP: If I want to become skillful at applying "The Program" to my life, I need to do more than go to an occasional meeting. I must make a commitment and practice, practice, practice.

"We are not saints. The point is that we are willing to grow along spiritual lines. The principles we have set down are guides to progress. We claim spiritual progress rather than spiritual perfection." -- Bill W., *Alcoholics Anonymous,* p.60.

"Change Is a Process, Not an Event"

Let us consider the term "spiritual experience" as used in Appendix II of *The Big Book*, *Alcoholics Anonymous*: "A spiritual experience is something that brings about a personality change. By surrendering our lives to God as we understand Him, we are changed. The nature of this change is not necessarily in the nature of a sudden and spectacular upheaval. We do not need to acquire an immediate and overwhelming God-consciousness, followed at once by a vast change in feeling and outlook. In most cases, the change is gradual."

According to William James, *The Varieties of Religious Experiences*, most of our "spiritual experiences" are of the educational variety, and they develop slowly over a period of time. Quite often friends of Newcomers are aware of the difference long before we are ourselves. We finally realize we have undergone a profound alteration in our reaction to life and such a change could hardly have been brought about by ourselves.

What often takes place in a few months could seldom have been accomplished by years of discipline. With few exceptions, we find we have tapped an unsuspected inner resource which we identify with our own conception of a Power greater than ourselves. Most of us think this awareness of a Power greater than ourselves is the essence of the spiritual experience. Some of us call it God-consciousness. In any case, willingness, honesty, and open-mindedness are the essentials of Recovery.

The LORD your God, who goes before you, He will fight for you, according to all He did for you in Egypt before your eyes, and in the wilderness where you saw how the LORD your God carried you, as a man carries his son, in all the way that you went until you came to this place. (Deuteronomy 1:30-32)

TODAY'S STEP: The Steps offer me a road map for living that leads to a spiritual awakening and beyond. I can't skip ahead to the end of the journey – which can at times be a challenging one – but I can put one foot in front of the other and follow the directions I've been given, knowing others who have gone before me have received more along the way than they had ever dreamed.

"Our consciences are littered like an old attic with the junk of sheer convictions." -- Wilfred O. Cross

"Don't Drink, Read The Big Book, and Go To Meetings"

The Twelfth Step of Alcoholics Anonymous, working with others, can be subdivided into five parts, five words beginning with the letter C – Confidence, Confession, Conviction, Conversion, and Continuance. The first part in trying to help other alcoholics is to get their **confidence.** We do this by telling them our own experiences with drinking, so they see we know what we're talking about. If we share our experiences frankly, they will know that we are sincerely trying to help them.

The second part is **confession.** By frankly sharing with Newcomers, we get them talking about their own experiences. They will open up and confess things to us they haven't been able to tell other people. And they feel better when this confession has been made. It's a great load off their minds to get these things out into the open. It's the things that are kept hidden that weigh on the mind.

The third part is **conviction.** Newcomers must be convinced they honestly want to stop drinking. They must see and admit that their life is unmanageable. They must face the fact they must do something about their drinking and that their life depends on this conviction.

The fourth part is **conversion.** Conversion means change. Newcomers must learn to change their way of thinking. They must see and admit they cannot overcome drinking by their own willpower, so they must turn to a Higher Power for help. They must start each day by asking their Higher Power for the strength to stay sober and thank Him at night for His help.

The fifth part is **continuance.** Continuance means our staying with Newcomers after they have started on the new way of living. We must stick with them and not let them down. We must encourage them to remember it's a simple program and to be successful all they have to do is – "Don't Drink, Read The Big Book, And Go To Meetings." Soon they will learn that keeping sober is a lot easier in the fellowship of others who are trying to do the same thing.

That there should be no division in the body, but that the members should have the same care for one another. And if one member suffers, all the members suffer with it; or if one member is honored, all the members rejoice with it. (1 Corinthians 12:25-26)

TODAY'S STEP: I allow myself to recognize and accept whatever feelings pass through me.

"Life is either a daring adventure or nothing. To keep our faces toward change and behave like free spirits in the presence of fate is strength undefeatable." -- Helen Keller

"N.U.T.S. = Not Using the Steps"

Power, greater than myself, as I understand You, I willingly admit that without Your help:

1. I am powerless over addiction and my life has become unmanageable.

2. I believe You can restore me to sanity.

3. I turn my life and my will over to You.

4. I have made a searching and fearless moral inventory of myself.

5. I admit to You, to myself, and to another the exact nature of my wrongs.

6. I am entirely ready to have You remove these defects of character.

7. I humbly ask You to remove my shortcomings.

8. I made a list of all persons I have harmed, and became willing to make amends to them all.

9. I have made direct amends to all persons I have harmed, except when to do so would injure them or others.

10. I will continue to take personal inventory and when I am wrong I will promptly admit it.

11. I seek through prayer and meditation to improve my conscious contact with You. I pray only for knowledge of Your will for me and the power to carry it out.

12. Grant me the grace to carry the message of Your help unto others and to practice the principles of the Twelve Steps in all my affairs.

Fear not, for I *am* with you; Be not dismayed, for I *am* your God. I will strengthen you, Yes, I will help you, I will uphold you with My righteous right hand. (Isaiah 41:10)

TODAY'S STEP: I have courage to go forward; to meet the new day, to handle whatever confronts me. Peace is coupled with courage, now and forever.

"Love is the will to extend one's self for the purpose of nurturing one's own or another's spiritual growth." -- M. Scott Peck, *The Road Less Traveled*

Suggestions for Spiritual Growth

Spiritual growth results from trusting God. "The righteous man shall live by faith" (Galatians 3:11). A life of faith enables us to trust God increasingly with every detail of our lives, and to practice the following"

G Go to God in prayer daily (John 15:7)

R Read God's Word daily (Acts 17:11) – you may want to begin with the Gospel of John.

O Obey God moment by moment (John 14:21).

W Witness for Christ by your life and words (Matthew 4:19; John 15:8).

T Trust God for every detail of your life (1 Peter 5:7).

H Holy Spirit – Allow Him to control and empower your daily life and witness (Galatians 5:16, 17; Acts 1:8).

As we continually and daily come to Him in prayer, He will build our faith. We will develop a trust relationship deeper than we have ever known before. We will learn the joy of an intimate communion with the living, loving God.

As our journey continues, we will look back, from time to time, and see how far we have come. One day we'll notice the old feelings of rejection just aren't triggered anymore. The pains of interference are gradually disappearing. We may not know exactly when or how, but we will know we are different. He has been working in our lives, our emotions and our relationships.

He who has My commandments and keeps them is the one who loves Me; and he who loves Me will be loved by My Father, and I will love him and will disclose Myself to him. (John 14:21)

TODAY'S STEP: Today, I will trust God's will is happening as it needs to in my life.

"If as Herod, we fill our lives with things, and again with things. If we consider ourselves so unimportant that we must fill every moment of our lives with action, when will we have time to make the long slow journey across the desert as did the magi? Or sit and watch the stars as did the shepherds? Or brood over the coming of the child as did Mary? For each one of us there is a desert to travel, a star to discover, and a being within ourselves to bring to life." – Author Unknown

A Child Is Born

According to Emmet Fox, author of **The Sermon on the Mount** and **Power Through Constructive Thinking**, there exists a mystic Power that is able to transform our lives so thoroughly, so radically, so completely, that when the process is completed our own friends will hardly recognize us, and, in fact, we will scarcely recognize ourselves. It can lift us out of an invalid's bed, and free us to go out into the world to shape our lives as we will. It can throw open the prison door and liberate us.

This power can do for us that which is probably the most important thing of all in our present stage: It can find our true place in life, and put us into it. This Power is really no less than the primal Power of Being, and to discover that Power is the divine birthright of all men.

> **. . . the kingdom of God is within you (Luke 17:21).**
> **. . . seek ye first the kingdom of God . . . (Matthew 6:33).**

But where is this wonderful Power to be contacted? The answer is simple – this Power is to be found within our own consciousness – the last place that most people would look for it. Within our own mentality there lies a source of energy stronger than electricity, more potent than high explosives; unlimited and inexhaustible. We only need to make conscious contact with it to set it working in all our affairs. This indwelling Power, the Inner Light, is spoken of in the Bible as a child. The conscious discovery by us that we
have the Power within us, and our determination to make use of it, is the birth of the child.

> **For unto us a child is born, unto us a son is given: And the government shall be upon His shoulder: And His name shall be called Wonderful Counselor, The Mighty God, The Everlasting Father, The Prince of Peace. (Isaiah 9:6)**

Now when Jesus was born in Bethlehem of Judaea in the days of Herod the king, behold, there came wise men from the east to Jerusalem. Saying, Where is he that is born King of the Jews? For we have seen his star in the east, and are come to worship him. (Matthew2:1-3)

TODAY'S STEP: I let consequences and responsibility fall where they belong.

"Our world is the place where our soul finds entry into us. The calamity that strikes may be our call to spiritual fulfillment." -- Ernest Lawrence Rossi

<u>Consequences of Unfaced Pain</u>

Living with emotional pain has very specific psychological and behavioral consequences. We need to learn to recognize them before we can begin the process of changing to a more pain-free and rewarding life.

DENIAL -- We pretend to ourselves that our condition doesn't exist, or doesn't affect us to the degree it really does, or it will go away if we ignore it. In other words, we deny our own reality.

DISHONESTY -- We evade the truth of our condition as we relate to others. We use half truths, distorted definitions, and constantly try to manage the impression we are making to maintain a charade.

INTOLERANCE -- We become so rigid in our need to control our environment and so centered on our problems we become intolerant, negative and critical.

SELF-PITY -- Our elaborate self-concern causes us to resent and reject others. We see ourselves and feel self-pity when others aren't as consumed with our problems as we are.

FALSE PRIDE -- False pride is pride based on the opinion of others. It develops when we reach for achievements and status that some people will judge as superior without regard to our own integrity, and also when we hide our weaknesses and vulnerabilities.

These five characteristics come from excessive self-involvement; yet, in another way, they keep us alienated from ourselves. Our cycles of emotional pain separate us from our real self and keep us insulated from friendship and intimacy. But we don't have to live this way. Our purpose in working the Steps is to expose the harmful emotions and character traits that we have developed and change them in a way that ensures our spiritual development.

O may Your loving kindness comfort me, according to Your word to Your servant. May Your compassion come to me that I may live, For Your will is my delight. (Psalm 119:76, 77)

TODAY'S STEP: I let go of denial and accept responsibility for myself and my life.

I Stand By the Door

I stand by the door.
I neither go too far in, nor stay too far out,
The door is the most important door in the world –
It is the door through which men walk when they find God.
There's no use my going way inside, and staying there,
When so many are still outside and they, as much as I,
Crave to know where the door is.
And all that so many ever find
Is only the wall where a door ought to be.
They creep along the wall like blind men,
With outstretched, groping hands.
Feeling for a door, knowing there must be a door,
Yet they never find it . . . So I stand by the door.
The most tremendous thing in the world
Is for men to find that door – the door to God.
The most important thing any man can do
Is to take hold of one of those blind, groping hands,
And put it on the latch – the latch that only clicks
And opens to the man's own touch.
Men die outside that door, as starving beggars die
On cold nights in cruel cities in the dead of winter –
Die for want of what is within their grasp.
They live, on the other side of it – live because they have not
found it.
Nothing else matters compared to helping them find it,
And open it, and walk in, and find Him . . . So I stand by the door.
You can go in too deeply, and stay in too long,
And forget the people outside the door.
As for me, I shall take my old accustomed place,
Near enough to God to hear Him, and know He is there,
But not so far from men as not to hear them,
And remember they are there, too. Where? Outside the door –
Thousands of them, millions of them.
But – more important for me –
One of them, two of them, ten of them,
Whose hands I am intended to put on the latch.
So I shall stand by the door and wait
For those who seek it.
"I had rather be a door-keeper . . ."
So I stand by the door.

The Reverend Sam Moor Shoemaker, "An Apologia for My Life" in Helen Smith Shoemaker, *I Stand By The Door*. New York, NY, Harper and Row, 1967

TODAY'S STEP: I let consequences and responsibility fall where they belong.

"Is sobriety all that we are to expect of a spiritual awakening? No, sobriety is only a bare beginning; it is only the first gift of the awakening. If more gifts are to be received, our awakening has to go on. As it does go on, we find that bit by bit we can discard the old life – the one that did not work – for a new life that can and does work under any conditions whatever." --- Bill W., *AA Grapevine,* December 1957

"Sometimes our light goes out, but is blown again into instant flame by an encounter with another human being." — Albert Schweitzer

"A Life Second to None"

Persons in Recovery often introduce themselves at meetings as "**grateful**" recovering alcoholics, addicts, adult children of alcoholics or codependents. They are not grateful for their addictive illnesses, but they are grateful for the relationship growth, the emotional healing, and the spiritual maturation that have been by-products (miracles or gifts) of Recovery.

Step Twelve is the **transcendence and evangelism Step,** in which we realize we have had – and will continue to have – a spiritual experience and wish to share that experience with others. We call this Step transcendent because now we have begun to transcend time and space. *Twenty-Four Hours A Day,* one of the first devotional books widely used by members of AA, talks about living and growing beyond the three dimensional bondage of our physical and material world.

Emancipation from addictions requires us to go beyond the confines of three-dimensional reality and enter the special healing realm of the spiritual fourth dimension. Throughout the New Testament, for instance, we are constantly reminded that God calls us to an eternal perspective, which breaks beyond the dimensions of space and time. We can have a foretaste of eternity right now, here on earth and we can experience a degree of peace and joy we never before thought possible.

For to everyone who has, more will be given, and he will have abundance; but from him who does not have, even what he has will be taken away. (Matthew 25:29)

TODAY'S STEP: Today, I will be grateful for the rewards of recovery. If I am new to recovery, I will have faith that I can achieve the long-term benefits; and, if I've been recovering for a while, I'll pause to reflect, and be grateful for The Program.

"It is certain that all recipients of spiritual experiences declare for their reality. The best evidence of that reality is in the subsequent fruits. Those who receive these gifts of grace are very much changed people, almost invariably for the better." -- Bill W., *Talk,* 1960

O Lord, How Many Are Thy Works

Shown below are a few of the many "works" the Lord can do in our lives if we have the "willingness" and "openness" to ask for help and to accept it.

Psalm	Lord, You . . .
3	. . . are a shield about me, the One who lifts my head.
	. . . listen to me and sustain me.
4	. . . relieve my distress.
	. . . put gladness in my heart.
5	. . . bless the righteous man.
6	. . . hear and receive my prayers.
7	. . . judge the peoples.
	. . . save the upright in heart.
8	. . . displayed Thy splendor above the heavens.
	. . . put the creatures under man's authority.
11	. . . test the righteous and the wicked.
13	. . . deal bountifully with me.
16	. . . counsel me.

Proverbs

2	. . . reveal the path of life to me.
	. . . give wisdom, knowledge and understanding.
	. . . shield those who walk in integrity.
	. . . preserve the way of Your godly ones.
3	. . . reprove and discipline those You love.
	. . . founded the earth, established the heavens, broke up the deeps and sent the rain.
	. . . keep my foot from being caught.
	. . . give grace to the afflicted.

Therefore by their fruits you will know them. Not everyone who says to Me, 'Lord, Lord,' shall enter the kingdom of heaven, but he who does the will of My Father in heaven. (Matthew 7:20-21)

TODAY'S STEP: When faced with difficult or painful situations, I remember a loving God is always here for me, always available as a source of comfort, guidance and peace.

"Life is an adventure in forgiveness." -- Norman Cousins
"Always forgive your enemies; nothing annoys them so much." — Oscar Wilde

Twelve Step Review

Identify a situation or condition in your life that is currently a source of resentment, fear, sadness, or anger. Use the following questions to apply the principles of the Twelve Steps:

Step One: In what ways are you powerless over this situation or condition, and how is it showing you the unmanageability of your life?

Step Two: How do you see your Higher Power assisting you in being restored to wholeness?

Step Three: How does being willing to turn your life over to the care of God assist you in dealing with this?

Step Four: What character traits have surfaced (e.g., fear of abandonment or authority figures, control, approval seeking, obsessive/compulsive behavior, rescuing, taking inappropriate responsibility)?

Step Five: Can you admit your wrongs to God, to yourself and to another human being?

Step Six: Are you entirely ready to work in partnership with God to remove your ineffective behaviors?

Step Seven: Can you humbly ask God for help in removing your shortcomings?

Step Eight: Make a list of the persons you have harmed?

Step Nine: What amends are necessary, and how will you make them?

Step Ten: Review the above Steps to be sure that you have not overlooked anything.

Step Eleven: Take a moment for prayer and meditation, asking for knowledge of God's will for you.

Step Twelve: How can your understanding and spiritual guidance assist you in dealing with this problem?

Blessed are the merciful: for they shall obtain mercy. (Matthew 5:7)

TODAY'S STEP: I ask God to free me from feelings of bitterness, resentment, anger, envy, and the desire for revenge in order that I receive the gift of forgiveness.

"Praise God, from whom all blessings flow! Praise Him, all creatures here below! Praise Him above, ye heavenly host! Praise Father, Son, and Holy Ghost! -- Thomas Ken, **Doxology**

"Be thankful for what you have; you'll end up having more. If you concentrate on what you don't have, you will never, ever have enough" — Oprah Winfrey

Count Your Blessings

When the year is nearing its close, it's a good time for us to take stock of the blessings we have received during the year.

As we look back over the year, we can see there was many a blessing "in disguise" which we would have recognized at the time had we gotten behind the appearance to the reality of God. In taking stock, we need not dwell on old difficulties, problems, and grievances; and we need not rehearse our past mistakes – rather, we need to count our blessings and inventory all the good we have received.

In business, a firm takes an inventory not only to find out what goods it has on hand, but also to see if it cannot improve its business through more judicious merchandising.

Likewise in our spiritual inventory, we should use it as a basis for making further progress. We can take a step forward by asking ourselves:

1.   When a problem arises do I "Golden Key" the situation? Do I stop thinking about the difficulty, no matter what it is, and think about God instead?

2.   Have I gotten rid of anger, fear, and resentment?

3.   Have I forgiven everyone whom I think has injured me? Jesus made this one of the cardinal points in the Lord's Prayer – we are to ask God to forgive us as we have forgiven others.

If we put these things into practice, then next year at this time our spiritual inventory will reflect the difference, for there will be many more blessings to count.

Taken from "**The Golden Key**" by Emmet Fox

Offer to God thanksgiving, and pay your vows to the Most High. (Psalm 50:14)

TODAY'S STEP: Thankfulness today will help me see the miracles at work in my life and in the lives of others on the road to Recovery.

APPENDIX A

THE TWELVE STEPS AND TWELVE TRADITIONS

THE TWELVE STEPS OF ALCOHOLICS ANONYMOUS*

1. We admitted we were powerless over alcohol – that our lives had become unmanageable.

2. Came to believe that a Power greater than ourselves could restore us to sanity.

3. Made a decision to turn our will and our lives over to the care of God **as we understood Him.**

4. Made a searching and fearless moral inventory of ourselves.

5. Admitted to God, to ourselves, and to another human being the exact nature of our wrongs.

6. Were entirely ready to have God remove all these defects of character.

7. Humbly asked Him to remove our shortcomings.

8. Made a list of all persons we had harmed, and became willing to make amends to them all.

9. Made direct amends to such people wherever possible, except when to do so would injure them or others.

10. Continued to take personal inventory and when we were wrong promptly admitted it.

11. Sought through prayer and meditation to improve our conscious contact with God **as we understood Him**, praying only for knowledge of His will for us and the power to carry that out.

12. Having had a spiritual awakening as a result of these steps, we tried to carry this message to alcoholics, and to practice these principles in all our affairs.

* The Twelve Steps are reprinted and adapted with permission of Alcoholics Anonymous World Services, Inc. Permission to reprint and adapt The Twelve Steps does not mean that AA has reviewed or approved the contents of this publication nor that AA agrees with the views expressed herein. AA is a program of Recovery from alcoholism – use of The Twelve Steps in connection with programs and activities which are patterned after AA, but which address other problems, does not imply otherwise.

THE TWELVE STEPS OF AL-ANON*

1. We admitted we were powerless over alcohol – that our lives had become unmanageable.

2. Came to believe that a Power greater than ourselves could restore us to sanity.

3. Made a decision to turn our will and our lives over to the care of God **as we understood Him.**

4. Made a searching and fearless moral inventory of ourselves.

5. Admitted to God, to ourselves, and to another human being the exact nature of our wrongs.

6. Were entirely ready to have God remove all these defects of character.

7. Humbly asked Him to remove our shortcomings.

8. Made a list of all persons we had harmed, and became willing to make amends to them all.

9. Made direct amends to such people wherever possible, except when to do so would injure them or others.

10. Continued to take personal inventory and when we were wrong promptly admitted it.

11. Sought through prayer and meditation to improve our conscious contact with God **as we understood Him**, praying only for knowledge of His will for us and the power to carry that out.

12. Having had a spiritual awakening as a result of these steps, we tried to carry this message to alcoholics, and to practice these principles in all our affairs.

* The Twelve Steps of Al-Anon are taken from ***Al-Anon Faces Alcoholism,*** 2nd ed., published by Al-Anon Family Group Headquarters, Inc., New York, N.Y. (pp. 236-37) Reprinted with permission of A.A. World Services, Inc.

<u>THE TWELVE STEPS FOR ADULT CHILDREN</u>*

1. We admitted we were powerless over **the effects of addiction** – that our lives had become unmanageable.

2. Came to believe that a Power greater than ourselves could restore us to **wholeness.**

3. Made a decision to turn our will and our lives over to the care of God **as we understood God.**

4. Made a searching and fearless moral inventory of ourselves.

5. Admitted to God, to ourselves, and to another human being the exact nature of our wrongs.

6. Were entirely ready to **work in partnership with God to remove our ineffective behavior.**

7. Humbly asked God to **help us** remove our shortcomings.

8. Made a list of all persons we had harmed, and became willing to make amends to them all.

9. Made direct amends to such people wherever possible, except when to do so would injure them or others.

10. Continued to take personal inventory and when we were wrong promptly admitted it.

11. Sought through prayer and meditation to improve our conscious contact with God **as we understood God**, praying only for knowledge of His will for us and the power to carry that out.

12. Having had a spiritual awakening as a result of these steps, we tried to carry this message to **others**, and to practice these principles in all our affairs.

*   The Twelve Steps for Adult Children were taken from ***The 12 Steps for Adult Children: From Addictive and Other Dysfunctional Families,*** Friends in Recovery, 1989, San Diego, CA: Recovery Publications, Inc.

<u>THE TWELVE TRADITIONS</u>*

1. Our common welfare should come first; personal recovery depends upon AA unity.

2. For our group purposes there is but one ultimate authority – a loving God as He may express Himself in our group conscience. Our leaders are but trusted servants; they do not govern.

3. The only requirements for AA membership is a desire to stop drinking.

4. Each group should be autonomous except in matters affecting other groups or AA as a whole.

5. Each group has but one primary purpose – to carry its message to the alcoholic who still suffers.

6. AA group ought never endorse, finance or lend the AA name to any related facility or outside enterprise, lest problems of money, property and prestige divert us from our primary purpose.

7. Every AA group ought to be fully self-supporting, declining outside contributions.

8. Alcoholics Anonymous should remain forever nonprofessional, but our service centers may employ special workers.

9. AA, as such, ought never be organized; but we may create service boards or committees directly responsible to those they serve.

10. Alcoholics Anonymous has no opinion on outside issues; hence the AA name ought never be drawn into public controversy.

11. Our public relations policy is based on attraction rather than promotion; we need always maintain personal anonymity at the level of press, radio and films.

12. Anonymity is the spiritual foundation of all our Traditions, ever reminding us to place principles before personalities.

(*The Twelve Traditions are reprinted and adapted with permission of Alcoholics Anonymous World Services, Inc. Permission to reprint and adapt the Twelve Traditions does not mean that AA has reviewed or approved the contents of this publication not that AA agrees with the views expressed herein. AA is a program of recovery from alcoholism – use of the Twelve Traditions in connection with programs and activities which are patterned after AA, but which address other problems, does not imply

APPENDIX B

<u>DAILY AFFIRMATIONS AND SELECTED PRAYERS</u>

<u>HOW TO USE AFFIRMATIONS:</u>

Affirmations are a powerful tool for changing negative beliefs and values. By speaking directly to ourselves in a positive and loving manner we can build attitudes, which act as a counterbalance to the conditioned reflex of our defensiveness.

Affirmations are done for a few minutes every day, at a regular time or whenever we feel tense or anxious. They can be written, spoken aloud or silently repeated.

Affirmations are designed particularly to combat a closed emotional stance. For example, Chuck, a recovering alcoholic, used the following affirmations daily:

> I, Chuck, am open and receptive.
> You, Chuck, are open and receptive.
> Chuck is open and receptive.
>
> I, Chuck, have value even when I'm wrong.
> You, Chuck, have value even when you're wrong.
> Chuck has value even when he is wrong.
> I, Chuck, am only human.
> You, Chuck, are only human.
> Chuck is only human.

Notice that each affirmation takes three forms: An "I" statement; a "you" statement; and a "name" statement. Hearing these statements from three different points of view help us make these open attitudes a reality. We can also use affirmations as a positive inner voice of strength and courage. For example:

1.   I (Your Name) am confident and strong and happy.

2.   I can face today's challenge.

3.   I feel loved and loving today.

4.   I feel happy and glad to be alive.

| **ACCEPTANCE:** | I let go of old ideas about myself and discover a new self through Recovery. |

| **ACHIEVEMENT:** | When I rely on my Higher Power's help I can achieve. |

| **ALCOHOLISM:** | I am finding the courage to face the truth about myself. |

| **ANGER:** | I am seeking a saner approach to everything I encounter. The slogans are a valuable source of sanity in chaotic situations. If I am tempted to act out of anger or frustration, I will remember "Easy Does It." |

| **ATTITUDES:** | There are so many ways in which I can improve the quality of my life. Instead of fretting about what I can't have or can't do, I'll take action to create something positive in my life today. |

| **BLAMING:** | I face my problems squarely and without blame. |

| **CHANGE:** | I visualize myself achieving my goal of changing for the better. |

| **CODEPENDENCY:** | God help me believe in myself and help me let go of old beliefs and feelings that are hurting me. |

| **COMMITMENT:** | If I want to become skillful at applying the Program to my life, I need to do more than go to an occasional meeting. I must make a commitment and practice, practice, practice. |

| **COURAGE:** | I have courage to go forward; to meet the new day, to handle whatever confronts me. Peace is coupled with courage, now and forever. |

| **DECISION-MAKING:** | With the help of a Higher Power, decision-making can be one of life's great adventures. Each crossroad brings a new challenge and I am capable of dealing with whatever comes my way. |

| **DENIAL:** | I let go of denial and accept responsibility for myself and my life. |

| **DETACHMENT:** | I avoid making excuses for my own or someone else's behavior. |

DISCIPLINE: I allow myself to recognize and accept whatever feelings pass through me.

DREAMS: I move confidently toward my ideal, knowing my steps are guided by my Higher Power.

FAITH: Faith is recognizing the longer I suffer under trying circumstances, the more certain I am to appreciate my deliverance.

FAILURE: By calling on my Higher Power for help daily I can turn failure into success.

FEAR: I am not afraid because God is my courage and my strength; He helps me face the Truth.

FORGIVENESS: I ask God to free me from feelings of bitterness, resentment, anger, envy, and the desire for revenge in order that I receive the gift of forgiveness.

GRATITUDE: Thankfulness today will help me see the miracles at work in my life and in the lives of others on the road to Recovery.

GUIDANCE: I move forward in confidence, knowing my steps are guided.

HEALING: I trust "The Program" works if I work it and I can be restored to wholeness with God's help.

HEALTH: Emotional health is from within not without.

HIGHER POWER: When faced with difficult or painful situations, I remember a loving God is always here for me, always available as a source of comfort, guidance and peace.

HONESTY: How do I feel today? How am I doing? If I can answer these questions truthfully, I am more likely to pursue the help I need and share the happy times with others as well.

HUMILITY: I understand the true nature of humility. I recognize that the ability to develop and practice it is the basic foundation of the Twelve Steps.

HUMOR: My sense of humor helps me carry – and to get – the message.

KNOWLEDGE: I pray my Higher Power will give me the courage and strength to recognize the Truth about myself, and help me accept I am powerless.

LETTING GO: I acknowledge my wants and needs, then turn them over to my Higher Power.

LOVE: I create a healthy atmosphere of love and nurturing around and within me. I accept the love and support of my sponsor and my group.

MEDITATION: My life is brightened, my burdens lifted and my hopes become realities whenever I look to my Higher Power for inspiration.

OBSTACLES: I avoid making excuses for my own or someone else's behavior.

PATIENCE: I focus on the power available to me by learning to wait.

PERSEVERANCE: There are many things I can do to improve my life and further my Recovery, but I cannot heal myself. I need to continually ask God's help in becoming free of all that blocks me from my true self.

POSITIVE EXPECTATIONS: I need to believe in myself and my dreams.

POWERLESSNESS: Day by day, I entrust my problems to a power greater than myself.

PRAYER: I connect with my Higher Power daily through prayer and meditation in the morning and at night.

PROSPERITY: I trust my truth, my instincts, and my ability to ground myself in reality.

| **RESPONSIBILITY:** | I do not run myself, my circumstances, or my feelings. I am open to myself, others, my Higher Power, and loving myself unconditionally. |

SELF-DETERMINATION: I have faith that daily work on myself will result in my becoming the best person I can be.

SELF-ESTEEM: I accept who I am, where I am, and I continue to push forward one day at a time.

SERENITY: My reward for practicing the principles of "The Program" in all my affairs is the priceless gift of serenity.

SPIRITUALITY: The Steps offer me a road map for living that leads to a spiritual awakening and beyond. I can't skip ahead to the end of the journey – which can at times be a hard one – but I can put one foot in front of the other and follow the directions I've been given, knowing that others who have gone before me have received more along the way than they had ever dreamed.

SUFFERING: God will strengthen me when life gets hard.

SURRENDER: I am beginning to understand that surrender is not defeat and I welcome my powerlessness.

TRANSFORMATION: I let consequences and responsibility fall where they belong.

TRUTH: I search for my own Truth, and I allow others to do the same.

TRUST: I trust that God will bring out the best in me and others.

VALUES: I practice the discipline of H.O.W. – Honesty, Open-mindedness and Willingness everyday.

WILLINGNESS: I am willing to turn my will and my life over to my Higher Power, to let go of willfulness and surrender myself to Recovery.

WISDOM: As I work the Steps, I grow in my capacity to be happy.

WORRY: I ask my Higher Power to help me let go of fear, doubt, and anxiety and fill me with faith, trust, and serenity.

THE LORD'S PRAYER

Our Father, Who art in heaven, hallowed be Thy Name. Thy kingdom come. Thy will be done, on earth as it is in heaven. Give us this day our daily bread. And forgive us our trespasses, as we forgive those who trespass against us. And lead us not into temptation, but deliver us from evil. For Thine is the kingdom and the power and the glory, forever and ever. Matthew :10

THE LORD'S PRAYER MODERN VERSION

Our Father in heaven, hallowed be your name, your kingdom come, your will be done, on earth as in heaven. Give us today our daily bread. Forgive us our sins as we forgive those who sin against us. Save us from the time of trial and deliver us from evil. For the kingdom, the power, and the glory are yours now and forever. Amen.

SANSKRIT PROVERB

Look to this day,
For it is life,
The very life of life.
In its brief course lies all
The realities and verities of existence,
The bliss of growth,
The splendor of action,
The glory of power.
For yesterday is but a dream,
And tomorrow is only a vision.
But today, well lived,
Makes every yesterday
A dream of happiness
And every tomorrow
A vision of hope.
Look well, therefore, to this day.

THIS I BELIEVE

Tomorrow is yet to be,
But should God grant me another day,
The Hope, Courage, and Strength
Through the working of the Twelve Steps
And Serenity Prayer,
I shall be sufficiently provided for to
Meet my every need.
This I believe.

THE TWELVE STEPS PRAYER

Power, greater than myself, as I understand You, I willingly
admit that without Your help I am powerless over alcohol
and my life has become unmanageable. I believe You
can restore me to sanity. I turn my life and my will
over to You. I have made a searching and fearless
moral inventory of myself and I admit to You, to myself,
and to another the exact nature of my wrongs. I am
entirely ready to have You remove these defects of
character. I humbly ask You to remove my shortcomings.
I have made direct amends to all persons I have harmed,
except when to do so would injure them or others. I
will continue to take personal inventory and when I am
wrong I will promptly admit it. I seek through prayer and
meditation to improve my conscious contact with You
and pray only for knowledge of Your will for me and
the power to carry it out.

Grant me the grace to carry the message of Your help
unto others and to practice the principles of the Twelve
Steps in all my affairs.

THE VICTIMS OF ADDICTION

O blessed Lord, You ministered to all who came to You.
Look with compassion upon all who through addiction
have lost their health and freedom. Restore to them the
assurance of Your unfailing mercy; remove from them the
fears that beset them; strengthen them in the work of their
Recovery; and to those who care for them, give patient
understanding and persevering love.

POSSIBILITIES PRAYER

I know, dear God, that my part in this Program is going
to be a thrilling and endless adventure. Despite all that
has happened to me already I know that I have just begun
to grow. I have just begun to open to Your love. I have
just begun to touch the varied live You are using me to change.
I have just begun to sense the possibilities ahead. And these
possibilities, I am convinced, will continue to unfold into ever
new and richer adventures, not only for the rest of my
reborn days, but through eternity.

Appendix C

<u>SUGGESTED READINGS</u>

Ackerman, Robert & Michaels, Judith A. *Recovery Resource Guide, Fourth Edition,* Deerfield Beach, FL: Health Communications, Inc. 1990.

Al-Anon's Twelve Steps & Twelve Traditions. New York, NY: Al-Anon Family Group Headquarters, Inc. 1988.

Alcoholics Anonymous, Third Edition. New York, NY: Alcoholics Anonymous World Services, Inc. 1976.

Beattie, Melody. *Codependent's Guide to the Twelve Steps.* New York, NY: Prentice Hall Press, 1990.

Codependent No More: How to Stop Controlling Others and Start Caring for Yourself. Center City, MN: Hazelden, 1987.

The Language of Letting Go: Daily Meditations for Codependents. New York, NY: HarperCollins Publishers, 1990.

Black, Claudia. *It Will Never Happen To Me.* New York, NY: Ballantine Books, 1981.

Bland, Glenn. *Legend of the Golden Scrolls: Ageless Secrets for Building Wealth.* Rocklin, CA: Prima Publishing, 1995.

Bradshaw, John. *Bradshaw On: The Family.* Deerfield Beach, FL: Health Communications, Inc., 1988.

Burns, John. *The Answer to Addiction: The Path to Recovery from Alcohol, Drug, Food and Sexual Dependencies.* New York, NY: Crossroad, 1990.

Butterworth, Eric. *Discover the Power Within You.* New York, NY: Harper Collins Publishers, 1989.

Carnegie, Dale. *How to Stop Worrying and Start Living.* New York, NY: Simon and Schuster, 1984.

Casey, Karen. *Each Day a New Beginning: Daily Meditations for Women.* Center City, MN: Hazeldon, 2006.

Cermak, Timmen L *Diagnosing and Treating Codependence.* Minneapolis, MN: Johnson Institute Books, 1986.

Conklin, Robert. *How to Get People To Do Things.* Chicago, IL: Contemporary
Books, 1979.

Covington, Stephanie & Beckett, Liana. *Leaving The Enchanted Forest: The
Path From Relationship To Intimacy.* San Francisco, CA: Harper &
Row Publishers, 1988.

Ellis, A., J.F. Mcinerney, *R.* DiGuiseppe, and *R.* Yeager. *Rational-Emotive Therapy
With Alcoholics and Substance Abusers.* Elmsford, New York: Pergammon,
1988.

Fishel, Ruth. *The Journey Within – A Spiritual Path To Recovery.* Deerfield
Beach, FL: Health Communications, Inc. 1987.

Fox, Emmet. *Power Through Constructive Thinking.* New York, NY:
HarperCollins Publishers, 1968.

    Stake Your Claim: Exploring the Gold Mine Within. New York, NY:
HarperCollins Publisher, 1992.

Fowler, Richard, et. Al. *Love Is A Choice: Recovery For Codependent
Relationships.* Nashville, TN: Thomas Nelson Publishers.

Friel, John & Friel, Linda. *Adult Children-The Secrets of Dysfunctional
Families.* Deerfield Beach, FL: Health Communications, Inc.

Friends in Recovery. *The 12 Steps for Adult Children.* San Diego, CA:
Recovery Publications, Inc.

    The Twelve Steps: A Spiritual Journey. San Diego, CA: Recovery
Publications, Inc., 1993.

    The Twelve Steps for Christians. San Diego, CA: Recovery Publications, Inc.,
1994.

Gannon, J. Patrick. *Soul Survivors: A New Beginning for Adults Abused as
Children.* New York, NY: Prentice Hall, 1989.

Gorski, Terence T. *Understanding the Twelve Steps.* New York, NY: Prentice
Hall Press, 1989.

Hill, Sally. *New Clothes from Old Threads: Daily Reflections for Recovering
Adults.* San Diego, CA: Recovery Publications, Inc., 1991.

Kritsberg, Wayne. *The Adult Children of Alcoholics Syndrome: From Discovery to Recovery.* Deerfield Beach, FL: Health Communications, Inc., 1986.

Larsen, Earnie and Hegarty, Carol. *Days of Healing-Days of Joy: Daily Meditations for Adult Children.* Center City, MN: Hazelden, 1987.

Lasater, Lane. *Recovery From Compulsive Behavior: How to Transcend Your Troubled Family.* Deerfield Beach, FL: Health Communications, Inc., 1988.

Lerner, Rokelle. *Daily Affirmations-For Adult Children of Alcoholics.* Deerfield, Beach, FL: Health Communications, Inc.

Maltz, Dr. Maxwell. *Creative Living for Today.* New York, NY: Trident Press, 1967.

Muller, Wayne. *Legacy of the Heart: The Spiritual Advantages of a Painful Childhood.* New York, NY: Simon & Schuster, 1992.

Peale, Dr. Norman Vincent. *You Can If You Think You Can.* Englewood Cliffs, NJ: Prentice-Hall, 1974

Pollard, Dr. John K., III. *Self-Parenting: The Complete Guide to Inner Conversations.* Malibu, CA: Generic Human Studies Publishing, 1987.

Rogers, Ronald *L.* and McMillin, Chandler Scott. *Under Your Own Power: A Secular Approach To 12-Step Programs.* New York, NY: The Putnam Publishing Group, 1992.

Ross, Ron. *When I Grow Up ... I Want To Be An Adult.* San Diego, CA: Recovery Publications, Inc.

Schuller, Robert H. *Tough Minded Faith For Tender Hearted People.* Nashville, TN: Thomas Nelson, Inc. 1982.

Sedgwick, Sherry. *The Good Sex Book: Recovering and Discovering Your Sexual Self.* Minneapolis, MN: CompCare Publishers, 1992.

Smith, *Ann W. Grandchildren of Alcoholics-Another Generation of Codependency.* Deerfield Beach, FL: Health Communications, Inc. 1988.

St. Roman, Philip. *Twelve Steps to Spiritual Wholeness: A Christian Pathway.* Liguori, MO: Liguori Publications.

12 Step Prayer Book: A Collection of Favorite 12 Step Prayers and Inspirational Readings. Seattle, WA: Lakeside Recovery Press, 1990.

Twelve Steps and Twelve Traditions. New York, NY: Alcoholics Anonymous World Services, Inc., 1990.

Waitley, Denis. *The Seeds of Greatness.* Nightingale Conant [sound recording], 1983.

Wegscheider-Cruse, Sharon. *Learning To Love Yourself.* Deerfield Beach, FL: Health Communications, Inc.

Whitfield, Charles. *Healing The Child Within.* Deerfield Beach, FL: Health Communications, Inc., 1983.

Woititz, Janet Geringer. *Adult Children of Alcoholics.* Deerfield Beach, FL: Health Communications, Inc. 1983.

Struggle For Intimacy. Pompano Beach, FL: Health Communications, Inc., 1987.

Yoder, Barbara. *The Recovery Resource Book: The Best Available Information on Addictions and Codependence.* New York, NY: Simon & Schuster, 1990.

Zink,   Muriel. *Step by Step: Daily Meditations for Living the Twelve Steps.* New York, NY: Ballantine Books.

INDEX OF QUOTES

TOPICAL INDEX: WHERE TO TURN FOR HELP

When you need help with:	Turn to:	Page
Acceptance	1 John 2:15-18	27
	Romans 12:21	55
	Luke 15:24	93
	Luke 6:41	154
	Hebrews 4:15	179
	2 Thessalonians 2:16,17	259
	1 Corinthians 13:11	377
Achievement	Proverbs 4:23	42
	Deuteronomy 33:27	100
	Psalm 84:7	214
	Romans 15:7	246
	Romans 11:33	277
	1 Timothy 6:17	353
	Ephesians 3:16, 20, 21	372
Alcoholism	Ephesians 5:14	10
	Proverbs 26::5	111
	Psalm 51:10	117
	1 Corinthians 6:19	119
	Ecclesiastes 4:10	120
	Matthew 6:30	121
	Romans 5:3,4	145
Anger	Deuteronomy 30:19	80
	James 1:19	103
	Matthew 6:14,15	167
	Proverbs 16:32	185

When you need help with:	Turn to:	Page
Guidance (cont)	1 Samuel 15:22	212
	Jeremiah 7:23	309
	Proverbs 4:11	347
	Romans 8:14-15	351
Healing	1 Peter 4:12-13	147
	Psalm 50:15	216
	Jeremiah 33:6	235
	Matthew 11:30	241
	Genesis 28:15	250
	1 Timothy 1:15-17	272
	Psalm 147:3-4	325
Health	Isaiah 40:31	50
	Job 34:32	115
	Romans 12:1	128
	Mark 11:25,26	183
	Isaiah 30:15	191
	John 6:28	220
	Isaiah 14:3	254
Higher Power	Proverbs 3:5-6	84
	Romans 12:2	109
	Psalm 130:1-6	173
	2 Chronicles 20:6	178
	Psalm 92:1-2	199
	Psalm 91:14-15	273
	Matthew 7:20-21	388
Honesty	Psalm 139:7-10	26
	Proverbs 4:25	118
	Psalm 89:23, 24	150
	Matthew 18:3	281
	Psalm 118:24	299
	Psalm 39:7	314
	Psalm 94:18-19	319
Humility	Jeremiah 42:2,3	151
	2 Corinthians 13:9	162
	Matthew 18:4	198
	1 Peter 5:5-7	226
	Matthew 5:23-25	278
	2 Corinthians 6:10	310
	Psalm 37:11	338

ABOUT THE AUTHOR

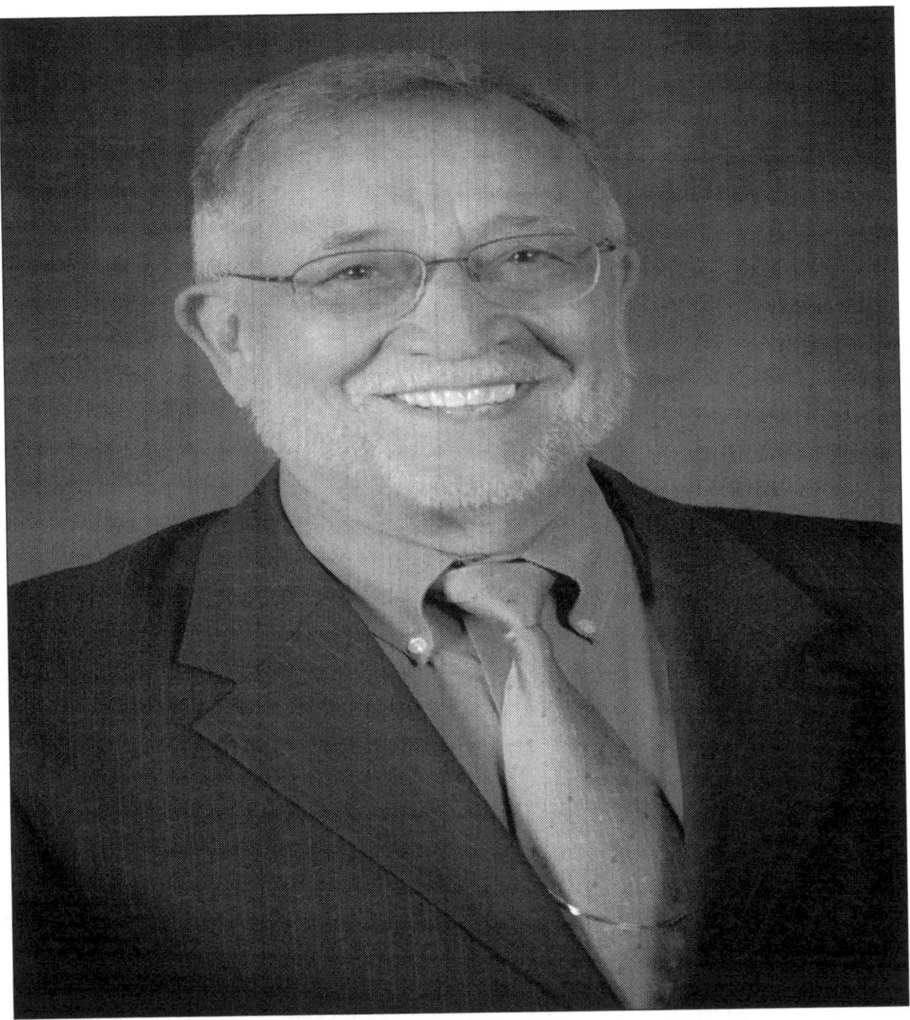

Anthony P. Caetano, M.Ed., C.A.G.S. is a retired Special Education Director, a Certified Grant Writer and Trainer and President of Five Star Consulting. He has been a grateful member of Al-Anon for over twenty-five years. He has served as a Group Rep for the Saturday Steps to Serenity Group in Sedona, AZ for the past three years.